# Advanced Immediate Loading

# Advanced Immediate Loading

**Georgios E. Romanos,** DDS, PhD, Prof Dr med dent

Professor and Associate Dean for Clinical Affairs
School of Dental Medicine
State University of New York at Stony Brook
Stony Brook, New York

Professor of Oral Surgery and Implant Dentistry
Dental School Frankfurt (Carolinum)
Johann Wolfgang Goethe University
Frankfurt, Germany

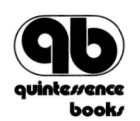

**Quintessence Publishing Co, Inc**

Chicago, Berlin, Tokyo, London, Paris, Milan, Barcelona, Istanbul,
São Paulo, New Delhi, Moscow, Prague, and Warsaw

**Library of Congress Cataloging-in-Publication Data**

Romanos, Georgios.
 Advanced immediate loading / Georgios E. Romanos.
    p. ; cm.
 Includes bibliographical references.
 ISBN 978-0-86715-491-7 (hardcover)
 I. Title.
 [DNLM: 1.  Immediate Dental Implant Loading–methods. 2.  Dental Implants.
3.  Dental Prosthesis, Implant-Supported.  WU 640]
 LC  Classification not assigned
 617.6'93–dc23
                                         2011046950

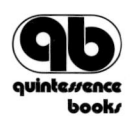

**qb**
quintessence
books

© 2012 Quintessence Publishing Co, Inc

Quintessence Publishing Co Inc
4350 Chandler Drive
Hanover Park, IL 60133
www.quintpub.com

5 4 3 2 1

All rights reserved. This book or any part thereof may not be reproduced, stored in a retrieval system, or transmitted in any form or by any means, electronic, mechanical, photocopying, or otherwise, without prior written permission of the publisher.

Editor: Bryn Grisham
Design: Ted Pereda
Production: Angelina Sanchez

Printed in China

# Contents

Dedication    ix
Foreword    x
Preface    xi
Contributors    xii

## 1 Bone Biology and Osseointegration of Dental Implants    1

Basic Bone Anatomy
Bone Remodeling
Bone Microvasculature
Bone Physiology
Strain Detection and Mechanotransduction
Bone Healing
Clinical Considerations
Conclusion

## 2 Basic Principles and Clinical Applications of Immediate Loading    11

Definition of Immediate Loading
Rationale for Immediate Loading
Clinical Treatment Concepts with Immediate Loading
Requirements for Successful Immediate Loading
Clinical Considerations
Conclusion

## 3 Role of the Implant Surface in Immediate Loading    27

Osseointegration and the Implant Surface
Testing of Implant Surface Designs
Surface Modification of Dental Implants
Conclusion

**4** **Role of Implant Design in Immediate Loading**  *39*
Types of Implant Stability
Micromovement at the Bone-Implant Interface
Conclusion

**5** **Histologic Evaluation of Immediately Loaded Implants**  *43*
Animal Studies
Human Studies
Conclusion

**6** **Immediate Loading in the Anterior Mandible Using Overdentures**  *55*
Immediate Loading in the Edentulous Patient
Immediate Loading with Telescopic Abutments in the Partially Edentulous Patient

**7** **Immediate Loading in Edentulous Jaws**  *63*
Case Reports
Guidelines for a Successful Immediate Loading Protocol in Edentulous Arches
Diet Protocol for Patients with Immediately Loaded Implants

**8** **Immediate Loading in Posterior Regions**  *79*
Posterior Maxilla
Posterior Mandible
Conclusion

**9** **Immediate Loading in Grafted Bone**  *89*
Case Reports

**10** **Immediate Loading in Immunocompromised Patients** *107*
Heavy Smokers
HIV-Positive Patients
Conclusion

**11** **Immediate Loading with Simultaneous Sinus Elevation** *121*
Case Reports

**12** **Immediate Loading of Single-Tooth Implants** *131*
Case Reports

**13** **Immediate Loading of Implants Placed in Fresh Extraction Sockets** *145*
Extraction Socket Healing and Tissue Preservation
Implant Placement in Fresh Extraction Sockets
Considerations for Clinical Application of the Protocol
Case Reports
Conclusion

**14** **Management of Immediate Loading Complications** *173*
Surgical Complications
Prosthetic Complications
Conclusion

**Index** *177*

# Dedication

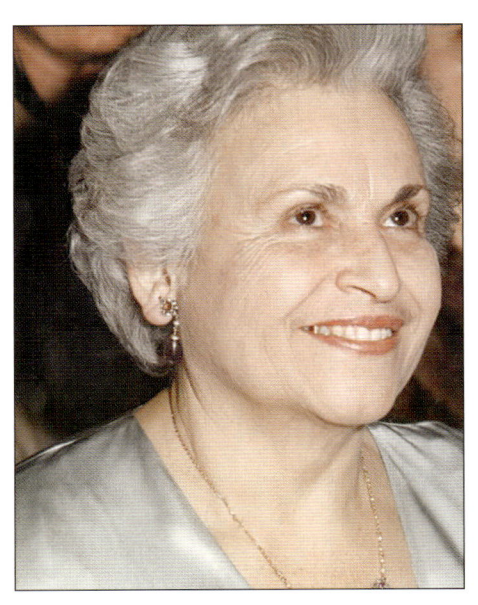

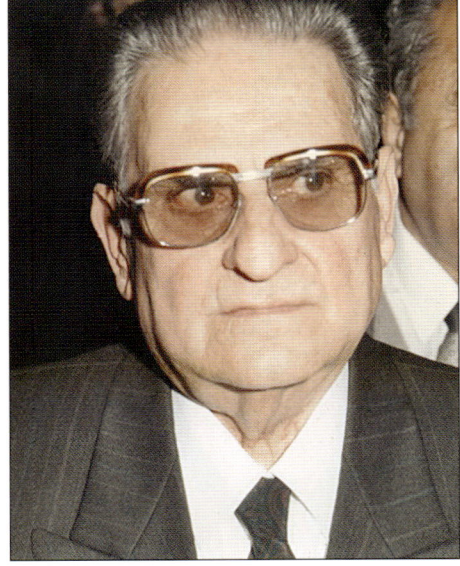

*In loving memory of my parents, Rallou and Evangelos Romanos,
who nurtured my passion for science and instilled in me the value of hard work.*

# Foreword

I am delighted to be asked to write the foreword for this new book on advanced immediate loading of dental implants. This book is greatly needed, and I am especially glad that Dr Georgios Romanos decided to undertake this work to provide the dental profession with an important resource on implant dentistry.

It is hard to believe that more than 30 years have gone by since the group at Harvard organized the landmark National Institutes of Health–Harvard Consensus Development Conference on Dental Implants. In June of 1978, a group of clinicians and investigators assembled in Boston to (1) examine the evidence that dental implants "work"; (2) determine the risks and benefits of placing dental implants; and (3) establish the rules for implant placement, postoperative wound healing, and implant loading. Although the conclusions reached during this conference were positive, those were nonetheless tentative days for the field of implant dentistry. We were still to some extent "flying by the seat of our pants" in the management of our patients with dental implants. But clearly the field of implant dentistry has come a long way since that time.

Over the ensuing 33 years, we have seen implant designs greatly change, such that now state-of-the-art root-form implants are standard practice. We have watched as biomaterials engineers have perfected implant surfaces to foster maximum osseointegration between device and bone. Periodontal and oral surgeons have taught us how to gain much-needed bone in sites prior to implant placement by using bone grafts, membranes, signaling molecules, and novel surgical techniques. But perhaps most surprisingly, restorative colleagues continue to teach us that, in certain clinical situations, dental implants can be restored and placed into function almost immediately, and if not immediately, then very soon after implant placement.

Now, to complicate things even more, we are learning that individuals with untreated periodontitis have a greater risk for certain systemic illnesses such as cardiovascular disease, diabetes, adverse pregnancy outcomes, and pulmonary disease. Thus, dentistry is asking at what point should a tooth with advanced periodontitis be extracted and replaced with a dental implant.

In the last 15 years, a number of excellent books on implant dentistry have been published. Written by outstanding clinicians, these books cover many aspects of dental implants, but it is evident that there has not been a good assembling of the evidence to show that, following implant placement in a variety of situations, implants may be immediately loaded. Clearly, this is something that has been on people's minds for some time. One cannot attend a conference on dental implants without hearing about the advantages, disadvantages, indications, and contraindications for immediate loading of implants. And so, Dr Romanos' book is very timely and much needed.

Dr Romanos has assembled an excellent group of players for this book. Equally noteable are the topics covered in this book; Dr Romanos covers the field thoroughly. This book is an excellent resource for patient management, with each chapter focusing on very specific issues that confront clinicians every day.

All told, I say "lucky us." We now have a first-rate book that provides another area in the multiple facets of management of our patients with dental implants; that is, the treatment planning and management of implants that are immediately loaded. I look forward to the coming years in the development of the field of implant dentistry knowing that clinicians such as Dr Romanos and his colleagues will help to continually advance this very exciting area of dentistry.

Ray C. Williams, DMD
Professor and Dean
School of Dental Medicine
State University of New York at Stony Brook
Stony Brook, New York

# Preface

Today, there are many books that cover the immediate loading of dental implants. This textbook and color atlas has a primary goal of providing clinicians and researchers with current information about the concepts of immediate functional loading when using different implant systems and surfaces.

I have tried to review the most significant studies in the current literature related to immediately loaded implants. The featured treatment protocols for immediate loading using the classical indications with cross-arch stabilization are demonstrated step by step. The histologic proof of this concept is the focus of a chapter that elaborates both previous animal studies as well as human histology to explain bone biology under occlusal loading forces. The reader is able to review the basic biology of the remodeling process and understand its role in immediate functional loading as well as in protocols for delayed and immunocompromised wound healing. I have also presented additional prosthetic concepts for the use of removable implant-supported restorations in conjunction with an immediate prosthesis, which is especially important for elderly patients and patients with special needs.

The inclusion of more advanced surgical techniques using lateral and vertical bone augmentation—including the sinus augmentation—with simultaneous implant placement and immediate functional loading illustrates one of the main areas of focus of this book. Long-term data is included as evidence of the viability of these advanced treatment protocols. The placement of implants in fresh extraction sockets and immediate restoration with simultaneous bone augmentations are illustrated in detail. The clinical scenarios are presented within the context of a biologic approach to both eliminate postoperative complications and further new principles in implant dentistry. The final chapter of this book addresses the complications with immediate loading concepts and discusses their solutions.

Because I am its primary author, this book presents clinical and research experience of the last 15 years of my clinical and academic career, throughout which I have been using advanced concepts of immediate functional loading in implant dentistry. I am also proud that I had the opportunity to work closely and collaborate with some of the best clinicians and researchers in Europe, Asia, South America, and the United States, many of whom have become my close friends and continue to inspire me in their work. Thus, I have also selected additional experts to contribute their advanced experience in the areas of wound healing and implant surfaces as well as to present representative clinical examples from their daily practice.

The production of this book has been performed with high precision and excellence by the group at Quintessence Publishing under the editorial guidance of Bryn Grisham and the leadership of Bill Hartman and Lisa Bywaters. I would also like to express special thanks to Christian Haase and his father, Dr h.c. Horst-Wolfgang Haase, who haved supported my vision from the first.

Finally, there is no doubt in my mind that a book like this would not be possible without the support, continuous encouragement, and patience of my wife, Dr Enisa Begic Romanos. I would like to thank her so much for her love and her vision to make my dream a reality.

—*Georgios E. Romanos, DDS, PhD, Prof Dr med dent*

# Contributors

**Camila Cinto Arita, DDS**
Private Practice
Ribeirao Preto, São Paulo, Brazil

**César Augusto Arita, DDS, MSc, PhD**
Private Practice
Ribeirao Preto, São Paulo, Brazil

**Estevam A. Bonfante, DDS, MSc, PhD**
Department of Prosthodontics
Bauru School of Dentistry
University of São Paulo
Bauru, São Paulo, Brazil

**Paulo G. Coelho, DDS, PhD**
Assistant Professor
Department of Biomaterials and Biomimetics
New York University College of Dentistry
New York, New York

**Jeffrey Ganeles, DMD**
Clinical Associate Professor
College of Dental Medicine
Nova Southeastern University
Fort Lauderdale, Florida

Private Practice
Boca Raton, Florida

**Jack E. Lemons, PhD**
Professor
Department of Prosthodontics
School of Dentistry
University of Alabama at Birmingham
Birmingham, Alabama

**Dittmar May, DMD, MD, Dr med dent**
Oral and Maxillofacial Surgeon
Practice Limited to Implant Surgery
Lunen, Germany

**Jose M. Navarro, DDS, MS**
Private Practice
Las Palmas, Spain

**Adriano Piattelli, DDS, MD, PhD**
Professor
Department of Oral Pathology and Medicine
School of Dentistry
University of Chieti-Pescara
Chieti, Italy

**Georgios E. Romanos, DDS, PhD, Prof Dr med dent**
Professor and Associate Dean for Clinical Affairs
School of Dental Medicine
State University of New York at Stony Brook
Stony Brook, New York

Professor of Oral Surgery and Implant Dentistry
Dental School Frankfurt (Carolinum)
Johann Wolfgang Goethe University
Frankfurt, Germany

**Nigel A. Saynor, BDS**
Private Practice
Stockport, England

**Karl Andreas Schlegel, MD, DDS, PhD, Prof Dr med dent**
Professor
Department of Oral and Maxillofacial Surgery
University of Erlangen-Nürnberg
Erlangen, Germany

**Nelson R. F. A. Silva, DDS, MS, PhD**
Assistant Professor
Department of Prosthodontics
Department of Biomaterials and Biomimetics
New York University College of Dentistry
New York, New York

**Tonino Traini, DDS, PhD**
Section of Prosthodontics
Department of Oral Sciences, Nano,
  and Biotechnologies
School of Dentistry
University of Chieti-Pescara
Chieti, Italy

Georgios E. Romanos, Tonino Traini, Adriano Piattelli

# Bone Biology and Osseointegration of Dental Implants

The term *osseointegration* refers to a direct connection between the implant surface and the surrounding bone. However, the directness of this connection cannot be well demonstrated under the electron microscope. There is an interaction between titanium oxide and bone via proteoglycans, as has been previously reported.[1] Bone collagen fibers contacting the implant surface have not been observed. At the soft tissue–implant interface, connective tissue fibers are in contact with the titanium surface; therefore, there is said to be soft tissue "adherence."

In order to explain the mechanisms of implant osseointegration, this chapter describes the basics of bone biology and, in particular, the kind of bone that can be formed after implant placement.

## Basic Bone Anatomy

Bone consists of a mineral phase enmeshed within organic fibers. It is generally accepted that both the minerals and the collagen fibers are involved in the mechanical resistance of the tissue. The orientation of the collagen fibers inside the bone matrix seems to be influenced by load.[2]

*Cortical bone* is found in both the maxilla and the mandible. It consists of concentric layers of matrix surrounding longitudinal vessels within the structure (haversian systems). Between these, mainly unremodeled interstitial bone is present. This type of bone consists of a framework of bone struts, which, although weaker than cortical bone, provide metabolically active lightweight support.

The relationship between mineral content and the strength of bone has been studied extensively. The elasticity of bone and thus its resistance to fracture is related to its degree of mineralization, ie, an increase in stiffness and brittleness of bone tissue follows the replacement of its water content by mineral. Nevertheless, increased mineralization density improves the ability of bone to absorb impact energy, although only up to a certain limit. For example, above an ash content of 60% by weight, femoral cortical bone becomes fragile, with microfractures more readily propagating through the highly mineralized bone.[3,4] There is a net increase in mineral density with age, reflected in reduced turnover and replacement.[5,6] The optimal mineralization density value for bone strength has not yet been determined.[7]

## Bone Remodeling

Bone remodeling is designed to maintain a mechanically competent skeleton[8] and to repair areas of microdamage.[9] It is achieved by an ongoing process of the removal of mature bone followed by replacement with new bone.[10] This involves a localized cycle of osteoclastic recruitment and activation followed by the subsequent initiation of osteoblast formation and repair of the resorption site. Within cortical bone, this process is achieved through osteonal remodeling, where a cutting cone of osteoclasts advances through the bone and is followed by osteoblasts making new bone.[10] In cancellous bone, a similar process occurs and has been described as *hemiosteonal remodeling*,[8] whereby a space is cut through the surface of individual trabeculae and filled in by osteoblast activity. Thus, bone turnover maintains the ability of the skeleton to withstand physiologic and mechanical demands.

## Osteoclasts

*Osteoclasts* are large, multinucleated cells that can penetrate 50 to 70 µm into compact bone and resorb a volume of bone equivalent to that formed by osteoblasts. Osteoclasts possess numerous mitochondria and an extensive Golgi system but have a sparse endoplasmic reticulum and few ribosomes. Contact with bone is through a ruffled border, where resorption occurs, and a peripheral clear zone, which acts as a seal that maintains an optimal acidic environment for the lysosomal enzymes involved in the degradation of both the mineral and organic phases of bone. This acidic environment is generated through the action of carbonic anhydrase type II and pumped across the ruffled border by a proton pump.[10] Contact with the bone surface is possibly through the integrin vitronectin receptor.[11]

Osteoclasts are formed from the hematopoietic mononuclear cells of the bone marrow, although the exact nature of the precursor cell is still a matter of debate. The regulation of osteoclast activity is complex, involving a variety of factors (including systemic hormones such as parathyroid hormone; 1,25-dihydroxyvitamin $D_3$; and calcitonin as well as numerous local factors).[12] A number of these factors act through the generation of secondary signals by osteoblasts, a mechanism that is believed to couple bone resorption with bone formation. The mechanism by which bone resorption is terminated includes activation of matrix-derived transforming growth factor β (TGF-β),[13,14] the presence of calcium sensors, and, finally, osteoclast apoptosis.[15]

## Osteoblasts

*Osteoblasts* are mononuclear, fibroblast-like cells[16] found in a single layer on bone surfaces. An osteoblast forms a volume of matrix equivalent to its own size every day. The bone matrix consists primarily of type I collagen and a number of noncollagenous proteins, such as sialoprotein, osteocalcin, and osteonectin.[17] High concentrations of growth factors, such as TGF-β and insulin-like growth factor (IGF), are also secreted into the matrix.

The control of osteoblast differentiation is poorly understood because a multiplicity of factors is involved.[18] Adaptation of bone in response to load has been in part elucidated.[19] Under compression, the cortex is thicker and has an increased osteon density but has smaller osteons and less turnover, while the cortex under tension is thinner and has a higher turnover with larger, less numerous osteons.[20,21] There are also differences in the degree of skeletal mineralization, with regions of bone that are under tension having a lower mineral density than those under compression.[6] Cortical porosity has been investigated in relation to the principal loading mode, compression or tension. Cortical bone remodeling varies in response to the loading environment so that analyzing small samples of bone may not present the true picture of the overall level of remodeling.[22] Furthermore, differing loading environments also affect the orientation of bone collagen fibers inside the bone matrix.[2] Around dental implants, bone under compression has oblique/transverse collagen fibers, while that under tension has longitudinal collagen fibers.[23-25]

## Osteocytes

*Osteocytes* are former osteoblasts that become trapped in the bone matrix during bone formation. They inhabit the lacunocanalicular system and communicate with other osteocytes and with the bone surface lining cells, in part, via gap junctions.

Osteocytes in the territory of a haversian capillary die if their blood supply is interrupted.[26] There is increasing evidence that osteocytes act as mechanoreceptors[27] and that they almost certainly sense rates of change of mechanical deformation (strain). A number of paracrine signals, including prostacyclin ($PGI_2$) and prostaglandin-$E_2$ ($PGE_2$), nitric oxide, and IGF, are stimulated in osteocytes following changes in skeletal loading. Moreover, the finding that expression of the glutamate transport is increased following loading[28] suggests that excitatory amino acids may play a role in the transduction of the loading signal. Recent studies have also raised the intriguing possibility that osteocyte apoptosis may be part of the mechanism whereby osteoclasts are targeted to sites of bone resorption[29] as bone is remodeled. Estrogen suppression, a known stimulant of bone resorption, increases osteocyte apoptosis, and changes in bone loading are also associated with osteocyte apoptosis.[30]

# Bone Microvasculature

Bone receives from 5% to 10% of cardiac output blood supply from four sources. Arterial supply of the cortex is *centrifugal* (from inside to outside). The direction is reversed in a displaced fracture, with disruption of the endosteal (nutrient) system. Venous flow is *centripetal*, with cortical capillaries draining to venous sinusoids to the emissary venous system. Blood flow within bone tissue is unique in two ways:

1. The blood circulates within a closed cavity in which pressure must remain constant, which is achieved in part through the distensibility of the intraosseous vessels and, above all, the veins.
2. The intraosseous circulation allows traffic of minerals between the blood and bone tissue and sends the blood cells produced within the bone marrow into the systemic circulation.

The intracortical vessels travel in canals located within the cortex, mainly haversian canals and secondarily Volkmann canals. Although the widest canals contain both an artery and a vein, most canals contain only a single capillary. This network undergoes continuous remodeling, as does the surrounding cortical bone. Intraosseous blood flow can adjust either through

**Fig 1-1** *(1)* If the stresses (strains) to which a bone is exposed are lowered, a net loss of bone will occur until a new equilibrium state is attained. *(2)* If the state of stress (strain) of bone is normal, neither a net resorption nor a net buildup of bone will take place. *(3)* If the stresses (strains) to which a bone is exposed are raised within physiologic limits, bone buildup will occur until a new equilibrium state is attained. *(4)* If bone is subject to extreme stresses (strains), it will be resorbed.

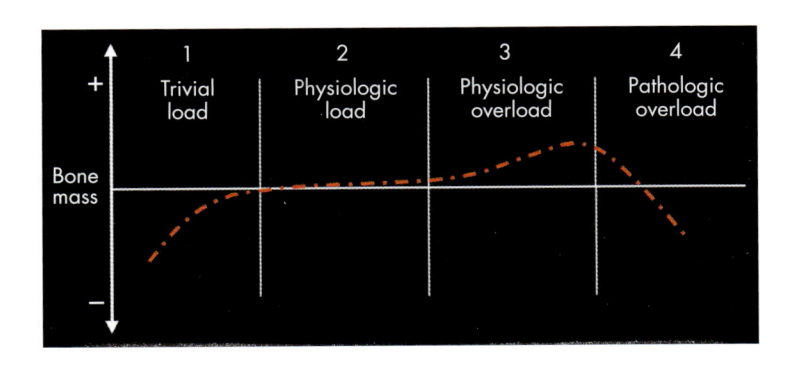

changes in the flow rate or through stimulation or inhibition of intraosseous angiogenesis (growth of new capillaries from preexisting capillaries). Blood supply is critical for the development, maintenance, and repair of most tissues, including bone.[31,32]

A close spatial correlation between angiogenesis and bone formation has been shown.[33] Blood vessels are an important component of bone formation and maintenance.[34] A reduction in bone blood flow and microvascular defects in the sinusoidal compartment have been reported in osteoporotic bone as well as in aplastic anemia.[35] Moreover, impairment of vascular supply results in the necrosis of bone, indicating the importance of angiogenesis for the maintenance of bone tissue.[36]

The formation of blood capillaries precedes the formation of new bone, with the perivascular loose connective tissue that accompanies the proliferating capillaries representing the source of osteoprogenitor cells.[33] Bone angiogenesis is an important event[37] in the process of bone remodeling because the remodeling tissues have higher metabolic needs.[34] The vascular endothelial growth factor (VEGF) receptor system also may be involved in both bone formation and bone remodeling.[38] In addition, VEGF has been shown to be important for the formation of osteoclasts.[39]

The three-dimensional bone vessel network around dental implants was investigated by Matsuo et al[40] in an animal model. The authors investigated the changes in the microvascular system produced by implant placement in 12 beagle dogs using the well-known vascular cast techniques for analyzing the morphology of the vessels network, while Traini et al[41] used a post fixation infiltrative method to investigate the vascular canal network organization in the bone tissue around immediately loaded implants in a canine model.

## Bone Physiology

Trehame[42] indicated three factors that govern the development of bone morphology:

1. Genetic programming
2. Hormonal activity
3. Loads to which the bone is exposed

Body weight and activity affect the size of bone.[43] In 1867, von Meyer[44] assessed that the orientation of the trabeculae of cancellous bone was correlated to the magnitude and the direction of the loads placed on it. Some years later, Wolff[45] reported that the remodeling of the bone, in response to the history of the mechanical loading, follows mathematic laws. Wolff's law can be summarized as: "Every change in the form and function of bones or of their function alone is followed by certain definite changes in their internal architecture and equally definite alteration in their external conformation, in accordance with mathematical laws."[45]

By 1930, it was generally assumed that osteoblasts and osteoclasts, ie, the bone effector cells, determine bone health and disease under the control of non-mechanical agents.[46] By 1960, those ideas became the "1960 paradigm" of bone physiology.[47] By 1964, following the Hard Tissue Workshops sponsored by the University of Utah, biomechanical and other functions at the tissue level, such as growth modeling, remodeling, and maintenance, were introduced in the "Utah paradigm" of skeletal physiology, which supplements the "1960 paradigm" and Wolff's law. The basic idea is that tissue-level mechanisms directly influence the bone effector cells to determine bone health and disease, with non-mechanical agents acting peripherally on both tissue-level mechanisms and effector cells. In this way, bone tissue was seen as achieving mechanical competence by the basic tissue-level biologic mechanisms.

By 1987, Frost's mechanostat theory had introduced a concept of dynamic interaction between form and function.[48] Mechanostat theory asserts that bone adapts by different biologic processes within four mechanical usage windows, with thresholds defined by the minimum effective strain that will activate an adaptive process (Fig 1-1).

Remodeling by basic multicellular units (BMUs) tends to remove or conserve bone and is activated by reduced mechanical usage in a trivial loading zone or microdamage in a pathologic overload zone but suppressed by a physiologic loading zone. Remodeling by BMUs can work in at least two modes:

1. Conservation mode (no significant gain or loss)
2. Disuse mode (less gain than loss but only next to or closest to marrow)

Remodeling can decrease the bone mass by way of disuse mode. In the pathologic overload zone, a rapid addition of woven bone to surfaces occurs in response to excessive loading. Modeling, which can add cortical and trabecular bone and reshape surfaces by resorption or lamellar formation drifts,[49] is activated in the physiologic overload zone and remains suppressed within or below the physiologic load zone. Modeling determines the cross-sectional size and shape of bone and trabeculae, which seems to be nature's preferred way of increasing bone strength.

# Strain Detection and Mechanotransduction

The cells ensconced throughout the mineralized matrix tissue of bone represent the living component of the tissue.[50] The cells provide the machinery for remodeling, allowing for adaptation of bone structure to fulfill dynamic functional demands. Osteocytes, osteoblasts, and, to some degree, osteoclasts form a functional syncytium, ie, an interconnected network allowing for communication and transport between cells deep within the tissue (osteocytes) and those located in the perivascular spaces and bone surface (osteoblasts and osteoclasts).[51]

The interconnection is intrinsic to both the cell structure (cytoskeleton) as well as the fluid presenting in the lacunocanalicular system and the intermatrix porosity. The pericellular fluid in the lacunocanalicular system is the coupling medium through which mechanical forces are translated into mechanobiologic, biochemical, mechanochemical, and electromechanical effects at the cellular level.

The structure of the lacunocanalicular system is dominated by the syncytium of cells, the majority of which are osteocytes.[52] Although it remains unknown how the mechanical load is transduced from the bone tissue to these cells, because the strains applied to whole bone in vivo are much smaller than the strains necessary to activate bone cell signaling in cell cultures,[53,54] the model proposed by You et al[54] assumes the existence of three basic components:

1. An organic matrix that fills the entire pericellular space surrounding the osteocyte body and the osteocytic process
2. Transverse elements that anchor and center the osteocytic process within its canaliculus
3. A cytoskeleton structure within the cell processes that resists hoop tension and bending deformation

The same authors also demonstrate the existence of the transverse tethering elements that connect the osteocytic process to the canalicular wall.[55]

# Quantum concept for bone formation

The mechanostat theory holds that loading produces different effects based on the peak strain magnitude; in an animal experiment, Forwood and Turner[56] reported that bone cells are also sensitive to frequency of loading. Each instance of loading activates a packet of cells that start forming osteoid approximately 4 days after activation. This delay period may reflect the 60-hour time sequence of osteoblast histogenesis.[57]

The increase of bone formation occurs by activating packets (quanta) of cells with each new occurrence of loading, the size of which is determined by the magnitude of the load. The strain rate determines the vigor of osteoblastic activity, while the recurrence of the strain determines recruitment in a "quantum fashion."

# Bone Healing

The result of rapid growth during healing is woven bone, while the slower bone formation that occurs during the remodeling process results in lamellar organization. It is evident that the early endosseous healing in peri-implant bone is crucial. For this reason, the formation of woven bone is of central importance. Nevertheless, no study has investigated the possibility of directly obtaining lamellar bone in the healing phase by application of immediate loading.

The microarchitecture of lamellar and woven bone differ (Figs 1-2 and 1-3). However, the histodynamics of the formation of these two distinct types of bone tissue are remarkably similar, with the same cells, nutrition, and pathway at work. The significant differences in the histologic appearances are mainly a result of the appositional rate.

Endosseous implant integration comprises three phenomenologically distinct mechanisms:

1. Osteoconduction
2. Appositional growth
3. Bone remodeling

However, these three phenomena are not unique to the peri-implant environment; they also occur during both bone remodeling and early events in bone wound healing. In fact, fracture and peri-implant healing exhibit many similarities,[58–60] although some authors have suggested that the presence of an implant may influence the healing process by acting as a "bioreactor."[61–64]

In recent reports, the new concepts of "static" and "dynamic" osteogenesis for intramembranous ossification were introduced.[65–67] They demonstrated the existence of cuboidal, polygonal cells, later identified as osteoblasts, which are always irregularly arranged in cords of two to three layers of cells. The osteoblasts are joined by gap junctions and appear polarized in different directions. Additionally, these osteoblasts appear to be stationary since they directly transform into osteocytes at the same site where they differentiate. In other words,

Bone Healing

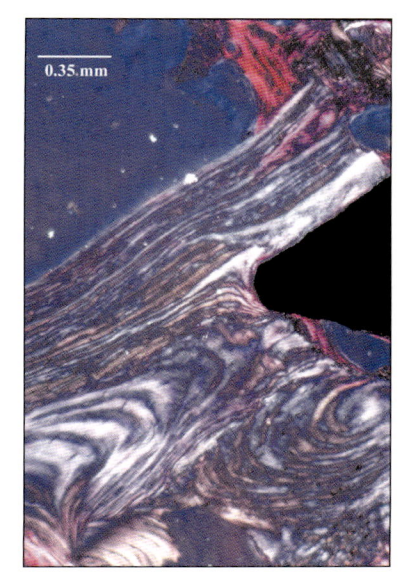

**Fig 1-2** Lamellar peri-implant bone viewed under a circularly polarized light microscope (unstained; original magnification ×100).

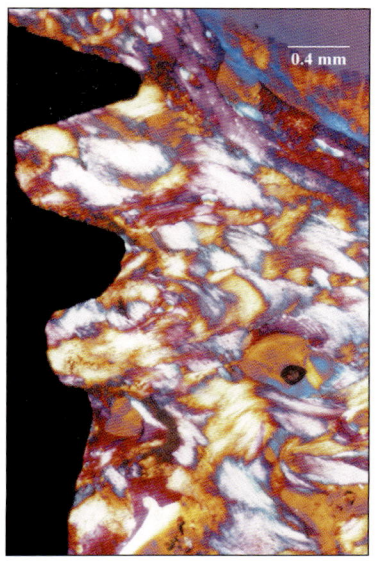

**Fig 1-3** Woven peri-implant bone viewed under a circularly polarized light microscope (unstained; original magnification ×100).

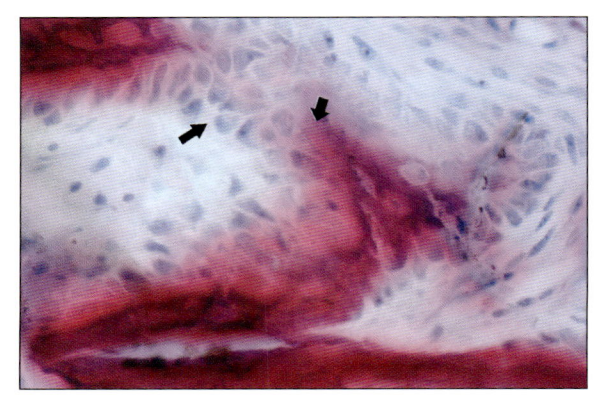

**Fig 1-4** Static osteogenesis in mandibular bone showing stationary osteoblasts *(left arrow)* as well as a preosseous mix *(right arrow)* (acid fuchsin and azure II-eosinate; original magnification ×430).

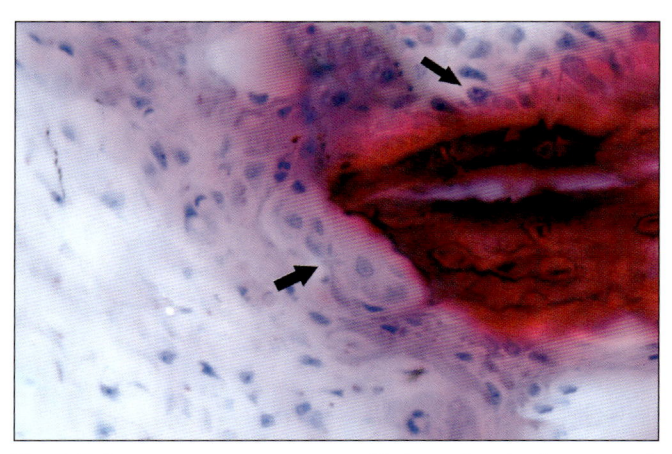

**Fig 1-5** Dynamic osteogenesis: mandibular trabecular bone growth showing movable osteoblastic laminae *(top arrow)* and osteoclasts *(bottom arrow)* (acid fuchsin and azure II-eosinate; original magnification ×430).

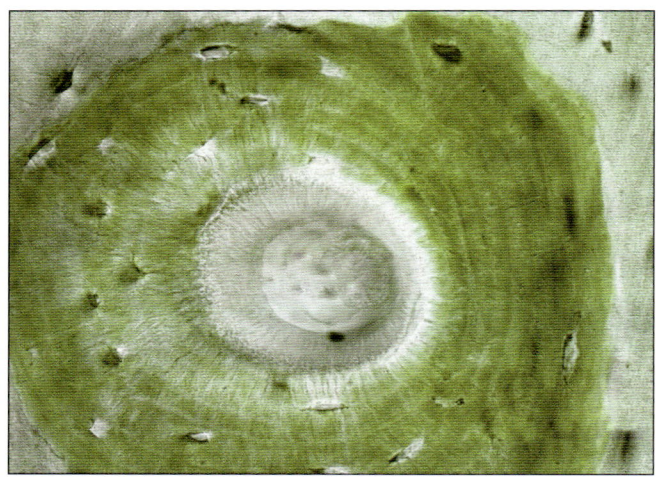

**Fig 1-6** Osteon in human maxillary bone observed with a confocal scanning laser microscope (unstained; original magnification ×200).

they remain self-entrapped by the mineralized matrix they produce. The osteocytes that originate this way appear irregularly grouped and globular and radiate a very short cytoplasmic process. This ossification process, called *static osteogenesis* (Fig 1-4), evolves into *dynamic osteogenesis* by the following sequence:

1. Differentiation of stationary osteoblasts irregularly arranged in cords around blood vessels
2. Secretion of osteoid and in situ transformation into osteocytes
3. Mineralization of the matrix with formation of thin (10- to 15-μm) bony trabeculae containing no more than two to three layers of osteocytes
4. Growth of thin trabeculae by dynamic osteogenesis (Fig 1-5), in which typical osteogenic laminae with movable osteoblasts, all polarized in the same direction, differentiate along the surface of the trabeculae previously laid down by stationary osteoblasts
5. Deposition of concentric layers of bone-forming osteons by osteoblasts (Fig 1-6)

Static osteogenesis is mainly devoted to the expansion of the ossification centers and consequently to increasing bone size, whereas dynamic osteogenesis is mainly involved in bone compaction or in thickening the primitive trabeculae. The main difference between these two types of osteogenesis concerns osteoblast arrangement and polarization. This means that in static osteogenesis the osteoblasts become osteocytes, whereas in dynamic osteogenesis the osteoblasts selected to transform into osteocytes are embedded within the bone matrix by secretory activity of the adjacent movable osteoblasts. The intramembranous ossification could be of interest in dentistry because the maxillary and mandibular bones are formed by this mechanism and probably maintain a genetic memory for regenerating processes.

During implant bed preparation, local bone tissue discontinuity and blood vessel network damage take place. The consequence of vessel interruption is redirection of blood circulation to the Volkmann canals,[68,69] which are sparsely distributed.

The healing of peri-implant sites is a process that involves a multitude of intra- and extracellular events, influenced by:

- Severity of trauma at the osteotomy site
- Degree of fixation during healing
- Age

Some authors[70,71] point out that bone tissue regenerates rather than repairs because, unlike all the other tissues, it heals without the formation of a scar.

Hemorrhage and hemostasis caused by the bone site preparation results in the formation of a blood clot. The clot normally lasts only a few days,[72] but sometimes it may persist for 2 weeks.[73] The clotting mechanism initiates a cellular cascade of wound healing that leads to the development of a fibrin clot. After clot formation, a transient vasoconstriction takes place at the ends of the truncated blood vessels. Activated platelets retract and condense the hemostatic plug through condensation of the fibrin strands, which reduces the wound site.[74–76] These very early healing events are of considerable importance in endosseous peri-implant wound healing because proteins and other macromolecules interact first with the implant surface rather than cells. It has been shown that the degranulating platelets release cytokines and growth factors stimulating regeneration.[77] Platelet-derived growth factor (PDGF) has been shown to be a mitogen for fibroblasts[78] and bone cells,[75] and TGF-β has been shown to be present in the thrombus and promote type I collagen formation in bone cells.[79] Several authors[80–82] have shown that substrate rugosity influences the number and degree of activation of platelets. The initial hematoma is replaced by a fibrous vascular tissue that typically lasts for 3 weeks.[83] The tissue, mainly composed of vessels (more than 60% of the mass), undergoes mineralization, forming woven bone.[84] Woven bone invades the healing site and grows over the resorbed bone surface.

Bone formation requires both the recruitment and/or migration of a potentially osteogenic cell population (osteoconduction) and the differentiation of this population into mature secretory cells that will initiate matrix synthesis (ie, appositional growth). Appositional growth, beginning with the arrival of differentiating cells at the reversal surface, initiates the secretion of a *cement line*,[85] an afibrillar mineralized matrix that is 0.5 μm thick and particularly rich in glycoprotein. It was von Ebner[86] who first reported that osteons were demarcated from the surrounding bone by a distinct matrix, which he called *cement lines*. However, there is considerable confusion with respect to usage of this term. Weinmann and Sicher[87] introduced the term *cementing lines* to define the two distinct matrices at resting and reversal lines in bone; McKee and Nanci[88] provided an operational definition that grouped all matrix interfaces in bone as cement lines.

The difference in microarchitecture between lamellar and woven bone is most likely a result of differences in the rate and coordination of the secretory activity of the cells. Lamellar bone is the result of slow and synchronous secretion, whereas woven bone is the result of rapid and asynchronous secretion. Osteoconduction as reported by Davies et al[85] is the recruitment and migration of osteogenic cells through a three-dimensional, transient, soft biologic matrix. Osteoconduction and appositional growth represent the growth of the filling cone during bone remodeling or bone growth along an implant surface during contact osteogenesis.

## Clinical Considerations

In order to have long-term success with dental implants, the surrounding bone has to be mechanically stable, bearing the occlusal loading forces. Initial mechanical stability of the implant with the surrounding lamellar bone is necessary during the implant insertion. This is clinically determined as *primary implant stability*.

The gentle osteotomy, without overheating or significant mechanical trauma, is necessary to get good primary contact between the implant and bone. Early cellular repair and increased vascularization are the first stages of the repair process in the injured implant-bone interface. The quality of the new bone is very weak, especially 3 to 5 weeks after implant insertion. This period is the most critical from the clinical standpoint, especially when implants are immediately loaded.[89] For this reason, a high bone-implant contact (BIC) percentage at the day of the surgery is of clinical importance and can positively influence the long-term success of the implant.

A narrow necrotic zone of 1 mm or more may be present at the interface due to surgical trauma.[90] Thermal or mechanical damage of the surrounding bone during the osteotomy may lead to osteonecrosis with granulation tissue formation and implant encapsulation.[91] Thermal damage (overheating) may occur because of insufficient sharpness of the drills, hardness of the bone, improper use (or non-use) of irrigation, inappropriate temperature of the irrigation solution, and inaccurate pressure of the instruments during drilling.

Mechanical damage may result when high insertion torque has been used. Implant insertion without bone tapping is recommended in bone with good or soft quality to provide increased BIC. Excessive torque, which

Clinical Considerations

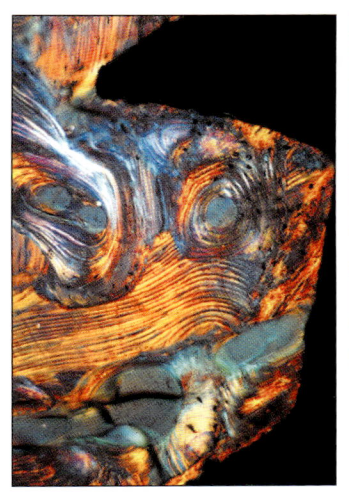

Fig 1-7 Lamellar bone contacting a dental implant, viewed with a circularly polarized light microscope (unstained; original magnification ×100).

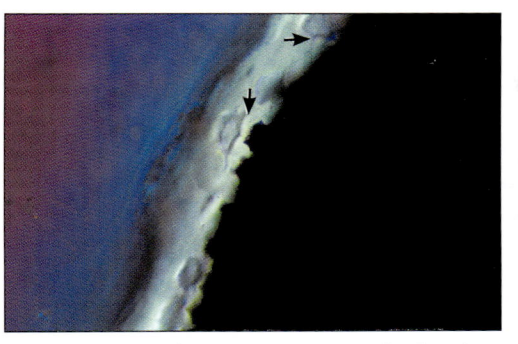

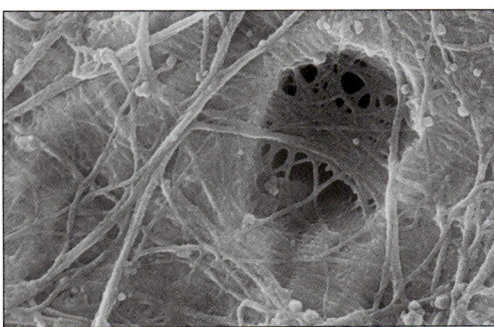

Fig 1-8 Osteoconduction *(arrows)* around a dental implant, observed using circularly polarized light microscopy (unstained; original magnification ×1,000).

Fig 1-9 Fibrin clot network over a dental implant surface viewed with a scanning electron microscope (original magnification ×30,000).

may damage the bone at the interface, must be avoided. Overcompression of the bone during implant insertion because of inadequate osteotomy size and the increased sharpness of the implant threads may be associated with implant failure because of necrosis at the implant interface.

Bone quality as defined by Lekholm and Zarb[92] is an important criterion for clinical implant success. Bone types 2 and 3 usually have the best healing capacity. However, this classification does not fully represent clinical reality because the implant-bone interface has different types of bone quality, depending on the location of the osteotomy site and whether monocortical or bicortical implant placement is used. The bone quality at the interface should be able to be classified in a three-dimensional way, ie, around the entire implant surface, giving the clinician the opportunity to make a better decision for the loading protocol.

In daily practice, different methods of measurement of primary stability, such as Periotest values using the Periotest device (Gulden Medizintechnik), resonance frequency analysis (RFA) with the Osstell device, and insertion torque, have been previously reported. Especially in areas with poor bone quality or compromised sites, the mechanical retention (immobilization) of the implant body in the osteotomy site is a prerequisite for later successful implant healing.

Implant design characteristics (tapered, threaded versus cylindric, nonthreaded), rough implant surface, and the correct implant bed preparation may promote the healing process. A cylindric implant with a smooth or polished surface will not osseointegrate. For example, the polished collar of tissue-level Straumann implants will not osseointegrate, and only connective tissue surrounds this area when these implants are placed subcrestally. In addition, long and narrow-diameter implants with primary stability may osseointegrate, and therefore, narrow-diameter implants may be used as successfully as standard-diameter implants.[93] Such implants heal when the primary contacts between the implant surface and the surrounding bone are high. Titanium-free (ie, stainless steel) implants can also heal and be functionally loaded successfully. Although the integration of the material presents a type of connective tissue formation and encapsulation of the implant, mechanical stability for long-term success is dependent on the implant shape. Areas for mechanical retention are important in order to have new bone formation around the implant and into the retention areas of the implant (Fig 1-7).

Threaded, conical implants allow for higher primary stability than do cylindric implants. The threaded design in association with the rough surface allows for better primary contact with the surrounding lamellar bone during implant placement. In case of mechanical anchorage, blood fills the grooves of the threaded implant, where the implant surface is not in close contact with the bone. In these areas, new immature bone is formed, with woven bone being the first type of bone formed (ie, distance osteogenesis). Later, composite bone will fill these areas. The migration of osteoblasts from the surrounding bone and osteoid production on the implant surface is necessary in this osteophyllic stage of bone healing. Later, carpet-like thin bone along the implant surface characterizes the phase of osteoconduction (Fig 1-8), in which the percentage of BIC increases significantly, with bone within 1 mm of the cervical margin in direct contact with the implant. This dense avascular bone is extensively remodeled and vital.

A rough implant surface has the additional advantage of increasing the affinity of the blood proteins for the osteotomy site, expediting blood clot formation (Fig 1-9), which leads to de novo and later to woven, composite, and lamellar bone formation.

In cases of mechanical anchorage of the implant with the surrounding bone, the primary contacts with the lamellar bone lead to further new bone formation (ie, contact osteogenenesis). The initial BIC increases during the healing process. However, an osseointegrated implant is characterized by a BIC percentage greater than 40%, whereas a mechanically (clinically) stable implant may also have approximately 25% BIC.[94,95]

An association between high stress concentrations due to lateral forces and high interface remodeling is observed. Under loading conditions, this bone will be reorganized, developing lamellae, which are responsible for the stability of the bone under occlusal masticatory forces. The BIC may not increase, but during loading conditions a characteristic thickening (ie, denser bone) is observed. This is the main characteristic of the osteoadaptive stage of implant healing. Dense trabecular bone may be formed 50% faster than dense cortical bone.[96]

The initial stage of healing is slower in older individuals but progresses normally thereafter.[97] Medical problems (eg, diabetes, metabolic bone diseases) are known to compromise healing potential. In addition, in the last few years special interest has been focused on bone healing during or after treatment with bisphosphonates in osteoporosis or tumor patients.[98] Clinicians should carefully consider medical parameters when determining the timing of implant loading or whether implant therapy is appropriate for a particular patient.

Of additional clinical interest is the biologic response of the bone when early or immediate loading has been used. Is osseointegration of an immediate implant possible? Considering the mechanisms of wound healing and the phenomenon of osseointegration, an implant placed in the fresh alveolar socket immediately after tooth extraction may heal if immobilization due to mechanical stability is present at the day of surgery. The gaps between the implant surface and the socket will close completely by woven bone if the gap is not too large.

Decisions regarding the use of flap elevation and membranes as well as the thickness of the bony buccal plate are very important criteria in immediate implant placement, especially in the esthetic areas, and should be considered in study protocols. Clinical protocols using multiple implants placed in fresh extraction sockets with immediate occlusal loading have been used previously[99,100] to avoid use of an interim prosthesis and to keep the treatment period short.

## Conclusion

To attain long-term success, initial mechanical implant stability immediately after placement in the osteotomy is very important and is dependent on implant configuration (shape) as well as factors such as sufficient cooling of the bone during drilling and avoidance of contamination of the insertion site or excessive placement torque, which may accelerate bone resorption and fibrous tissue formation, thereby jeopardizing new bone formation at the interface and leading to implant loss. For these reasons, correct implant site preparation, standards of hygiene, and adequate removal of inflamed granulation tissue in sites with periapical cystic lesions, granulomas, or previous periodontal disease should be considered very carefully. However, these considerations are of heightened importance when implants are to be immediately loaded.

## References

1. Listgarten MA, Buser D, Steinemann SG, Donath K, Lang NP, Weber HP. Light and transmission electron microscopy of the intact interfaces between non-submerged titanium-coated epoxy resin implants and bone or gingiva. J Dent Res 1992;71:364–371.
2. Riggs CM, Lanyon LE, Boyde A. Functional associations between collagen fibre orientation and locomotor strain direction on cortical bone of the equine radius. Anat Embryol (Berl) 1993;187:231–238.
3. Currey JD. The mechanical consequences of variation in the mineral content of bone. J Biomechanics 1969;2:1–11.
4. Zioupos P, Currey JD. The relationship between the microstructure of bone and its mechanical stiffness [comment]. J Biomech 1994;27:993–995.
5. Vose GP, Kubala AL. Bone strength—Its relationship to X-ray determined ash content. Hum Biol 1959;31:262–270.
6. Currey JD, Brear K, Zioupos P. The effects of ageing and changes in mineral content in degrading the toughness of human femora. J Biomech 1996;29:257–260.
7. Reid SA, Boyde A. Changes in the mineral density distribution in human bone with age: Image analysis using backscattered electrons in SEM. J Bone Miner Res 1987;2:13–22.
8. Parfitt AM. Osteonal and hemi-osteonal remodeling: The spatial and temporal framework for signal traffic in adult human bone. J Cell Biochem 1994;55:273–286.
9. Burr D, Forwood M, Fyhrie D, Martin R, Schaffler M, Turner C. Bone microdamage and skeletal fragility in osteoporotic and stress fractures. J Bone Miner Res 1997;12:6–15.
10. Baron R. Molecular mechanisms of bone resorption. An update. Acta Orthop Scand Suppl 1995;266:66–70.
11. Helfrich MH, Nesbitt SA, Lakkakorpi PT, et al. Beta 1 integrins and osteoclasts function: Involvement in collagen recognition and bone resorption. Bone 1996;19:317–328.
12. Mundy GR. Bone resorbing cells. In: Favus MJ (ed). Primer on Metabolic Bone Diseases and Disorders of Mineral Metabolism, ed 2. New York: Raven, 1993:25–33.
13. Pfeilschifter J, Seyedin SM, Mundy GR. Transforming growth factor beta inhibits bone resorption in fetal long bone cultures. J Clin Invest 1988;82:680–685.
14. Kameda T, Mano H, Yamada Y, et al. Calcium-sensing receptor in mature osteoclasts, which are bone resorbing cells. Biochem Biophys Res Commun 1998;245:419–422.
15. Hughes DE, Dai A, Tiffee JC, Li HH, Mundy GR, Boyce BF. Estrogen promotes apoptosis of murine osteoclasts mediated by TGF-beta. Nat Med 1996;2:1132–1136.
16. Rodan GA, Martin TJ. Role of osteoblasts in hormonal control of bone resorption—A hypothesis. Calcif Tissue Int 1981;33:349–351.
17. Rodan G, Harada S. The missing bone. Cell 1997;89:677–680.
18. Reddi AH. Bone morphogenetic proteins: An unconventional approach to isolation of first mammalian morphogens. Cytokine Growth Factor Rev 1997;8:11–20.
19. Rubin CT, Lanyon LE. Kappa Delta Award paper. Osteoregulatory nature of mechanical stimuli: Function as a determinant for adaptive remodeling in bone. J Orthop Res 1987;5:300–310.

20. Skedros JG, Mason MW, Bloebaum RD. Differences in osteonal micromorphology between tensile and compressive cortices of a bending skeletal system: Indication of potential strain-specific differences in bone microstructure. Anat Rec 1994;239:405–413.
21. Skedros JG, Bloebaum RD, Mason MW, Bramble DM. Analysis of a tension/compression skeletal system: Possible strain-specific differences in the hierarchical organization of bone. Anat Rec 1994;239:396–404.
22. Lanyon LE. Using functional loading to influence bone mass and architecture: Objectives, mechanisms, and relationship with estrogen of the mechanically adaptive process in bone. Bone 1996;18(1 suppl):37S–43S.
23. Traini T, Degidi M, Strocchi R, Caputi S, Piattelli A. Collagen fiber orientation near dental implants in human bone: Do their organization reflect differences in loading? J Biomed Mater Res B Appl Biomater 2005;74:538–546.
24. Traini T, Degidi M, Caputi S, Strocchi R, Di Iorio D, Piattelli A. Collagen fiber orientation in human peri-implant bone around immediately loaded and unloaded titanium dental implants. J Periodontol 2005;76:83–89.
25. Traini T, Neugebauer J, Thams U, Zöller JE, Caputi S, Piattelli A. Peri-implant bone organization under immediate loading conditions: Collagen fiber orientation and mineral density analyses in the minipig model. Clin Implant Dent Relat Res 2009;11:41–51.
26. Jee WS. The influence of reduced local vascularity on the rate of internal reconstruction in adult long bone cortex. In: Frost HM (ed). Bone Biodynamics. Boston: Little Brown, 1968:259–277.
27. Rubin C, Gross T, Qin YX, Fritton S, Guilak F, McLeod K. Differentiation of the bone-tissue remodeling response to axial and torsional loading in the turkey ulna. J Bone Joint Surg Am 1996;78:1523–1533.
28. Mason DJ, Suva LJ, Genever PG, et al. Mechanically regulated expression of a neural glutamate transporter in bone: A role for excitatory amino acids as osteotropic agents? Bone 1997;20:199–205.
29. Noble BS, Stevens H, Mosley JR, Pitsillides AA, Reeve J, Lanyon LE. Bone loading changes the number and distribution of apoptotic osteocytes in cortical bone [abstract]. J Bone Miner Res 1997;12(1 suppl):111S.
30. Skerry TM, Bitensky L, Chayen J, Lanyon LE. Early strain-related changes in enzyme activity in osteocytes following bone loading in vivo. J Bone Miner Res 1989;4:783–788.
31. Klagsbrun M, D'Amore PA. Regulators of angiogenesis. Ann Rev Physiol 1991;53:217–239.
32. Folkman J, Shing Y. Angiogenesis. J Biol Chem 1992;267:10931–10934.
33. Schmid J, Wallkamm B, Hämmerle CH, Gogolewski S, Lang NP. The significance of angiogenesis in guided bone regeneration. Clin Oral Implants Res 1997;8:244–248.
34. Lakey LA, Akella R, Ranieri JP. Angiogenesis: Implications for tissue repair. In: Davies JE (ed). Bone Engineering. Toronto: EM Squared, 2000:137–142.
35. Burkhardt B, Kettner G, Bohm W, et al. Changes in trabecular bone, hematopoiesis and bone marrow vessels in aplastic anemia, primary osteoporosis, and old age: A comparative histomorphometric study. Bone 1987;8:157–164.
36. Cruess RL. Osteonecrosis of bone. Current concepts as to etiology and pathogenesis. Clin Orthop Relat Res 1986;208:30–39.
37. Esbrit P, Alvarez-Arroyo MV, De Miguel F, Martin O, Martinez ME, Caramelo C. C-terminal parathyroid hormone-related protein increases vascular endothelial growth factor in human osteoblastic cells. J Am Soc Nephrol 2000;11:1085–1092.
38. Wang DS, Miura M, Demura H, Sato K. Anabolic effects of 1,25-dihydroxyvitamin $D_3$ on osteoblasts are enhanced by vascular endothelial growth factor produced by osteoblasts and by growth factors produced by endothelial cells. Endocrinology 1997;138:2953–2962.
39. Zheng MH, Xu J, Robbins P, et al. Gene expression of vascular endothelial growth factor in giant cell tumors of bone. Hum Pathol 2000;31:804–812.
40. Matsuo M, Nakamura T, Kishi Y, Takahashi K. Microvascular changes after placement of titanium implants: Scanning electron microscopy observations of machined and titanium plasma-sprayed implants in dogs. J Periodontol 1999;70:1330–1338.
41. Traini T, Assenza B, San Roman F, Thams U, Caputi S, Piattelli A. Bone microvascular pattern around loaded dental implants in a canine model. Clin Oral Investig 2006;10:151–156.
42. Trehame RW. Review of the Wolff's law and its proposed means of operation. Orthop Rev 1981;10:35–47.
43. Galileo G. Discorsi e dimotrazioni matematiche intorno a due nuove scienze. In: Bourne GH (ed). The Biochemistry and Physiology of Bone, ed 2. Vol 3: Development and Growth. New York: Academic, 1971:311–352.
44. von Meyer HV. Die Architektur der Spongiosa. Arch Anat Physiol Wissen Med 1867;34:615–628.
45. Wolff J. Das Gesetz der Transformation der Knochen. Berlin: Hirschwald, 1892.
46. Luck JV. Bone and joint disease. In: Weinmann JP, Sicher H (eds). Bone and Bones, ed 2. St Louis: Mosby, 1955:137.
47. Frost HM. The Utah paradigm of skeletal physiology: An overview of its insights for bone, cartilage and collagenous tissue organs. J Bone Miner Metab 2000;18:305–316.
48. Frost HM. Bone "mass" and the "mechanostat": A proposal. Anat Rec 1987;219:1–9.
49. Jee WS. The skeletal tissues. In: Weiss L (ed). Cell and Tissue Biology. A Textbook of Histology. Baltimore: Urban and Schwartzenberg, 1989:211–259.
50. Junqueira LC, Carneiro J, Kelley RO. Bone. In: Junqueira LC, Carneiro J, Kelley RO (eds). Basic Histology. Norwalk, CT: Appleton & Langer, 1995:132–151.
51. Aarden EM, Burger EH, Nijweide PJ. Function of osteocytes in bone. J Cell Biochem 1994;55:287–299.
52. Knothe Tate ML. "Whither flows the fluid in bone?" An osteocyte's perspective. J Biomech 2003;36:1409–1424.
53. Fritton SP, McLeod KJ, Rubin CT. Quantifying the strain history of bone: Spatial uniformity and self-similarity of low-magnitude strains. J Biomech 2000;33:317–325.
54. You L, Cowin SC, Schaffler MB, Weinbaum S. A model for strain amplification in the actin cytoskeleton of osteocytes due to fluid drag on pericellular matrix. J Biochem 2001;34:1375–1386.
55. You L, Weinbaum S, Cowin SC, Schaffler MB. Ultrastructure of the osteocyte process and its pericellular matrix. Anat Rec A Discov Mol Cell Evol Biol 2004;278:505–513.
56. Forwood MR, Turner CH. Skeletal adaptation to mechanical usage: Results from tibial loading studies in rat. Bone 1995;17(4 suppl):197S–205S.
57. Roberts WE, Morey ER. Proliferation and differentiation sequence of osteoblast histogenesis under physiological conditions in rat periodontal ligament. Am J Anat 1985;174:105–118.
58. Schenk RK, Herrmann RW. Histologic studies on the incorporation of uncemented implants. In: Morscher E (ed). The Cementless Fixation of Hip Endoprostheses. Berlin: Springer, 1984:52–58.
59. Gross UM. Biocompatibility—The interaction of biomaterials and host response. J Dent Educ 1988;52:798–803.
60. Plenk H Jr, Zitter H. Material consideration. In: Watzek G (ed). Endosseous Implant: Scientific and Clinical Aspects. Chicago: Quintessence, 1996:63–99.
61. Schwartz Z, Boyan BD. Underlying mechanisms at the bone-biomaterial interface. J Cell Biochem 1994;56:340–347.
62. Kieswetter K, Schwartz Z, Dean DD, Boyan BD. The role of implant surface characteristics in the healing of bone. Crit Rev Oral Biol Med 1996;7:329–345.

63. Schwartz Z, Kieswetter K, Dean DD, Boyan BD. Underlying mechanisms at the bone-surface interface during regeneration [review]. J Periodontal Res 1997;32:166–171.
64. Steflik DE, Corpe RS, Lake FT, et al. Ultra-structural analyses of the attachment (bonding) zone between bone and implanted biomaterials. J Biomed Mater Res 1998;39:611–620.
65. Marotti G, Ferretti M, Palumbo C, Benincasa M. Static and dynamic bone formation and the mechanism of collagen fiber orientation. Bone 1999;25:156.
66. Ferretti M, Palumbo C, Contri M, Marotti G. Static and dynamic osteogenesis: Two different types of bone formation. Anat Embryol (Berl) 2002;206:21–29.
67. Palumbo C, Ferretti M, Marotti G. Osteocyte dendrogenesis in static and dynamic bone formation: An ultrastructural study. Anat Rec A Discov Mol Cell Evol Biol 2004;278:474–480.
68. Ham AW. Some histophysiological problems peculiar to calcified tissue. J Bone Joint Surg Am 1952;24-A-3:701–728.
69. Harris WR, Ham AW. The mechanism of nutrition in bone and how it affects its structure, repair and transplantation. In: Wolstenholme GEW, O'Connor CM (eds). Ciba Foundation Symposium—Bone Structure and Metabolism. London: J&A Churchill, 1956:135–147.
70. Brighton CT. Principles of fracture healing. In: Murry JA (ed). Instructional Course Lectures. St Louis: Mosby, 1984:60–82.
71. Walter JB, Talbot IC. Wound healing. In: General Pathology, ed 7. New York: Churchill Livingstone, 1996:165–180.
72. Halkier T. Blood coagulation. In: Halkier T (ed). Mechanisms in Blood Coagulation, Fibrinolysis and the Complement System. Cambridge, England: Cambridge University, 1991:1–127.
73. Cormack DH. Bone. In: Cormack DH, Ham AW (eds). Ham's Histology, ed 9. Philadelphia: Lippincott Williams & Wilkins, 1987:273–323.
74. Chao FC, Shepro D, Tullis JL, Belamarich FA, Curby WA. Similarities between platelet contraction and cellular motility during mitosis: Role of platelet microtubules in clot retraction. J Cell Sci 1976;20:569–588.
75. Canalis E. Effect of growth factors on bone cell replication and differentiation. Clin Orthop Relat Res 1985;193:246–263.
76. Colman RW, Marder VJ, Salzman EW, Hirsch J. Overview of hemostasis. In: Colman RW, Hirsch J, Marder VJ, Salzman EW (eds). Hemostasis and Thrombosis: Basic Principles and Clinical Practice, ed 2. Philadelphia: Lippincott Williams & Wilkins, 1987:3–17.
77. Einhorn TA, Majeska RJ, Bosch CG, Rush EB, Horowitz MC. The production of cytokines by fracture. Presented at the Orthopedic Research Society 37th Annual Meeting, Anaheim, 4–7 March 1991.
78. Scher CD, Shepard RC, Antoniades HN, Stiles CD. Platelet-derived growth factor and regulation of the mammalian fibroblast cell cycle. Biochim Biophys Acta 1979;560:217–241.
79. Joyce ME, Jingushi S, Bolander ME. Transforming growth factor-beta in the regulation of fracture repair. Orthop Clin North Am 1990;21:199–209.
80. Nygren H, Tengvall P, Lundström I. The initial reactions of $TiO_2$ with blood. J Biomed Mater Res 1997;34:487–492.
81. Nygren H, Eriksson C, Lausmaa J. Adhesion and activation of platelets and polymorphonuclear granulocyte cells at $TiO_2$ surfaces. J Lab Clin Med 1997;129:35–46.
82. Hong J, Andersson J, Ekdahl KN, et al. Titanium is a highly thrombogenic biomaterial: Possible implication for osteogenesis. Thromb Haemost 1999;82:58–64.
83. Kanagaraja S, Lundström I, Nygren H, Tengvall P. Platelet binding and protein adsorption to titanium and gold after short time exposure to heparinized plasma and whole blood. Biomaterials 1996;17:2225–2232.
84. Winet H, Bao JY, Moffat R. A control model for tibial cortex neovascularization in the bone chamber. J Bone Miner Res 1990;5:19–30.
85. Davies JE, Ottensmeyer P, Shen X, Hashimoto M, Peel SA. Early extracellular matrix synthesis by bone cells. In: Davies JE (ed). The Bone-Biomaterial Interface. Toronto: University of Toronto, 1991:214–228.
86. von Ebner (Ritter von Rosenheim) V. Über den feineren Bau der Knochensubstanz. SB Akad Wiss Math Nat Kl Abt III 1875;72:49–138.
87. Weinmann JP, Sicher HS. Bone and Bones: Fundamentals of Bone Biology, ed 2. St Louis: Mosby, 1955.
88. McKee MD, Nanci A. Osteopontin and the bone remodeling sequence. Colloidal-gold immunocytochemistry of an interfacial extracellular matrix protein. Ann N Y Acad Sci 1995;760:177–189.
89. Buchs AU, Levine L, Moy P. Preliminary report of immediately loaded Altiva Natural Tooth Replacement dental implants. Clin Implant Dent Relat Res 2001;3:97–106.
90. Roberts WE, Smith RK, Zilberman Y, Mozsary PG, Smith RS. Osseous adaptation to continuous loading of rigid endosseous implants. Am J Orthod 1984;86:95–111.
91. Eriksson A, Albrektsson T, Grane B, McQueen D. Thermal injury to bone. A vital-microscopic description of heat effects. Int J Oral Surg 1982;11:115–121.
92. Lekholm U, Zarb GA. Patient selection and preparation. In: Brånemark P-I, Zarb GA, Albrektsson T (eds). Tissue-integrated prostheses: Osseointegration in Clinical Dentistry. Chicago: Quintessence, 1985:199–209.
93. Froum SJ, Simon H, Cho SC, Elian N, Rohrer MD, Tarnow DP. Histologic evaluation of bone-implant contact of immediately loaded transitional implants after 6 to 27 months. Int J Oral Maxillofac Implants 2005;20:54–60.
94. Roberts WE, Garetto LP, DeCastro RA. Remodeling of devitalized bone threatens periosteal margin integrity of endosseous titanium implants with threaded or smooth surfaces: Indications for provisional loading and axially directed occlusion. J Indiana Dent Assoc 1989;68:19–24.
95. Albrektsson T, Johansson C. Quantified bone tissue reactions to various metallic materials with reference to the so-called osseointegration concept. In: Davies JE (ed). The Bone-Biomaterial Interface. Toronto: University of Toronto, 1991:357–363.
96. Plenk H Jr, Danhel-Mayrhauser M, Matejka M, Watzek G. Experimental comparison of Brånemark and Ledermann titanium dental screw implants in sheep. Presented at the World Congress on Implantology and Biomaterials, Paris, 8–11 March 1989.
97. Tonna EA, Cronkite EP. Changes in the skeletal cell proliferative response to trauma concomitant with aging. J Bone Joint Surg 1962;44:1557–1568.
98. Migliorati CA, Casiglia J, Epstein J, Jacobsen PL, Siegel MA, Woo SB. Managing the care of patients with bisphosphonate-associated osteonecrosis: An American Academy of Oral Medicine position paper. J Am Dent Assoc 2005;136:1658–1668.
99. Grunder U. Immediate functional loading of immediate implants in edentulous arches: Two-year results. Int J Periodontics Restorative Dent 2001;21:545–551.
100. Cooper LF, Rahman A, Moriarty J, Chaffee N, Sacco D. Immediate mandibular rehabilitation with endosseous implants: Simultaneous extraction, implant placement, and loading. Int J Oral Maxillofac Implants 2002;17:517–525.

# Basic Principles and Clinical Applications of Immediate Loading

Implant survival is associated with implant stability during loading. Implant osseointegration is a prerequisite to establishing long-term stability. This may be promoted by using implant designs that allow primary anchorage of the implant in the surrounding bone as well as minimizing inflammatory reactions during healing.

According to empiric methods, healing periods of 3 months for the mandible and 6 months for the maxilla are required prior to loading an implant; however, this has not been confirmed by experiments.[1-3] A period without loading is considered part of the standard protocol for successful osseointegration. Initial biomechanical forces exerted on implants are linked to the formation of connective tissue at the bone-implant interface.[4-7] If implants are initially stable but have not yet undergone osseointegration and are stabilized later, the peri-implant connective tissue can be differentiated and new bone formed.[8] This clinical situation is similar to the immobilization of mobile fractured bone fragments by osteosynthesis plates in orthopedics.

## Definition of Immediate Loading

There is no standardized terminology for immediate loading of dental implants in the recent literature. Even early studies showed a splinting of the placed implants using a bar in the first 3 to 4 days of healing.[9-11] The loading of implants may be performed in two ways: *(1)* by provisional crowns or partial dentures having occlusal contacts (direct immediate or occlusal, functional loading) or *(2)* by using a removable prostheses without occlusal contacts (indirect or nonocclusal, nonfunctional loading).

Several papers present the exact terminology currently associated with immediate loading.[12-15] Van Steenberghe et al[12] differentiated *early* from *immediate* loading in their paper, presenting a concept of treatment in the maxilla in which a custom template was used and the definitive prosthesis was placed immediately after surgery. The definitive prosthesis was fabricated before surgery using precise three-dimensional planning software. Although this concept requires the use of innovative technology and advanced experience and cannot be used in daily practice by every clinician, it establishes the concept of *immediate loading* as referring to placing a definitive prosthesis with occlusal contacts immediately (within the first day) after surgery.

Degidi and Piattelli[14] defined *immediate functional* and *immediate nonfunctional loading* as the placement of provisional restorations the same day or within a few days of surgery with (functional) or without (nonfunctional) occlusal contacts. When the provisional prostheses are placed between 4 days and 3 weeks after implant placement, the approach should be defined as *early loading* according to these authors.

According to studies performed by Misch,[16,17] bone density in the bone-implant interface may be increased if the implant is loaded progressively. This is a treatment concept used when implants are placed in sites with poor bone quality. The implants are connected to their abutments without any occlusal contacts and are loaded only during chewing. Provisional crowns or partial dentures without contacts may promote bone regeneration at the interface and enhance implant stability. Bone-implant contact (BIC) can increase, and fine woven bone trabeculae can mature into coarser lamellar trabeculae, with an increase in mineral content.[17] This concept should be referred to as *progressive bone load-*

*ing* or *immediate provisionalization*, but not *immediate loading*. To avoid misunderstanding and to allow more critical and accurate evaluation, the occlusal condition of implants loaded immediately after surgery has to be clarified more precisely in the literature. Unfortunately, many authors do not provide details about the occlusal concept at the provisional stage immediately after implant placement.

## Rationale for Immediate Loading

Immediate loading is beneficial because it reduces the treatment period significantly, which has positive social and psychologic effects for the patient.[18] This is the reason that various methods were developed to reduce the healing period of implants.

The surgical and prosthetic requirements for ensuring that immediately loaded dental implants heal without complications have been described previously in several treatment protocols.[9,14,18–30] Recent studies demonstrate the use of modern technology for placement and immediate loading of implants using computer technology and medical imaging.[12,31–33]

Brunski et al[5] used histologic methods to examine the alveolar bone–implant interface that formed during immediate and delayed functional loading in dogs. Direct bone apposition was observed on the implants that had undergone delayed functional loading, while immediate functional loading resulted in the formation of fibrous, nonmineralized connective tissue in the interface. This bone was *repaired* when the implants were loaded immediately and was *regenerated* when implants were loaded after a healing period. Other studies produced similar results.[34–39] These findings are different than the histologic observations in the dog model by Sagara et al,[40] who demonstrated complete bone apposition and nonconnective tissue or fibrous encapsulation around immediately loaded implants. In contrast, less BIC was found in the implants subjected to delayed loading.

Implant stability, ie, a lack of micromotion along the interface, during healing can be achieved by delaying the time point at which functional loading is initiated and by increasing the total amount of BIC in order to compensate for the loading forces around the implants, which can be achieved, regardless of the biomaterial used, by the roughness of the implant surface (microinterlocking), proper implant thread design, and/or increasing the length of the implant (macrointerlocking). If certain requirements are considered, screw-type implants can be loaded immediately and osseointegrated successfully because of the high initial stability.[9,18,21,25,41,42]

## Clinical Treatment Concepts with Immediate Loading

Clinical experience has shown that high long-term success rates of implants loaded immediately after placement depends on bone quality and other specific conditions. In a systematic review of survival rates for more than 10,000 immediately loaded dental implants placed in approximately 3,000 patients with a maximum follow-up period of 13 years, the authors concluded that implant micromorphology and careful patient selection affect treatment outcomes. The overall implant survival rate for the included studies was 96.39%.[43]

For a better analysis of the literature and to demonstrate the important parameters for achieving a predictable result in different clinical protocols, this section presents the clinical application of immediate loading based on the type of the prosthetic restoration. The final part of this section discusses immediate loading of immediate implants (ie, implants placed in fresh extraction sockets).

### Overdentures

Ledermann[9,44] placed four implants in the interforaminal area in the mandible and loaded them immediately after surgery using a bar-retained restoration. This treatment concept enables patients to be provided with a restoration quickly and efficiently immediately after implant placement and without having to wait for the osseointegration period to elapse (Figs 2-1 and 2-2). The concept of an immediately loaded bar-supported restoration on four Ledermann threaded implants in the anterior mandible has been proven scientifically and clinically over more than 20 years of experience.[45] The study, involving 411 patients and 1,523 immediately loaded implants, in situ for an average of 7.23 years, produced a cumulative success rate of 92%.

Using a similar treatment concept with four screw-type implants, Babbush et al[10] showed that immediate loading can be successful when the implants are immobilized with a rigid splint, which safeguards the implant-bone interface against masticatory forces. Between 2 and 3 days after placement, the implants were splinted with a Dolder bar; the denture supported on it was relieved to accommodate the bar and adapted with a soft liner. Because the bone in the anterior mandible is relatively dense, a success rate of 88% was documented in this prospective study.

A further study carried out by Bijlani and Lozada[46] over a period of 6 years showed that Brånemark implants can also be exposed to full masticatory loading immediately after surgery if they are splinted during the initial stages of healing. The highly functional implant stability achieved with this treatment concept pleases patients and benefits both them and surgeons.

Clinical Treatment Concepts with Immediate Loading

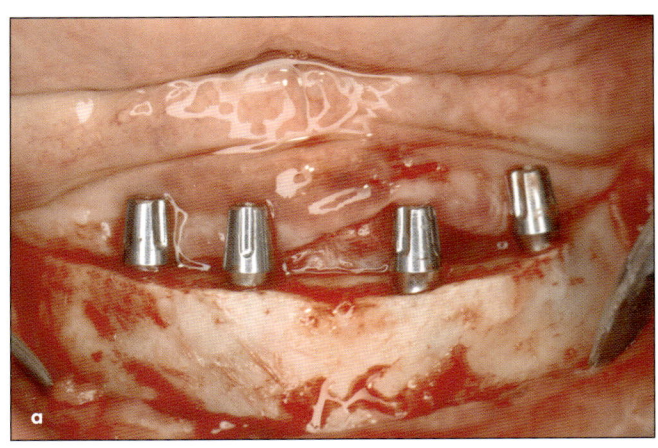

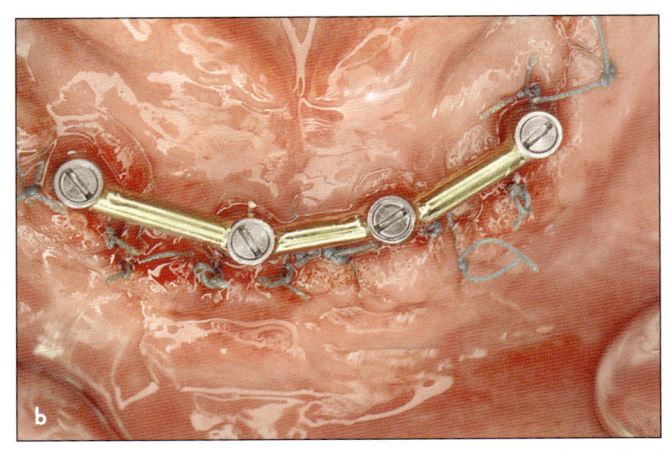

**Fig 2-1** *(a)* Implants placed in the anterior mandible for immediate loading splinted with a bar according to the Ledermann concept. *(b)* Occlusal view weeks after placement and splinting.

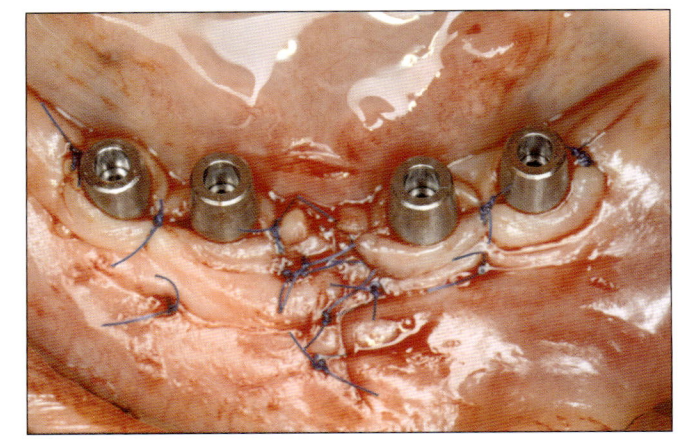

**Fig 2-2** Four implants with a progressive thread design in the interforaminal area connected with prefabricated conical abutments immediately after surgery. The implants were connected secondarily by the denture.

The multicenter study carried out by Chiapasco et al,[11] involving 226 patients and 776 immediately loaded implants splinted with a bar and loaded for a mean period of 6.4 years, produced a failure rate of approximately 3.1%.

Spiekermann et al[47] documented cases (11 patients) of mandibular overdentures fixed to three implants with rough surfaces splinted together with a Dolder bar and loaded immediately. The survival rate of the 36 implants documented in this study was 97.3% after 5 years.

Another clinical study was performed by Dietrich et al,[48] who used two different implant systems: *(1)* IMZ-TwinPlus (Dentsply Friadent) for submerged healing and *(2)* delayed conventional loading and titanium plasma-sprayed (TPS) implants for bar splinting and immediate loading. Five years after surgery, 83.6% of the immediately loaded implants and 94.6% of the submerged healed implants were in function. The overall survival rate in this study was 92.5% for 421 immediately loaded implants over a follow-up period of 6 months to 5 years.

Gatti et al[49] presented data for 21 patients with four tissue-level Straumann implants in the interforaminal area of the mental symphysis (84 implants in total), which were placed and splinted together with a bar for immediate loading with an overdenture. After a mean follow-up of 37 months (range: 25 to 60 months), the cumulative survival rate was 96%.

In a randomized clinical trial (RCT), Gatti and Chiapasco[50] documented a cumulative survival rate of 100% for immediately loaded implants with machined surfaces (ad modum Brånemark) placed in the mandible and restored with an overdenture in 10 patients (four implants per patient) after 24 months of loading. Similar results were observed by Romeo et al[51] in another RCT using implants with rough surfaces (tissue-level Straumann system) in the anterior mandible after 2 years of loading. In another study with 82 patients and 328 immediately loaded implants restored with overdentures, a survival rate of 97.6% was found after 36 to 96 months of loading.[52]

Further studies indicate that implants with increased primary stability placed in the interforaminal region can be loaded immediately not only using a bar but also with prefabricated telescopic crowns. Using this technique, the complete denture provides indirect splinting immediately after placement of the implants, eliminating micromotions, but only when a precise fit between abutment and secondary copings is guaranteed.[53]

May and Romanos[53] showed in a clinical study that implants (N = 204) placed in the anterior mandible can be successfully loaded when they are indirectly connected using an overdenture with telescopic abutments (see Fig 2-2). Immediately after surgery, the implants were connected to the prefabricated telescopic abutments (with 4- to 6-degree angulation), which were placed on the endosteal implants. Telescopic secondary copings were placed in the denture base using cold-curing resin and attached to the telescopic abutments. Using

13

this treatment concept, the authors presented a survival rate of 97.54% after 2 years of loading (see chapter 6).

A recent clinical study followed a similar concept but with a longer loading period of 79 ± 29.8 months (range: 17 to 129 months) and placement of 488 implants in the anterior mandible of 122 patients using prefabricated telescopic abutments with an angle of 4 to 6 degrees. A survival rate of 94.06% was observed.[54]

In another clinical protocol in which two implants with rough surfaces were placed in the anterior mandible of 10 patients and loaded 1 day after surgery using overdentures, the authors showed only a 20% survival rate after a mean of 29.8 months (range: 4 to 36 months) of loading.[55]

## Fixed restorations

A further study completed by Schnitman et al[56] indicated that a fixed restoration can be placed on immediately loaded threaded implants in the mandible using a provisional restoration during the healing period and without compromised osseointegration. In each patient, five to six implants were inserted in the anterior mandible, and two additional implants were placed distally. The authors loaded three implants immediately after surgery and evaluated the implant survival rate after 10 years. The failed implants in this study were all in the posterior mandible and were 7 mm in length. The authors pointed out that the primary reason for implant failure was the compromised bone quality in the region of the implant site, which was distal to the mental foramen. The 5-year results for this treatment concept did not indicate any significant differences between immediately loaded implants and those that were not immediately loaded.[57] The 10-year study, which involved a higher number of patients, produced a success rate of 85.7%.[58]

A study by Tarnow et al[20] that involved 10 edentulous patients with immediately loaded threaded implants also produced good clinical results (97% survival rate). The failed implants were from the posterior region of the mandible. The authors established that osseointegration took place after 5 years in cases in which the implants had been splinted with a provisional restoration. To prevent compromise of implant integration by shear forces, the authors suggested that the provisional restoration not be removed for a period of 4 to 5 months, during which there should be frequent checkups to control fractures of the resin partial dentures.

More recent clinical cases involving immediately loaded root-form implants splinted with provisional fixed partial dentures immediately after implant placement also report that it is only advisable to use the immediate loading protocol under certain conditions.[18,59] In an older publication, Salama et al[18] recommended the following criteria/prerequisites for successful immediate loading:

- High-density bone in the implant site (It is only advisable to place the implant in the anterior region of the mandible, where the bone is of relatively high quality.)
- Implant design that increases mechanical retention
- Rough implant surface to increase primary stability
- Bicortical implant placement for increased stabilization (if possible)
- Avoidance or reduction of distal cantilevers
- Occlusal scheme that guarantees that the implants are loaded axially and protected against overloading

A clinical study carried out by Randow et al[21] using self-tapping Brånemark implants appears to show that immediate loading is possible in humans when five to six machined titanium implants are placed bicortically in the interforaminal region of edentulous mandibles and immediately loaded with fixed partial dentures. The authors fully recommended the immediate loading concept and were able to prove that 18 months after implant placement no more peri-implant alveolar bone resorption had taken place than would have occurred using the traditional loading protocol. However, the implants were loaded after 10 days of healing using only soft-relined original dentures and 20 days after surgery using definitive fixed restorations. According to the current definition, this is not immediate loading. Nevertheless, this report may be found in Pubmed using the search term *immediate loading*.

Balshi and Wolfinger[19] recommended placing at least 10 implants in edentulous mandibles for fixed restorations and preferred bone height of at least 7 mm in the posterior region when implants have to be loaded immediately.

Glauser et al[24] examined 127 immediately loaded Brånemark implants in different clinical indications in 41 patients 1 year after loading. All implants, which were newly restored with fixed restorations, were loaded for a period of 1 year by means of provisional crowns or partial dentures. The cumulative success rate after 1 year of loading was 82.7%. For most implants placed in this study (66%), a guided bone regeneration technique was used because fenestrations, dehiscences, and intraosseous defects were present at the time of the implant placement and at the start of loading. The most failures were observed in the posterior part of the maxilla or in patients with bruxism.

Horiuchi et al[22] presented data on immediate loading of 140 Brånemark implants placed in the maxilla and mandible. The implant insertion torque was more than 40 Ncm, and the abutments were connected immediately after surgery. No grafting procedures were used. Temporary cylinders were incorporated into the provisional prosthesis using autopolymerizing resin. The provisional prostheses were screw retained and lingually/palatally reinforced with cobalt-chromium alloy. In each patient, 8 implants were placed in the maxilla and 10 were placed in the mandible. The healing period was 4 months for the mandibular implants and 6 months for the maxillary implants. During this healing period, provisional prostheses were not removed. According to the data, 44 implants were loaded immediately in the maxilla and 96 in the mandible. From these implants, 42 (95.5%) in the maxilla and 94 (97.9%) in the mandible were osseointegrated during a loading period of 8 to 24 months.

According to previous studies, posterior implant placement in association with immediate loading should be avoided because of the poor bone quality in the implant site and the resulting high failure rate. According to Schnitman et al,[60] factors associated with the survival of immediately loaded implants include intimacy of initial fit, percentage of implant in contact with cortical bone, density of the cortical bone, and elimination of micromovements during the bone remodeling period.

Horiuchi et al[22] recommended the use of 4-mm-diameter standard implants without tapping in areas with poor-quality (soft) bone. In addition, primary stability in the maxilla may be maximized when implants are placed in contact with the floor of the sinus or nasal cavity (ie, bicortical fixation). Micromotions during the healing period may disturb the remodeling phase and result in overloading. This can be more critical when unilateral partial dentures have to be used because of the high bending moments at the interface. Screw-retained provisional prostheses that rigidly splint the implants together may significantly minimize the micromovements.[22]

In general, cross-arch implant-supported fixed restorations may decrease overload because of loading force decompensation when implant position is optimized and the occlusal scheme is appropriate. An excellent treatment plan is therefore necessary.

Degidi and Piattelli[14] studied the prognosis of 646 immediately loaded implants placed in 152 patients. Only six failures were reported in the first 6 months of loading. A soft diet was recommended for the initial stages of the healing. Different implant systems with various geometries were used. The authors presented different survival rates depending on the implant site. Specifically, the survival rate was very high in the anterior mandible, in full-arch restorations of the mandible, and in the posterior maxilla (100%). Of great importance is the significantly lower survival rate presented in the posterior mandible (91%), in complete restoration of the maxilla (98.5%), and in the anterior maxilla (87.5%). All failures in this study had the same implant design placed in different bone qualities.

A recent multicenter study presented by Testori et al[28] showed no differences in crestal bone loss around immediately loaded and delayed loaded implants in the mandible. Implants with a rough surface (Osseotite, Biomet 3i) were placed in 64 patients. The implants (N = 325) were splinted 4 hours after surgery using provisional partial dentures; the provisional full-arch screw-retained restorations had occlusal contacts. The definitive partial dentures were placed 6 months after surgery. A cumulative success rate of 99.4% was found at the four clinical centers involved after a loading period of 28.6 months.

The precise morphologic changes that take place in the tissue when endosseous dental implants are functionally loaded under various biomechanical principles and factors that may improve the bone-implant interface should be examined in greater detail. Various authors have appealed to dental researchers to collect data on immediately loaded implants with different designs and surfaces so that the immediate loading treatment concept can become established in daily dental practice in the future.[61,62]

In the Brånemark Novum system for the anterior mandible, four Brånemark implants are placed according to the standard surgical protocol and loaded immediately after surgery using prefabricated components. In the preliminary clinical study, 50 patients with 150 implants were followed for 6 months to 3 years; three implants were lost, representing a survival rate of 98%.[63] In addition, the "all-on-four" concept for the mandible was used by different international centers and presented high survival rates.[64] However, in these case series, there is no critical discussion about the long-term peri-implant soft tissue quality nor esthetic considerations of the restorations.

For the Brånemark Novum treatment protocol, there are specific patient selection criteria, including alveolar ridge height of more than 11 mm and width of 6 to 7 mm. In addition, the shape and interrelationship of the jaws must meet certain requirements for surgery,[65] and bicortical fixation in the interforaminal area is recommended. At the moment, this surgical protocol may be used successfully only in the anterior mandible, which represents a relatively rare clinical condition; for example, only 3.5% of the Swedish population belongs to this group.

Maló et al[66] used this concept to treat 44 patients with 176 machined-surface implants with a cumulative survival rate of 97.2% after a 6-month loading period. A provisional acrylic-reinforced metal prosthesis was placed within 2 hours after surgery and replaced with the definitive restoration (Procera Implant Bridge, Nobel Biocare) 6 months after surgery.

In another report of cases with maxillary implants restored the same day after their placement with fixed full prostheses (388 immediately loaded implants in 43 patients), a cumulative survival rate of 98% was observed after 60 months of loading.[67] These data are similar to the observations of Balshi et al,[68] with 522 immediately loaded implants in the maxilla presenting a 99% survival rate after a mean loading period of 2.8 years.

An additional treatment protocol using Brånemark implants and immediate loading is the splinting of implants using provisional partial dentures.[69] This method was established in Hong Kong and is known as the *Hong Kong Bridge Protocol*. In a report of 14 patients, the authors placed four Brånemark implants in each patient and connected them with the final abutments. The length of the implants varied between 13 and 18 mm. Bicortical anchorage was used to maximize mechanical primary stability. The authors do not discuss the exact timing of definitive partial denture placement nor the possibility of problems like fractures of the provisional prosthesis. However, to be included, patients had to be nonbruxers and were required to adhere to a consistent follow-up schedule.

Transitional implants have been used for the rehabilitation of edentulous jaws when adjacent implants are placed and have to be loaded after healing. The small-diameter transitional implants can be loaded immediately after their insertion and, upon histologic examination, showed bone growth at the interface and osseointegration. Specifically, the BIC achieved with transitional implants was similar to that documented in the literature for conventional turned, machined-surface implants.[70,71]

## Partial dentures

The immediate loading concept has not been studied extensively in partially edentulous patients. Biomechanically, immediately loaded implants placed in partially edentulous patients are at higher risk because of bending moments applied during occlusal loading. Cross-arch stabilization and immobilization reduce and effectively control micromotions, keeping them below the critical threshold at which implant success is jeopardized. Therefore, immediate loading concepts in partially edentulous patients frequently involve placement of implants without occlusal contacts (immediate nonfunctional loading).

Rocci et al[72] tested immediate loading of Brånemark implants with two different surfaces (machined versus TiUnite [Nobel Biocare]) in the posterior mandible. The authors documented 10% higher success rates when the implants had a TiUnite surface rather than a machined surface (95.5% versus 85.5%).

Calandriello et al[73] placed 50 Brånemark machined-surface implants in the posterior maxilla and mandible with high primary stability of 40 Ncm, supporting 30 fixed partial dentures, and reported a survival rate of 98% after 1 year of loading. Even though primary stability was relatively high, the authors avoided normal occlusion in the provisionalization phase. They allowed only light occlusal contacts, and no contacts in lateral movements or cantilevers were used. A soft diet was advised for the first month of healing. Impressions were taken in the mandible and maxilla 3 and 5 months after surgery, respectively. The cumulative success rate after 18 months of functional loading was 98%.

Bogaerde et al[74] presented data for early and immediately loaded implants placed in areas with poor bone quality, namely the posterior mandible and maxilla. The study included 21 patients with 69 Neoss implants. Within the first 3 weeks of healing, provisional prostheses with narrow occlusal platforms, flat cusps, and light occlusal contacts were placed. An overall survival rate of 96.8% after 18 months was reported. This study concluded that the early or immediate loading protocol is a predictable method of treatment comparable to the traditional two-stage protocol.

However, Testori et al[27] used an immediate nonocclusal loading concept in partially edentulous jaws and compared the prognosis of 52 implants with early loaded implants. The authors recommended this treatment concept for daily practice because of the high predictability of the immediately loaded implants. According to this study, the cumulative survival rate was almost 96% after 19 months of loading.

In addition, excellent prognosis for implants placed using an immediate versus a delayed loading protocol in the posterior part of the mandible has been reported in a series of 12 cases using an implant system with a progressive thread design, a conical implant-abutment connection, and an abutment collar that is narrower than the implant diameter (ie, platform switching).[29,30] The success rate after 2 years of loading was 100% without cervical bone loss around the immediately loaded implants. The authors included an extensive discussion of the role of initial primary stability and its dependence on bone quality, surgical technique, and implant design, as well as the importance of splinting and a soft diet in controlling loading forces.

## Single-tooth implants

Studies on the immediate loading of single-tooth implants have been performed by different groups using various implant systems.[75–79]

Ericsson et al[77] used immediate functional loading of Brånemark single-tooth implants placed anterior to the molars and restored them with provisional crowns for 6 months. The definitive restoration was performed after this period. The authors reported 2 failures out of 14 implants (86% survival rate) and only minor bone changes after a mean loading period of 18 months. These data were also confirmed at a 5-year follow-up.[80]

In 14 consecutive case reports of immediate provisionalization of single-tooth implants, Wöhrle[76] showed maintenance of hard and soft tissues after a period of 6 months.

Chaushu et al[81] compared immediately loaded single-tooth implants placed in healed bone with those placed in fresh extraction sockets (ie, immediate implants). The survival rate was 82.4% for the immediate implants compared with 100% for the immediately loaded implants placed in healed ridges. For maxillary implants, they found a 75% survival rate in the immediate implant group compared to 100% for the implants placed in the healed sockets.

Kupeyan and May[82] reported on a series of 10 immediately restored implants in the maxillary anterior region. All implants were clinically integrated and remained stable for the 3-year observation period.

Other case series documented 100% survival of immediately loaded single-tooth implants replacing teeth in the anterior maxilla. A treatment protocol that includes long implants and the elimination of occlusal contacts in centric and excursive movements of the mandible has resulted in a high success rate.[83–85]

Other authors emphasize the diet protocol and the role of a liquid diet for the first 2 weeks postoperatively, followed by a soft diet for 5 months.[86] Following this protocol, a group of 35 threaded hydroxyapatite-coated immediate implants, which were provisionalized immediately after placement, showed an esthetic outcome and a survival rate of 100% after 1 year of follow-up.

In a case series study, Abboud et al[87] reported placement of single-tooth implants in the maxilla as well as in the mandible and restoration at the same day of insertion. Twenty implants with a progressive thread design and a rough surface were placed in 20 patients, and a cumulative survival rate of approximately 95% was found after 12 months of loading.

## Immediate implants

Grunder[26] showed data on the prognosis of immediate implants in the maxilla and mandible (66 sites) that were loaded immediately after their placement. No grafting techniques were used during surgery. The number of implants placed was 8 to 11 per jaw. The implants were splinted together with provisional metal-reinforced partial dentures for 6 months. Two years after loading, a success rate of 92.31% (87.50% in the maxilla and 97.26% in the mandible) was found.

Good experience using this concept has been reported in previous studies, in which periodontally involved teeth with poor prognosis were extracted and immediate implants were placed in combination with augmentation of the surrounding tissues if necessary. A cross-arch provisional restoration without contact in the lateral movements of the mandible was used. A soft or liquid diet was advised for the first stages of the healing in order to avoid overloading the immediate implants.[15,88] The provisional partial denture was replaced with the definitive fixed or removable implant-supported restoration after complete healing and evaluation of the peri-implant soft and hard tissue condition (3 to 5 months after surgery). Statistical evaluation of the 126 immediately placed and loaded implants showed a success rate of 97.62% after 15 months of loading. Replication of such results is dependent on patient compliance as well as the experience of the clinician.[89]

# Requirements for Successful Immediate Loading

Healing of immediately loaded implants depends on the initial implant stability, the type of splinting, and the occlusal forces (loading). Initial stability is influenced by the implant design and surface as well as the osteotomy site and the immobilization; the biomechanics are influenced by the type and magnitude of occlusal forces and the type of restoration. Many authors have recommended a soft or liquid diet to avoid overloading and implant failure in immediate loading protocols.[14,15,23,25,29]

## Implant design

The geometry of the implant, which includes the implant length and design, influences the micromotion and initial retention of the implant in the bone. Micromotion along the interface has a tolerance limit of 50 to 150 μm.[90–92] Movements exceeding 150 μm lead to connective tissue encapsulation resembling the healthy periodontal ligament of teeth.[93,94]

Several authors have recommended that the implant be at least 10 mm long.[10,11,20,21,23,95] In general, threaded implants should be used for immediate loading because their mechanical retention may be far superior immediately after placement.[61] The design of the implant can provide for extremely high initial stability and introduce the loading into the bone. This was confirmed in anatomical[96] and photoelastic[97] studies using an implant with progressive thread geometry. The designs of both the thread flank and back as well as the thread profile, which increases toward the apical aspect, ensure that the implant is retained particularly firmly, even in the soft cortical bone in the posterior mandible. However, current studies recommend replacing single molars with two or three implants or an implant with a wide diameter to avoid bending moments and reduce complications involving the restorations, such as screw loosening or implant fracture.[98–100]

In contrast to these studies, Romanos and Nentwig[101] found that a single molar may be replaced successfully with a single small-diameter implant (3.5 mm) when the implant-abutment connection is conical (Morse taper) and the implant has a progressive thread design. Using this implant system, a successful immediate loading concept is possible using partial restorations[29,30] as well as full-arch, implant-supported prostheses.[102,103] However, tapered implants have a higher primary stability compared with conventional cylindric implants.[104] In general, tapered implants present higher insertion torque levels and/or immediate removal torque values compared with cylindric implants. The use of tapered implants has been recommended over cylindric implants for functional or nonfunctional immediate loading. The tapered implants seem to have higher resonance frequency analysis values compared with cylindric implants.[27] Therefore, implants with tapered designs implants should be used in immediate loading protocols.

## Implant surface

The implant surface influences osseointegration[105] and initial stability.[106] Cylindric and porous implants have a better prognosis than threaded implants with smooth surfaces[107]; implants with porous surfaces may be loaded successfully after only 6 weeks[108] if two of them are splinted together. The role of splinting was also documented when ceramic implants splinted to adjacent teeth in monkeys presented successful loading after only 4 weeks.[109] TPS single implants were loaded 30 days after placement and compared with nonloaded implants at a later date, and no significant difference in the bone was found between the two groups.[110] During other studies, it was noted that TPS implants undergo osseointegration in the maxilla and mandible if they are allowed to remain nonloaded for 2 months.[111] Immediately loaded hydroxyapatite-coated blade implants splinted with adjacent teeth in rhesus monkeys also underwent osseointegration. However, the same treatment concept with uncoated blade implants resulted in connective tissue healing.[7]

Other clinical studies found a worse prognosis for Brånemark implants (failure rate: 35%) and Osseotite implants (failure rate: 34.4%) than for porous IMZ implants (failure rate: 4.3%) if they were placed in relatively thin and weak structured trabecular bone.[112–114] Quirynen et al[115] produced an even higher percentage of failures with Brånemark implants in the posterior max-

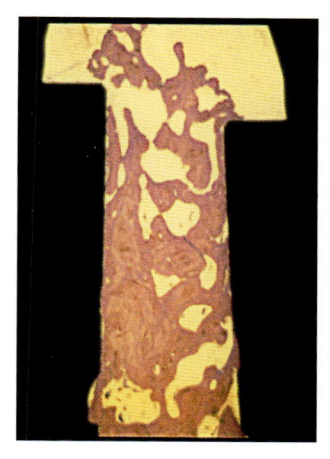

**Fig 2-3a** Histologic demonstration of two immediately loaded implants with a progressive thread design placed in the monkey posterior mandible showed a connection with the alveolar bone in the interface. No bone loss was found in the interface. The implants were covered by newly formed bone without any gaps of connective tissue (original magnification ×1.63).

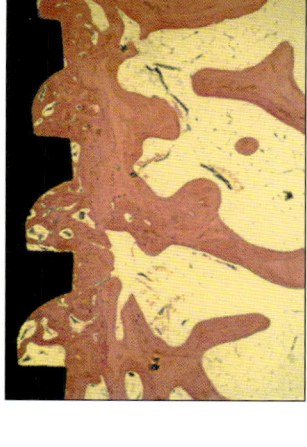

**Fig 2-3b** Firm connection of the immediately loaded implant (monkey posterior mandible) with the bone in the interface. Lamellar bone with thick bone trabeculae as oriented parallel to the implant surface. Some distance away from the implant surface, the bone presented marrow spaces with connective, especially fat, tissue and a weak consistency in comparison with the interfacial bone (original magnification ×25).

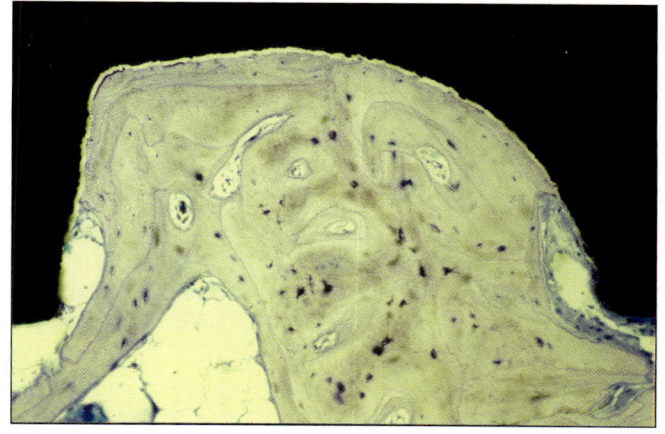

**Fig 2-3c** Well-organized bony tissue with healthy haversian systems and osteocyte lacunae were found within the threads of an immediately loaded implant in the monkey posterior mandible (original magnification ×50).

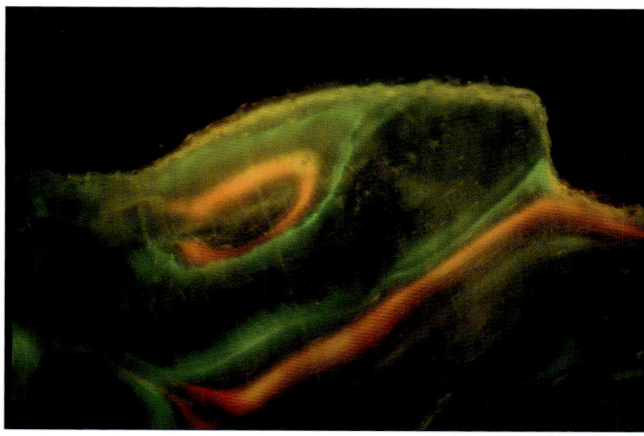

**Fig 2-3d** Fluorescent labeling of an immediately loaded implant in the posterior mandible showed well-marked stained bands of newly formed bone in close contact with the implant surface (original magnification ×20).

illa. The role of implant surface roughness on immediately loaded implants in the maxilla versus the mandible was demonstrated by Jaffin et al,[23] who found lower success rates when implants with machined surfaces were used in comparison with those with rough surfaces, especially in poor-quality bone.

## Bone quality

The quality of the bone is a decisive factor in the success of immediate loading because implant integration is based on the bone quality of the osteotomy site. Misch[16] divided bone quality in the maxilla and mandible into four classes (D1 to D4). He pointed out the different trabecular structure in the denser, clinically harder bone in the anterior mandible (D1) in comparison with the cancellous, poor-quality bone in the posterior region (D4). The density in the premolar region was similar to that in the molar region and lower than that in the interforaminal region. Jaffin and Berman[112] determined an association between implant failure and fine trabecular bone (D4). There appear to be significant inter-individual differences in bone density in humans, depending on various local and systemic factors (eg, osteoporosis).[116–119] Implants that had osseointegrated while submerged in regions with thin cortical layers were subject to much higher failure rates.[111,120–123]

Although many reports of successful immediate loading were performed in the anterior mandible, where the bone density is usually increased, according to the author's studies,[15,29,124–127] this loading concept also can be successful in the relatively weak-in-structure posterior mandibular bone. This has been proven clinically and histologically (Figs 2-3 and 2-4).

The quality of maxillary bone is considerably lower than that of mandibular bone. Maxillary bone has a very thin cortical layer and extensive areas with loose connective tissue.[128] This is the reason that long-term prognosis of maxillary implants is lower than that of mandibular implants.[129,130] A study involving implant-supported overdentures indicated a failure rate of 3.3% in the mandible and 27.6% in the maxilla during an observation period of 3 years.[123] A study carried out by Jaffin et al[23] confirmed that the failure rate in the maxilla is higher than that in the mandible. For these reasons the authors recommended only the use of rough-surfaced implants for immediate loading in the maxilla. Other studies recommended that tapping be avoided when implants have to be loaded immediately in areas with poor bone quality.[15,18,56,58]

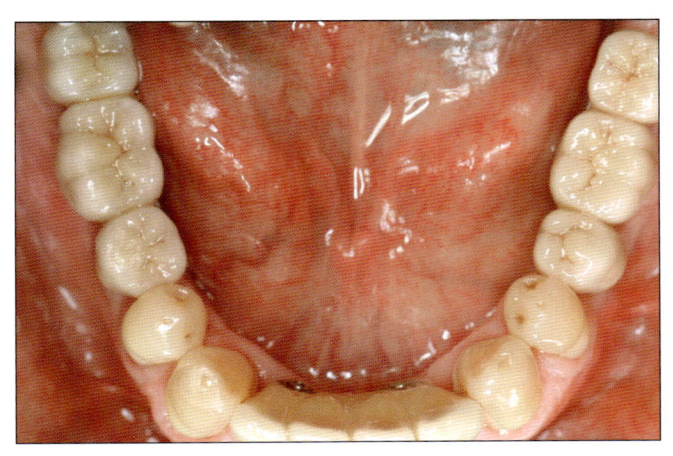

**Fig 2-4a** Clinical situation of the two implant-supported restorations in the posterior mandible 3 years after loading. The implants placed in the left side of the mandible were loaded immediately.

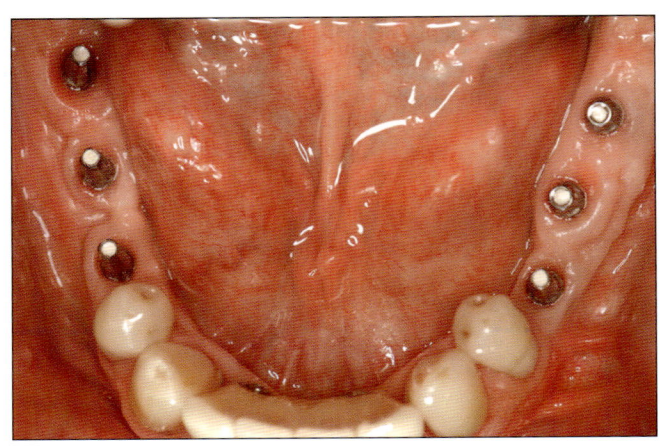

**Fig 2-4b** Clinical situation of the soft tissue healing 3 years after loading and following removal of the prosthetic restorations. The soft tissue was without any signs of inflammation in the delayed *(right side)* as well as immediately *(left side)* loaded implants.

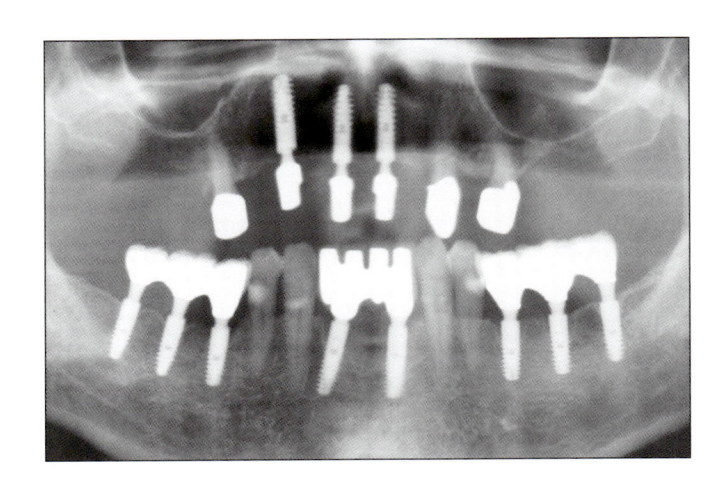

**Fig 2-4c** Radiologic examination of the delayed *(right side)* and immediately *(left side)* loaded implants showed no signs of bone loss 3 years after loading. The mandibular implants (delayed and immediately loaded) were loaded with a removable prosthesis in the maxilla.

## Biomechanics and bone remodeling

The role played by primary splinting and biomechanics in early or immediate loading of splinted implants[40,44,45,131] or implants splinted to teeth[7,61,109] has been discussed previously. The turning moments caused by masticatory loading are reduced considerably by splinting a higher number of implants.[132] This keeps the micromotion along the interface and below the critical level. A minimum of four implants splinted with a bar is optimal.[133]

Because osseointegration of an implant is comparable with the healing process of a fracture, mechanical stimulation of the bone, as when treating a fracture, is of particular interest. In orthopedics, it is often recommended that fractured, immobilized, splinted bone fragments be loaded at an early stage. Relatively early mechanical loading is considered advisable for the spinal column and conventional fractures of tubular bones[134,135] to accelerate the healing process.[136,137] Loading the bone increases vascularization and osteon formation significantly and leads to active remodeling.[138] To achieve this effect, it is essential that the load is applied not continuously but rather intermittently by exerting compressive and tensile forces on the bone.

Another study showed that quantitative mechanical parameters are closely linked to modeling and remodeling.[139] An annual remodeling rate of approximately 30% has been established for the interface of functionally loaded implants.[140] Generally speaking, the mechanical surroundings in the mandible are completely different after placing an implant. Most changes in mechanical parameters occur in the interface region.[141] Despite these research results, it remains unknown which biomechanical factor induces the initial bone or cell activity. Whereas some studies indicate that bone forms faster in areas exposed to severe compression, other studies consider the tensile forces as the stimulating factor for osteogenesis.[142,143] Currently, finite-element models are able to explain functional bone remodeling processes[144–147] but sometimes lead to entirely different results. Compressing the bone around implants may cause resorption[148]; expansion or inactivity of the peri-implant bone is also associated with bone loss.[149] Therefore, only in vivo studies are of significance.

## Splinting

The issue of micromotion at the bone-implant interface as an important parameter that jeopardizes osseointegration and forms connective tissue around implants has been studied extensively in the past. Cameron et al[91] reported that motions of approximately 200 µm resulted in fibrous tissue integration rather than bone formation. When micromotions occur, the bone formation is dependent on the surface roughness and does not necessarily lead to fibrous encapsulation. Maniatopoulos et al[150] showed that under the same amount of micromotion only porous endodontic implants osseointegrated.

Many authors have stated that the threshold of acceptable micromotion is important in association with the implant design and implant surface characteristics for bone growth.[93,94,150] The threshold level of tolerated micromotion was between 50 and 150 µm for bioinert materials.[151] Micromotions over 150 µm should be considered excessive and consequently deleterious for osseointegration. However, the presence of calcium phosphate layers on the implant surface enhances the threshold level of tolerated micromotions.[7,152,153]

Other authors also recommended in their immediate loading protocols that tapping be avoided or reduced in order to provide the best primary stability.[18,56,58]

To eliminate micromotions at the implant-abutment interface, immobilization of the implants through rigid splinting is necessary. For example, an implant-supported bar restoration immobilizes the implants. In addition, a fixed cross-arch prosthesis is able to immobilize the abutments and therefore the implants in order to control micromovements. The immobilization has to be secured if the primary stability of the placed implant is not excellent, especially if the peri-implant area is augmented, the residual lamellar bone is insufficient and weak, and if there is concern regarding the biomechanical components (ie, the magnitude of the occlusal forces).

## Implant-abutment connection

Based on the prosthetic protocol of the different implant systems, there is a variety of final torque levels recommended for connecting the abutment to the implant. There is no doubt that adequate final torque is necessary to allow fixation of the final abutment on an implant when implants are to be loaded immediately after their insertion. This eliminates micromovements so that the implant-abutment assembly behaves like a one-piece implant.

The variation in the required torque is dependent on the mechanical connection between implant and abutment, which differs among implant systems. This is important to reduce the microgap and to control micromovements between the abutment and implant. However, because of the high abutment torque, the immediate loading is not always successful in poor-quality bone.

In general, conical abutment connections need lower torque levels compared with other implant-abutment connections, which is of importance for immediate loading protocols, especially in weak cancellous bone.

## Clinical Considerations

The role of loading as a mechanical stimulus of bone that induces remodeling was introduced to implant dentistry by Linkow and Mahler.[154] Further experiments were carried out by Schroeder et al[155] and showed that the physicochemical bone-implant bond is strengthened by functional loading. The fresh bone accumulates on the rough surface and probably propagates as a result of the forces transferred directly to the bone.

Ledermann[44] was the first to immediately load TPS implants. Babbush et al[10] and Ledermann[45] recommended placing four implants interforaminally, in areas where the bone is at least 11 mm in height, splinting them with a bar and loading them immediately with a bar-retained restoration. These studies achieved a success rate exceeding 90%. Studies performed by Lozada et al[95] indicated that a success rate of virtually 100% can be achieved if the implants are at least 14 mm in length and the bone density is D1 or D2. This treatment protocol has clinical advantages for the patient because the surgical trauma is minimal and the total duration of the treatment curtailed considerably.

The results produced with provisional fixed restorations in the mandible indicated that the implants had a survival rate of only 84.7% because implants placed in the soft bone of the distal region failed.[58] Other studies indicated that immediately loaded implants in the posterior mandible failed at an even earlier stage. The general reason for these implant failures appears to be the relatively weak structure of the bone in this part of the mandible.[60,156]

Because bone quality differs, Tarnow et al[20] and Horiuchi et al[22] recommended leaving the provisional restorations in situ for 4 to 6 weeks. If the provisional restoration is to be removed, the authors recommend using screw retention to prevent creating stresses in the peri-implant bone while removing it. Tarnow et al[20] also applied this immediate loading concept to the maxilla and mandible. Splinting the immediately loaded implants temporarily and then connecting them to osseointegrated implants produces good results when restoring edentulous jaws. Distal cantilevers in the provisionalization stage must be avoided.[18,22]

When provisional crowns were delivered immediately after single-tooth implant placement in the maxilla, the occlusal contacts were eliminated in centric as well as eccentric excursions.[75,77]

Clinical, radiologic, histologic, and histomorphometric results indicate that a provisional restoration is an especially useful alternative for enhancing osseointegration. These findings were demonstrated when provisional restorations were placed in monkeys and screw-retained to ensure that no force had to be applied to remove them, which was required frequently. Because the Periotest values deteriorated continually during the loading period[126] and the histomorphometric data showed increases in mineralized bone,[157] further clinical examinations were carried out to transfer this treatment concept to daily clinical practice. Clinical examination using the same immediate loading treatment concept in the posterior mandible showed similar clinical and radiologic results for the implants with immediate and delayed loading. That means that implants can be immediately loaded also in areas with a relatively weak quality of bone if some requirements are considered.[29,30]

Optimum initial implant stability is a prerequisite for long-term success. Adequate initial splinting improves the prognosis, especially where the bone is of inadequate quality. Critical evaluation of the literature shows that a nonloaded healing period is no longer essential.

# Conclusion

Today, the surgeon is able to achieve high success rates if an implant system with good properties (design and surface) is selected and loaded immediately. Modern industry and its innovative technology produce numerous quality-assured implant designs and surfaces that promote osteogenesis and rigid bone-implant bonding. Selecting an implant system with good thread design and rough surface is a reliable means of assuring the quality of the immediate loading concept, even in areas with poor-quality bone. If the correct implant system is selected, bicortical fixation and placement of long implants can be avoided.

That which Salama et al[18] and Randow et al[21] previously recommended is no longer required. These authors had selected implant systems with smooth (machined) surfaces, which therefore permitted relatively large micromotions along the interface immediately after surgery. These authors assumed that a high number of implants were needed in order to compensate for the masticatory forces.[18,21]

As micromotions have to be controllable, some authors do not place the fixed restoration until the initial 20-day healing period has been completed[21] or the provisional acrylic restorations have been placed and the implants loaded for 4 to 6 months.[22] In these studies, the implants are not placed and loaded immediately in the maxilla or in areas where the bone quality is inadequate.[23] If implants are placed in the mandible, the interforaminal region is preferred for immediate loading.[21,56]

To prevent bending moments, many authors recommend the use of long-span partial prostheses with bilateral loading in edentulous jaws.[20–23]

Naturally, the surgeon's experience is especially significant if an immediate loading concept is used. Optimum handling of the soft and hard tissues, intraoperative condensation of the implant site with condensers and adequate cooling of the bone prevent injury to the tissue and enhance the quality of the bone-implant bond. In this way, postoperative complications can be minimized and failures reduced significantly. The implants should be placed parallel to each other to prevent incorrect loading. The occlusal contact areas can be checked to neutralize functional overloading and harmful eccentric forces.

Implants can be loaded immediately after placement if the implant system and the site preparation comply with all the requirements for optimum initial stability. The surgeon should produce a systematic presurgical diagnosis for every clinical case and carry out the treatment very carefully. The patient should be examined prior to the surgical procedure and the possible risks explained to him or her in detail. This is essential for ensuring that the patient gains maximum benefit from this treatment concept, ie, the duration of the treatment is curtailed considerably and long-term success is guaranteed. The surgeon must adhere strictly to the general principles of oral surgery, prosthodontics, and periodontology. The patient must maintain oral hygiene and comply with the surgeon's instructions. Optimum results can only be achieved if the entire team (surgeon, restorative dentist, and dental technician) is highly committed and takes an interdisciplinary approach.

# References

1. Brånemark PI, Hansson BO, Adell R, et al. Osseointegrated implants in the treatment of the edentulous jaw. Experience from a 10-year period. Scand J Plast Reconstr Surg 1977;16:1–132.
2. Brånemark PI, Zarb GA, Albrektsson T (eds). Tissue-Integrated Prostheses: Osseointegration in Clinical Dentistry. Chicago: Quintessence, 1985.
3. Cochran D. Implant therapy. I. Ann Periodontol 1996;1:707–791.
4. Ducheyne P, De Meester P, Aernoudt E. Influence of a functional dynamic loading on bone ingrowth into surface pores of orthopedic implants. J Biomed Mater Res 1977;11:811–838.
5. Brunski JB, Moccia AF, Pollack SR, Korostoff E, Trachtenberg DI. The influence of functional use of endosseous dental implants on the tissue-implant interface. I. Histological aspects. J Dent Res 1979;58:1953–1969.
6. Akagawa Y, Hashimoto M, Kondo N, Satomi K, Takata T, Tsuru H. Initial bone-implant interfaces of submergible and supramergible endosseous single-crystal sapphire implants. J Prosthet Dent 1986;55:96–100.
7. Lum LB, Beirne OR, Curtis DA. Histologic evaluation of hydroxylapatite-coated versus uncoated titanium blade implants in delayed and immediately loaded applications. Int J Oral Maxillofac Implants 1991;6:456–462.
8. Uhthoff HK, Germain JP. The reversal of tissue differentiation around screws. Clin Orthop Relat Res 1977;123:248–252.
9. Ledermann PD. Sechsjährige klinische Erfahrung mit dem titanplasmabeschichteten ITI-Schraubenimplantat in der Regio interforaminalis des Unterkiefers. Schweiz Monatsschr Zahnheilkd 1983;93:1070–1089.
10. Babbush CA, Kent JN, Misiek DJ. Titanium plasma-sprayed (TPS) screw implants for the reconstruction of the edentulous mandible. J Oral Maxillofac Surg 1986;44:274–282.
11. Chiapasco M, Gatti C, Rossi E, Haefliger W, Markwalder TH. Implant-retained mandibular overdentures with immediate loading. A retrospective multicenter study on 226 consecutive cases. Clin Oral Implants Res 1997;8:48–57.

12. van Steenberghe D, Naert I, Andersson M, Brajnovic I, Van Cleynenbreugel J, Suetens P. A custom template and definitive prosthesis allowing immediate implant loading in the maxilla: A clinical report. Int J Oral Maxillofac Implants 2002;17:663–670.
13. Aparicio C, Rangert B, Sennerby L. Immediate/early loading of dental implants: A report from the Sociedad Española de Implantes World Congress consensus meeting in Barcelona, Spain, 2002. Clin Implant Dent Relat Res 2003;5:57–60.
14. Degidi M, Piattelli A. Immediate functional and non-functional loading of dental implants: A 2- to 60-month follow-up study of 646 titanium implants. J Periodontol 2003;74:225–241.
15. Romanos GE. Surgical and prosthetic concepts for predictable immediate loading of oral implants. J Calif Dent Assoc 2004;32:991–1001.
16. Misch CE. Density of bone: Effect on treatment plans, surgical approach, healing, and progressive bone loading. Int J Oral Implantol 1990;6:23–31.
17. Misch CE. Progressive bone loading. In: Misch CE (ed). Contemporary Implant Dentistry. St Louis: Mosby, 1999:595–609.
18. Salama H, Rose LF, Salama M, Betts NJ. Immediate loading of bilaterally splinted titanium root-form implants in fixed prosthodontics—A technique reexamined: Two case reports. Int J Periodontics Restorative Dent 1995;15:344–361.
19. Balshi TJ, Wolfinger GJ. Immediate loading of Brånemark implants in edentulous mandibles: A preliminary report. Implant Dent 1997;6:83–88.
20. Tarnow DP, Emtiaz S, Classi A. Immediate loading of threaded implants at stage 1 surgery in edentulous arches: Ten consecutive case reports with 1- to 5-year data. Int J Oral Maxillofac Implants 1997;12:319–324.
21. Randow K, Ericsson I, Nilner K, Petersson A, Glantz PO. Immediate functional loading of Brånemark dental implants. An 18-month clinical follow-up study. Clin Oral Implants Res 1999;10:8–15.
22. Horiuchi K, Uchida H, Yamamoto K, Sugimura M. Immediate loading of Brånemark implants following placement in edentulous patients: A clinical report. Int J Oral Maxillofac Implants 2000;15:824–830.
23. Jaffin RA, Kumar A, Berman CL. Immediate loading of implants in partially and fully edentulous jaws: A series of 27 case reports. J Periodontol 2000;71:833–838.
24. Glauser R, Rée A, Lundgren AK, Gottlow J, Hämmerle C, Schärer P. Immediate loading of Brånemark implants applied in various jawbone regions: A prospective, 1-year clinical study. Clin Implant Dent Relat Res 2001;3:204–213.
25. Ganeles J, Rosenberg MM, Holt RL, Reichman LH. Immediate loading of implants with fixed restorations in the completely edentulous mandible: Report of 27 patients from a private practice. Int J Oral Maxillofac Implants 2001;16:418–426.
26. Grunder U. Immediate functional loading of immediate implants in edentulous arches: Two-year results. Int J Periodontics Restorative Dent 2001;21:545–551.
27. Testori T, Bianchi F, Del Fabbro M, Szmukler-Moncler S, Francetti L, Weinstein RL. Immediate non-occlusal loading vs. early loading in partially edentulous patients. Pract Proced Aesthet Dent 2003;15:787–794.
28. Testori T, Meltzer A, Del Fabbro M, et al. Immediate occlusal loading of Osseotite implants in the lower edentulous jaw. A multicenter prospective study. Clin Oral Implants Res 2004;15:278–284.
29. Romanos GE. Immediate loading of endosseous implants in the posterior mandible: Animal and clinical studies. Berlin: Quintessence, 2005.
30. Romanos GE, Nentwig GH. Immediate versus delayed functional loading of implants in the posterior mandible: A 2-year prospective clinical study of 12 consecutive cases. Int J Periodontics Restorative Dent 2006;26:459–469.
31. Tardieu PB, Vrielinck L, Escolano E. Computer-assisted implant placement. A case report: Treatment of the mandible. Int J Oral Maxillofac Implants 2003;18:599–604.
32. Balshi SF, Wolfinger GJ, Balshi TJ. Surgical planning and prosthesis construction using computer technology and medical imaging for immediate loading of implants in the pterygomaxillary region. Int J Periodontics Restorative Dent 2006;26:239–247.
33. Rosenfeld AL, Mandelaris GA, Tardieu PB. Prosthetically directed implant placement using computer software to ensure precise placement and predictable prosthetic outcomes. Part 1: Diagnostics, imaging, and collaborative accountability. Int J Periodontics Restorative Dent 2006;26:215–221.
34. Brånemark PI, Adell R, Breine U, Hansson BO, Linström J, Ohlsson Å. Intra-osseous anchorage of dental prostheses. I. Experimental studies. Scand J Plast Reconstr Surg 1969;3:81–100.
35. Piliero SJ, Schnitman P, Pentel L, Cranin AN, Dennison TA. Histopathology of oral endosteal metallic implants in dogs. J Dent Res 1973;52:1117–1127.
36. Listgarten MA, Lai CH. Ultrastructure of the intact interface between an endosseous epoxy resin dental implant and the host tissues. J Biol Buccale 1975;3:13–28.
37. Gourley IM, Richards LW, Cordy DR. Titanium endosteal dental implants in the mandibles of beagle dogs: A 2 year study. J Prosthet Dent 1976;36:550–566.
38. Young FA, Spector M, Kresch CH. Porous titanium endosseous dental implants in Rhesus monkeys: Microradiography and histological evaluation. J Biomed Mater Res 1979;13:843–856.
39. Albrektsson T, Brånemark PI, Hansson HA, et al. The interface zone of inorganic implants in vivo: Titanium implants in bone. Ann Biomed Eng 1983;11:1–27.
40. Sagara M, Akagawa Y, Nikai H, Tsuru H. The effects of early occlusal loading on one-stage titanium alloy implants in beagle dogs: A pilot study. J Prosthet Dent 1993;69:281–288.
41. Buser D, Nydegger T, Hirt HP, Cochran DL, Nolte LP. Removal torque values of titanium implants in the maxilla of miniature pigs. Int J Oral Maxillofac Implants 1998;13:611–619.
42. Buser D, Weber HP, Brägger U. The treatment of partially edentulous patients with ITI hollow-screw implants: Presurgical evaluation and surgical procedures. Int J Oral Maxillofac Implants 1990;5:165–175.
43. Del Fabbro M, Testori T, Francetti L, Taschieri S, Weinstein R. Systematic review of survival rates for immediately loaded dental implants. Int J Periodontics Restorative Dent 2006;26:249–263.
44. Ledermann PD. Stegprothetische Versorgung des zahnlosen Unterkiefers mit Hilfe von plasmabeschichteten Titanschraubenimplantaten. Dtsch Zahnärztl Z 1979;34:907–911.
45. Ledermann PD. Über 20jährige Erfahrung mit der sofortigen funktionellen Belastung von Implantatstegen in der Regio interforaminalis. Z Zahnärztl Implantol 1996;12:123–136.
46. Bijlani M, Lozada J. Immediately loaded dental implants—Influence of early functional contacts on implant stability, bone level integrity, and soft tissue quality: A retrospective 3- and 6-year clinical analysis. Int J Oral Maxillofac Implants 1996;11:126–127.
47. Spiekermann H, Jansen VK, Richter EJ. A 10-year follow-up study of IMZ and TPS implants in the edentulous mandible using bar-retained overdentures. Int J Oral Maxillofac Implants 1995;10:231–243.
48. Dietrich U, Lippold K, Dirmeier T, Behneke W, Wagner W. Statistical 13-year results for implant prognosis based on 2,017 IMZ implants in different indications [in German]. Z Zahnärztl Implantol 1993;9:9–18.

# References

49. Gatti C, Haefliger W, Chiapasco M. Implant-retained mandibular overdentures with immediate loading: A prospective study of ITI implants. Int J Oral Maxillofac Implants 2000;15:383–388.
50. Gatti C, Chiapasco M. Immediate loading of Brånemark implants: A 24-month follow-up of a comparative prospective pilot study between mandibular overdentures supported by conical transmucosal and standard MK II implants. Clin Implant Dent Relat Res 2002;4:190–199.
51. Romeo E, Chiapasco M, Lazza A, et al. Implant-retained mandibular overdentures with ITI implants. Clin Oral Implants Res 2002;13:495–501.
52. Chiapasco M, Gatti C. Implant-retained mandibular overdentures with immediate loading: A 3- to 8-year prospective study on 328 implants. Clin Implant Dent Rel Res 2003;5:29–38.
53. May D, Romanos GE. Immediate implant-supported mandibular overdentures retained by conical crowns: A new treatment concept. Quintessence Int 2002;33:5–12.
54. Romanos GE, May S, May D. Treatment concept of the edentulous mandible with prefabricated telescopic abutments and immediate functional loading. Int J Oral Maxillofac Implants 2011;26:593–597.
55. Stricker A, Gutwald R, Schmelzeisen R, Gellrich NG. Immediate loading of 2 interforaminal dental implants supporting an overdenture: Clinical and radiographic results after 24 months. Int J Oral Maxillofac Implants 2004;19:868–872.
56. Schnitman PA, Wöhrle PS, Rubenstein JE. Immediate fixed interim prostheses supported by two-stage threaded implants: Methodology and results. J Oral Implantol 1990;16:96–105.
57. Wöhrle PS, Schnitman PA, DaSilva JD, Wang NH, Koch GG. Brånemark implants placed into immediate function: 5-year results [abstract]. J Oral Implantol 1992;18:382.
58. Schnitman PA, Wöhrle PS, Rubenstein JE, DaSilva JD, Wang NH. Ten-year results for Brånemark implants immediately loaded with fixed prostheses at implant placement. Int J Oral Maxillofac Implants 1997;12:495–503.
59. Levine RA, Rose L, Salama H. Sofortige Belastung von wurzelförmigen Implantaten: zwei Fallberichte drei Jahre nach Belastung. Int J Parodontol Restaurative Zahnheilkd 1998;18:307–317.
60. Schnitman PA, Rubenstein JE, Wöhrle PS, DaSilva JD, Koch GG. Implants in partial edentulism. J Dent Educ 1988;52:725–736.
61. Brunski JB. Biomechanical factors affecting the bone-dental implant interface. Clin Mater 1992;10:153–201.
62. Piattelli A, Paolantonio M, Corigliano M, Scarano A. Immediate loading of titanium plasma-sprayed screw-shaped implants in man: A clinical and histological report of two cases. J Periodontol 1997;68:591–597.
63. Brånemark PI, Engstrand P, Ohrnell LO, et al. Brånemark Novum: A new treatment concept for rehabilitation of the edentulous mandible. Preliminary results from a prospective clinical follow-up study. Clin Implant Dent Relat Res 1999;1:2–16.
64. Brånemark PI. The Brånemark Novum Protocol for Same-Day Teeth: A Global Perspective. Chicago: Quintessence, 2001.
65. Lekholm U. Patient selection for Brånemark Novum treatment. Appl Osseointegration Res 2001;2:36–39.
66. Maló P, Rangert B, Nobre M. "All-on-Four" immediate-function concept with Brånemark System implants for completely edentulous mandibles: A retrospective clinical study. Clin Implant Dent Relat Res 2003;5(suppl 1):2–9.
67. Degidi M, Piattelli A, Felice P, Carinci F. Immediate functional loading of edentulous maxilla: A 5-year retrospective study of 388 titanium implants. J Periodontol 2005;76:1016–1024.
68. Balshi SF, Wolfinger GJ, Balshi TJ. A prospective study of immediate functional loading, following the Teeth in a Day protocol: A case series of 55 consecutive edentulous maxillas. Clin Implant Dent Relat Res 2005;7:24–31.
69. Chow J, Hui E, Li D, Lui J. Immediate loading of Brånemark System fixtures in the mandible with a fixed provisional prosthesis. Appl Osseointegration Res 2001;2:30–35.
70. Zubery Y, Bichacho N, Moses O, Tal H. Immediate loading of modular transitional implants: A histological and histomorphometric study in dogs. Int J Periodontics Restorative Dent 1999;19:343–353.
71. Froum SJ, Simon H, Cho SC, Elian N, Rohrer, MD, Tarnow DP. Histologic evaluation of bone-implant contact of immediately loaded transitional implants after 6 to 27 months. Int J Oral Maxillofac Implants 2005;20:54–60.
72. Rocci A, Martignoni M, Gottlow J. Immediate loading of Brånemark System TiUnite and machined-surface implants in the posterior mandible: A randomized open-ended clinical trial. Clin Implant Dent Relat Res 2003;5(suppl 1):57–63.
73. Calandriello R, Tomatis M, Vallone R, Rangert B, Gottlow J. Immediate occlusal loading of single lower molars using Brånemark System Wide-Platform TiUnite implants: An interim report of a prospective open-ended clinical multicenter study. Clin Implant Dent Relat Res 2003;5(suppl 1):74–80.
74. Bogaerde LV, Pedretti G, Sennerby L, Meredith N. Immediate/early function of Neoss implants placed in maxillas and posterior mandibles: An 18-month prospective case series study. Clin Implant Dent Relat Res 2010;12(suppl 1):83–94.
75. Gomes A, Lozada JL, Caplanis N, Kleinman A. Immediate loading of a single hydroxyapatite-coated threaded root form implant: A clinical report. J Oral Implantol 1998;24:159–166.
76. Wöhrle PS. Single-tooth replacement in the aesthetic zone with immediate provisionalization: Fourteen consecutive case reports. Pract Periodontics Aesthet Dent 1998;10:1107–1114.
77. Ericsson I, Nilson H, Lindh T, Nilner K, Randow K. Immediate functional loading of Brånemark single tooth implants. An 18 months' clinical pilot follow-up study. Clin Oral Implants Res 2000;11:26–33.
78. Hanisch O, Yildirim M, Höfer S, Spiekermann H. Sofortbelastung von Einzelzahnimplantaten—Experimentelle und klinische Ergebnisse. Implantologie 2000;2:163–172.
79. Malo P, Rangert B, Dvärsäter L. Immediate function of Brånemark implants in the esthetic zone: A retrospective clinical study with 6 months to 4 years of follow-up. Clin Implant Dent Relat Res 2000;2:138–146.
80. Ericsson I, Nilson H, Nilner K. Immediate functional loading of Brånemark single tooth implants. A 5-year clinical follow-up study. Appl Osseointegration Res 2001;2:12–17.
81. Chaushu G, Chaushu S, Tzohar A, Dayan D. Immediate loading of single-tooth implants: Immediate versus non-immediate implantation. A clinical report. Int J Oral Maxillofac Implants 2001;16:267–272.
82. Kupeyan HK, May KB. Implant and provisional crown placement: A one-stage protocol. Implant Dent 1998;7:213–219.
83. Andersen E, Haanaes HR, Knutsen BM. Immediate loading of single-tooth ITI implants in the anterior maxilla: A prospective 5-year pilot study. Clin Oral Implants Res 2002;13:281–287.
84. Touati B, Guez G. Immediate implantation with provisionalization: From literature to clinical implications. Pract Proced Aesthet Dent 2002;14:1699–1707.
85. Lorenzoni M, Pertl C, Zhang K, Wimmer G, Wegscheider WA. Immediate loading of single-tooth implants in the anterior maxilla. Preliminary results after one year. Clin Oral Implants Res 2003;14:180–187.
86. Kan JY, Rungcharassaeng K, Lozada J. Immediate placement and provisionalization of maxillary anterior single implants: 1-year prospective study. Int J Oral Maxillofac Implants 2003;18:31–39.

87. Abboud M, Koeck B, Stark H, Wahl G, Paillon R. Immediate loading of single-tooth implants in the posterior region. Int J Oral Maxillofac Implants 2005;20:61–68.
88. Nentwig GH, Romanos GE. Sofortversorgung von enossalen Implantaten. Literaturübersicht und eigene Erfahrungen. Implantologie 2002;10:53–66.
89. Romanos GE, Nentwig GH. Immediate loading of immediate implants for complete jaw restoration [abstract 276]. Presented at the 82nd Meeting of the International Association for Dental Research, Honolulu, 11 March 2004.
90. Cameron H, Macnab I, Pilliar R. Porous surfaced Vitallium staples. S Afr J Surg 1972;10:63–70.
91. Cameron HU, Pilliar RM, Macnab I. The effect of movement on the bonding of porous metal to bone. J Biomed Mater Res 1973;7:301–311.
92. Brunski JB. Avoid pitfalls of overloading and micromotion of intraosseous implants [interview]. Dent Implantol Update 1993;4:77–81.
93. Pilliar RM, Lee JM, Maniatopoulos C. Observations on the effect of movement on bone in-growth into porous-surfaced implants. Clin Orthop Relat Res 1986;208:108–113.
94. Szmukler-Moncler S, Salama H, Reingewirtz Y, Dubruille JH. Time of loading and effect of micromotion on bone-dental implant interface: Review of experimental literature. J Biomed Mater Res 1998;43:192–203.
95. Lozada JL, Tsukamoto N, Farnos A, Kan J, Rungcharassaeng K. Scientific rationale for the surgical and prosthodontic protocol for immediately loaded root form implants in the completely edentulous patient. J Oral Implantol 2000;26:51–58.
96. Bade H, Günes Y, Koebke J. Untersuchungen zur Primärstabilität von Dentalimplantaten. Z Zahnärztl Implantol 2000;16:33–39.
97. Nentwig GH, Moser W, Knefel T, Ficker E. Dreidimensionale spannungsoptische Untersuchungen der NM-Implantatgewindeform im Vergleich mit herkömmlichen Implantatgewinden. Z Zahnärztl Implantol 1992;8:130–135.
98. Becker W, Becker BE. Replacement of maxillary and mandibular molars with single endosseous implant restorations: A retrospective study. J Prosthet Dent 1995;74:51–55.
99. Bahat O, Handelsman M. Use of wide implants and double implants in the posterior jaw: A clinical report. Int J Oral Maxillofac Implants 1996;11:379–386.
100. Balshi TJ, Hernandez RE, Pryszlak MC, Rangert B. A comparative study of one implant versus two replacing a single molar. Int J Oral Maxillofac Implants 1996;11:372–378.
101. Romanos GE, Nentwig GH. Single molar replacement with a progressive thread design implant system: A retrospective clinical report. Int J Oral Maxillofac Implants 2000;15:831–836.
102. Romanos GE, Nentwig GH. Immediate loading in edentulous jaws [abstract 363]. J Clin Periodontol 2003;30(Suppl 4):92.
103. Romanos GE. Treatment of advanced periodontal destruction with immediately loaded implants and simultaneous bone augmentation. A case report. J Periodontol 2003;74:255–261.
104. O'Sullivan D, Sennerby L, Meredith N. Measurements comparing the initial stability of five designs of dental implants: A human cadaver study. Clin Implant Dent Relat Res 2000;2:85–92.
105. Thomas KA, Cook SD, Renz EA, et al. The effect of surface treatments on the interface mechanics of LTI pyrolytic carbon implants. J Biomed Mater Res 1985;19:145–159.
106. Hansson HA, Albrektsson T, Brånemark PI. Structural aspects of the interface between tissue and titanium implants. J Prosthet Dent 1983;50:108–113.
107. Pilliar RM. Porous-surfaced endosseous dental implants—Design/tissue response. In: Kawahara H (ed). Oral Implantology and Biomaterials. New York: Elsevier, 1989:151–161.
108. Deporter DA, Watson PA, Pilliar RM, Howley TP, Winslow J. A histological evaluation of a functional endosseous, porous-surfaced, titanium alloy dental implant system in the dog. J Dent Res 1988;67:1190–1195.
109. Hashimoto M, Akagawa Y, Nikai H, Tsuru H. Single-crystal sapphire endosseous dental implant loaded with functional stress—Clinical and histological evaluation of peri-implant tissues. J Oral Rehabil 1988;15:65–76.
110. Piattelli A, Ruggeri A, Franchi M, Romasco N, Trisi P. An histologic and histomorphometric study of bone reactions to unloaded and loaded non-submerged single implants in monkeys: A pilot study. J Oral Implantol 1993;19:314–320.
111. Corigliano M, Quaranta M, Scarano A, Piattelli A. Bone reactions to early loaded plasma-sprayed titanium implants [abstract 275]. J Dent Res 1995;74(special issue):435.
112. Jaffin RA, Berman CL. The excessive loss of Brånemark fixtures in type IV bone: A 5-year analysis. J Periodontol 1991;62:2–4.
113. Fugazzotto PA, Wheeler SL, Lindsay JA. Success and failure rates of cylinder implants in type IV bone. J Periodontol 1993;64:1085–1087.
114. Sullivan DY, Sherwood RL, Mai TN. Preliminary results of a multicenter study evaluating a chemically enhanced surface for machined commercially pure titanium implants. J Prosthet Dent 1997;78:379–386.
115. Quirynen M, Naert I, van Steenberghe D, et al. The cumulative failure rate of the Brånemark system in the overdenture, the fixed partial and then fixed full prostheses design: A prospective study on 1273 fixtues. J Head Neck Pathol 1991;10:43–53.
116. Atwood DA. Reduction of residual ridges: A major oral disease entity. J Prosthet Dent 1971;26:266–279.
117. Tillmann B, Härle F, Schleicher A. Biomechanik des Unterkiefers. Dtsch Zahnärztl Z 1983;38:285–293.
118. von Wowern N, Storm TL, Olgaard K. Bone mineral content by photon absorptiometry of the mandible compared with that of the forearm and the lumbar spine. Calcif Tissue Int 1988;42:157–161.
119. Ulm CW, Kneissel M, Hahn M, Solar P, Matejka M, Donath K. Characteristics of the cancellous bone of edentulous mandibles. Clin Oral Implants Res 1997;8:125–130.
120. Saadoun AP, Le Gall ML. Clinical results and guidelines on Steri-Oss endosseous implants. Int J Periodontics Restorative Dent 1992;12:486–495.
121. Jemt T. Implant treatment in resorbed edentulous upper jaws. A three-year follow-up in 70 patients. Clin Oral Implants Res 1993;4:187–194.
122. Truhlar RS, Morris HF, Ochi S, Winkler S. Second-stage failures related to bone quality in patients receiving endosseous dental implants: DICRG interim report no. 7. Implant Dent 1994;3:252–255.
123. Hutton JE, Heath MR, Chai JY, et al. Factors related to success and failure rates at a 3-year follow-up in a multicenter study of overdentures supported by Brånemark implants. Int J Oral Maxillofac Implants 1995;10:33–42.
124. Romanos GE, Toh CG, Siar CH, Swaminathan D. Histologic and histomorphometric evaluation of peri-implant bone subjected to immediate loading: An experimental study with Macaca fascicularis. Int J Oral Maxillofac Implants 2002;17;44–51.
125. Romanos GE, Toh CG, Siar CH, Wicht, H, Yacoob H, Nentwig GH. Bone-implant interface around titanium implants under different loading conditions: A histomorphometrical analysis in the Macaca fascicularis monkey. J Periodontol 2003;74:1483–1490.
126. Toh CH, Romanos GE, Siar CH, Swaminathan D, Ong AH. Immediate loading of implants with splinted crowns: A clinical and radiographic evaluation in a monkey model [abstract]. J Dent Res 2000;79:337.

127. Romanos GE, Toh CG, Siar CH, et al. Peri-implant bone reactions to immediately loaded implants. An experimental study in monkeys. J Periodontol 2001;72:506–511.
128. Razavi R, Khan Z, Zena R, Gould A. Anatomic evaluation of edentulous maxillae for placement of endosseous implants [abstract]. J Dent Res 1990;69:305.
129. Adell R, Lekholm U, Rockler B, Brånemark PI. A 15-year-study of osseointegrated implants on the treatment of the edentulous jaw. Int J Oral Surg 1981;10:387–416.
130. Adell R, Eriksson B, Lekholm U, Brånemark PI, Jemt T. Long-term follow-up study of osseointegrated implants in the treatment of totally edentulous jaws. Int J Oral Maxillofac Implants 1990;5:347–359.
131. Akagawa Y, Ichikawa Y, Nikai H, Tsuru H. Interface histology of unloaded and early loaded partially stabilized zirconia endosseous implant in initial bone healing. J Prosthet Dent 1993;69:599–604.
132. Skalak R. Stress transfer at the implant interface. J Oral Implantol 1988;13:581–593.
133. Rungcharassaeng K, Kan JY. Immediately loaded mandibular implant bar overdenture: A surgical and prosthodontic rationale. Int J Periodontics Restorative Dent 2000;20:71–79.
134. Sarmiento A, Schaeffer JF, Beckerman L, Latta LL, Enis JE. Fracture healing in rat femora as affected by functional weight bearing. J Bone Joint Surg Am 1977;59:369–375.
135. Goodman S, Aspenberg P. Effects of mechanical stimulation on the differentiation of hard tissues. Biomaterials 1993;14:563–569.
136. Goodship AE, Kenwright J. The influence of induced micromovement upon the healing of experimental tibial fractures. J Bone Joint Surg Br 1985;67:650–655.
137. Kenwright J, Richardson JB, Cunningham JL, et al. Axial movement and tibial fractures. A controlled randomized trial of treatment. J Bone Joint Surg Br 1991;73:654–659.
138. Hert J, Pribylová E, Lisková M. Reaction of bone to mechanical stimuli. 3. Microstructure of compact bone of rabbit tibia after intermittent loading. Acta Anat (Basel) 1972;82:218–230.
139. Brown TD, Pedersen DR, Gray ML, Brand RA, Rubin CT. Toward an identification of mechanical parameters initiating periosteal remodeling: A combined experimental and analytic approach. J Biomech 1990;23:893–905.
140. Roberts WE, Marshall KJ, Mozsary PG. Rigid endosseous implant utilized as anchorage to protract molars and close an atrophic extraction site. Angle Orthod 1990;60:135–152.
141. Chen J, Lu X, Paydar N, Akay HU, Roberts WE. Mechanical simulation of the human mandible with and without an endosseous implant. Med Eng Phys 1994;16:53–61.
142. Frost HM. Skeletal structural adaptations to mechanical usage (SATMU): 1. Redefining Wolff's law: The bone modeling problem. Anat Rec 1990;226:403–413.
143. Oda J, Sakamoto J, Aoyama K, Sueyoshi Y, Tomita K, Sawaguchi T. Mechanical stresses and bone formation. In: Hayashi K, Kamiya A, Ono K (eds). Biomechanics: Functional Adaptation and Remodeling. Tokyo: Springer, 1996:123–140.
144. Hart RT, Davy DT, Heiple KG. A computational method for stress analysis of adaptive elastic materials with a view toward applications in strain-induced bone remodeling. J Biomech Eng 1984;106:342–350.
145. Carter DR, Fyhrie DP, Whalen RT. Trabecular bone density and loading history: Regulation of connective tissue biology by mechanical energy. J Biomech 1987;20:785–794.
146. Hart RT, Hennebel VV, Thongpreda N, Van Buskirk WC, Anderson RC. Modeling the biomechanics of the mandible: A three-dimensional finite element study. J Biomech 1992;25:261–286.
147. Meyer U, Vollmer D, Homann C, et al. Experimentelle und Finite-Elemente-Analyse der Biomechanik des Unterkiefers unter Belastung. Mund Kiefer Gesichts Chir 2000;4:14–20.
148. Soltész U, Siegele D, Riedmüller J, Schulz P. Stress concentration and bone resorption in the jaw for dental implants with shoulders. In: Lee AJC, Albrektsson T, Brånemark PI (eds). Clinical Applications of Biomaterials. New York: John Wiley & Sons, 1982:115–122.
149. Cook SD, Weinstein AM, Klawitter JJ. Parameters affecting the stress distribution around LTI carbon and aluminum oxide dental implants. J Biomed Mater Res 1982;16:875–885.
150. Maniatopoulos C, Pilliar RM, Smith DC. Threaded versus porous-surfaced designs for implant stabilization in bone-endodontic implant model. J Biomed Mater Res 1986;20:1309–1333.
151. Søballe K, Hansen ES, B-Rasmussen H, Jørgensen PH, Bünger C. Tissue ingrowth into titanium and hydroxyapatite-coated implants during stable and unstable mechanical conditions. J Orthop Res 1992;10:285–299.
152. Geesink RG, de Groot K, Klein CP. Chemical implant fixation using hydroxylapatite coatings. The development of a human hip prosthesis for chemical fixation to bone using hydroxylapatite coatings on titanium substrates. Clin Orthop Relat Res 1987;225:147–170.
153. Søballe K, Hansen ES, Brockstedt-Rasmussen H, Bünger C. The effects of osteoporosis, bone deficiency, bone grafting and micromotion on fixation of porous-coated hydroxylapatite-coated implants. In: Geesink RGT, Manley MT (eds). Hydroxylapatite coatings in orthopaedic surgery. New York: Raven, 1993:107–136.
154. Linkow LI, Mahler MS. Implants for fixed and removable prostheses. Dent Clin North Am 1977;21:443–458.
155. Schroeder A, Stich H, Straumann F, Sutter F. Über die Anlagerung von Osseozement an einen belasteten Implantatkörper. SSO Schweiz Monatsschr Zahnheilkd 1978;88:1051–1058.
156. DaSilva JD, Wöhrle P, Rubenstein JE, Koch G, Schnitman PA. Four-year survival for 137 two-stage implants in partially edentulous patients [abstract]. J Dent Res 1990;69:268.
157. Romanos GE, Toh CG, Siar CH, Swaminathan D, Ong AH, Nentwig GH. Immediate loading on implants in the posterior mandible of M. fascicularis monkeys [abstract]. J Clin Periodontol 2000;27(suppl 1):27.

Paulo G. Coelho, Estevam A. Bonfante, Nelson R. F. A. Silva,
Jose M. Navarro, Georgios E. Romanos, and Jack E. Lemons

# Role of the Implant Surface in Immediate Loading 3

In immediate or early loading of endosseous implants, it has been speculated that alterations in surgical and restorative procedures as well as in implant design may significantly affect short- and long-term outcomes. From the perspective of implant design, two approaches based on the emerging fields of biomaterials and biomechanics have been most used: *(1)* implant body design and *(2)* surface modifications.

In this chapter, the different methods used for increasing surface roughness ($R_a$) and applying osseoconductive physicochemical modifications to titanium alloys used in dental implants are discussed. Surface treatments, such as titanium plasma spraying, grit blasting, acid etching, anodizing, and calcium phosphate coatings, and their corresponding surface morphologies and properties are presented. The majority of these surfaces are commercially available and have shown clinical efficacy.[1]

The objective of the present chapter is to describe critically the potential effects of current biomaterial and biomechanical engineering in implant dentistry, as well as their limitations and future trends. Because in-depth discussion of the covered topics is beyond the scope of this book, the interested reader is referred to the literature cited for more detailed information.

## Osseointegration and the Implant Surface

The osseointegration rate of dental implants is related to their composition and surface characteristics. Surfaces with highly osseoconductive surfaces may promote bone healing and apposition, leading to rapid biologic fixation of implants to bone.[1] Surface modifications have been extensively employed in commercially available systems in an attempt to accelerate bone-healing kinetics, allowing practitioners immediate and early loading of dental implants. Rough-surface implants have shown to favor both bone anchoring and biomechanical stability.[2-4]

Immediately following implant placement, a series of events occurs between the host and the surface of endosseous implants.[5] This sequence of events progresses from the initial interaction between blood and the implant surface, where proteins and ligands are dynamically adsorbed onto and released from the implant surface, through an inflammatory process, which is followed by initial bone formation around the implant (modeling), and through several remodeling cycles, where bone, in intimate contact with the implant, achieves its highest degree of organization and mechanical properties.[5] Because of the dynamic nature of the bone-biomaterial interface in terms of implantation time, endosseous dental implant biomaterials must have short- and long-term biocompatible and biofunctional properties.[6]

From a physics perspective, a *surface* may be defined as the sudden interruption of the crystallographic atomic arrangement. This sudden interruption results in differences between surface and bulk electronic properties, leading to different physicochemical behavior in the two regions of the material.[7] Therefore, theoretically, different modification methods applied in implant surface engineering may lead to different and unique surface properties. Because different physicochemical properties are achieved through surface modifications, potentially leading to changes in the host-implant response, new surface treatments should be tested as new biomaterials. Among surface modifications, the alteration of surface topography and the incorporation of bioactive ceramics as coatings have been investigated and used on a large scale by implant dentistry practitioners.[2-5,8-12]

# Testing of Implant Surface Designs

Despite the extensive literature accumulated over the past decades concerning the host-biomaterial response, several considerations should be taken into account concerning the real effect of endosseous dental implants' surface modifications during and after the process of osseointegration. Biologic concerns, such as the effect of surface modifications on the overall biocompatibility and osseoconductivity of the implant, should be considered. In addition, specific surface effects on initial bone-healing kinetics and the evolution of mechanical properties as implantation time elapses in vivo, as well as the in vivo stability of the surface (often regarded as one of the leading factors in long-term osseointegration), should be hierarchically investigated to rationalize modification of surgical and/or prosthetic implant therapy protocol following the introduction of new commercial surface designs.

This hierarchical approach, in which in vitro testing is followed by laboratory animal research, which leads to subsequent controlled prospective and/or retrospective clinical trials, often has been neglected prior to the introduction of new commercial surface designs. Therefore, treatment protocol changes, such as a decrease in the time allowed for osseointegration of immediately or early loaded dental implants, have been empirically or market driven.

A general description of the different surface treatments that are or will soon be commercially available is provided in the following sections. In order to facilitate the understanding of professionals not involved in basic or clinical research, a brief critical overview of the classic methodologies used for in vitro and in vivo performance assessment of endosseous implants is included.

## Biocompatibility of biomaterials

Prior to clinical trials, new biomaterials (including surface modifications, as these potentially change the interaction scenario between implant and host) should undergo in vitro and in vivo evaluation.[13] This type of evaluation typically follows a hierarchical approach, in which in vitro testing leads to in vivo laboratory experiments and then to clinical trials in humans. The hierarchical testing approach is useful in cases where surface modifications are compared with surfaces that have been in function successfully for several years. In simple terms, if in vitro and in vivo laboratory models do not show the new surface or biomaterial to have performance at least equivalent to existing surfaces/biomaterials, time-consuming and complex clinical research protocols may be avoided.

## In vitro testing

In vitro laboratory models often consist of evaluating the effects of novel surfaces versus control surfaces (in the case of dental implant surfaces, machined or surface-modified commercially pure titanium [cpTi] or titanium alloys) on cell cultures.[14] Cell culture studies attempt to track cell morphology, adhesion, migration, proliferation, or cellular death as a function of potentially toxic agents derived from the biomaterial.[5] While in vitro cell culture evaluation may be useful for preliminary evaluation of a biomaterial's biocompatibility with respect to controls, results obtained in cell cultures have not yet been appropriately correlated to in vivo performance.[14] Cell cultures by no means represent the dynamic bone-biomaterial environment that exists following implant placement, and any conclusions concerning the potential in vivo behavior based on in vitro testing should be seen as speculation and must be validated in animal models and subsequently in clinical trials. Nonetheless, this methodology has been useful as a first assessment of biocompatibility of novel biomaterial designs.[14] It may not be general consensus, but it has been suggested that the term *biocompatibility* may be more adequately employed for in vivo testing, whereas *cytocompatibility* should be used for in vitro characterization.[15]

## In vivo testing

Following in vitro laboratory testing of new biomaterial surfaces, laboratory in vivo models are the next stage in biocompatibility testing. Various animal models and surgical protocols have been used to evaluate the host response to endosseous implants.[2,4,16–24] Despite the development of extensive literature in the field, variations in wound healing and physiologic bone kinetics of different surgical sites and animal species have not been sufficiently characterized to enable direct comparisons between animal models or data extrapolation to clinical scenarios.[19] Nonetheless, animal models are extremely useful when novel biomaterial design is compared with older designs of known clinical performance. A potential advantage is the possibility of testing materials under loading scenarios over different evaluation periods and in different tissue qualities (eg, osteoporotic bone).[13]

Considering the variation in animal models, surgical sites, time periods in vivo, and control biomaterials among the many in vivo studies reported in the literature, direct comparison between previously published results is practically impossible with respect to which implant surface has the best physicochemical configuration to increase early wound-healing kinetics.

In vivo controlled laboratory studies are extremely valuable in cases where measurable indicators of the host-implant response are under comparison for two different surface designs. However, in order to decrease the degree of speculation with respect to the governing mechanism of the host-implant response between surface designs, the highest number of biologic response indicators (static and dynamic histomorphometric parameters, as well as biomechanical testing) should be evaluated and correlated.

Substantial data have been published concerning different surfaces' bone-biomaterial interface. Yet, whether the increased mechanical stability of different surfaces is due to an increased mechanical locking of tissue within the surface roughness, increased bone-implant contact (BIC), increased surrounding bone density, biologically modified bone bonding, or the interplay between such variables is still controversial or unknown.[5,25]

In vivo comparisons between different implant surface designs typically have a histomorphometric and/or a biomechanical component. The histomorphometric part of the study typically evaluates static parameters such as the amount of BIC, bone density, amount of cellular content, and bone area fraction occupancy (BAFO), among others, and dynamic parameters such as mineral apposition rate (MAR). Three-dimensional observations including the use of microcomputed tomography imaging have also been used to temporally quantify bone formation around implants and have been shown to statistically correlate with two-dimensional histologic observations.[26] The biomechanical testing component usually evaluates the push-out force,[27] pull-out force,[28] torque-to-interface failure[2,29] of implants in bone, and more recently, the evaluation of the surrounding bone mechanical properties by means of nanoindentation testing.[30]

While general tissue response to implants, biocompatibility, and osseoconductivity information may be obtained through static histomorphometric measurements, any one of the previously mentioned parameters alone does not address the tissue-healing events that lead to the parameters evaluated at a given time period in vivo.[31] For example, if a given surface resulted in higher BIC percentage relative to another at early implantation times, it is not possible to conclude whether this occurred because of higher osseoconductivity positively influencing healing kinetics or relative surface chemistry differences. It is possible that lower degrees of BIC from one surface relative to the other, derived from increased bone modeling/remodeling, may also lead to higher bone mechanical properties and improved biomechanical fixation. In this case, if no bone dynamic measurement or mechanical testing was carried out to support that the implant with lower BIC possibly presented better clinical performance, data misinterpretation would likely lead researchers away from an improvement in implant surface engineering.

Studies concerning the effect of different surfaces in bone-healing kinetics have been successful in indicating relationships between MAR and static parameters like density.[14,15,27] Unfortunately, the literature concerning bone-healing dynamics around different implant surfaces are not only sparse but contradictory,[32-34] and comprehensive studies using both static and dynamic histomorphometric parameters are desirable for better characterizing the evolution of the bone-biomaterial interface around different implant surfaces. It is also recommended that biomechanical testing of the bone-biomaterial interface is performed to support histomorphometric findings.

Standard ex vivo biomechanical tests (ie, torque, pull-out, push-out)[2,6,24–26,30,31] usually measure the amount of force or torque to failure of the bone-biomaterial interface surrounding different implant surfaces. While information concerning the relative degree of biomechanical fixation between different surfaces is obtained, these tests do not provide accurate information about inherent mechanical properties of the bone-biomaterial interface. In addition, these test methods tend to favor rough implant surfaces, making it challenging to evaluate different implant surfaces' effect on the evolution of the healing and mechanical properties of bone.

Recently, nanoindentation successfully evaluated the effect of different surface textures on bone mechanical properties as a function of implantation time.[17] While inherent mechanical property as a function of time may be assessed through nanoindentation, the value of relative changes in modulus as a function of healing time around implants is still subjective. For example, it is not possible to predict by simple mechanical property assessment if, over a given loading range, stress pattern or microstrain threshold for bone maintenance or loss[35,36] would significantly affect the overall biomechanical response as a function of implant surface and implantation time. Thus, biomechanical experimental designs taking into consideration bone mechanical properties and morphology around the implant as a function of implant surface and time are desirable for future design of improved dental implant systems.

Several factors that influence the phenomena of osseointegration remain under active investigation (eg, implant/biofluid interactions, the elemental chemistry and structure of surfaces, and the overall mechanisms and kinetics of bone response to implants). Therefore, careful interpretation of the literature, along with definitive characterization of bone physiology and kinetics of healing (eg, MAR, bone mechanical properties) around implants of different surfaces through evaluation of the highest possible number of host-implant response parameters should be considered in future research. This approach would allow a better understanding of bone-healing mechanisms around different implant surfaces, providing an informed design rationale of future implant systems that deliver decreased osseointegration time frames and therefore minimizing failures of immediately and early loaded implants.

## Clinical evaluation of implant surfaces

Clinical evaluation comprises the most complex type of biomaterial testing. While clinical data collection may illustrate the interaction between human tissues and different implant surfaces, from a statistical standpoint, any data collected from clinical trials should be interpreted with extreme caution. Clinical evaluation of different implant surfaces may be a challenge because large numbers of subjects must be analyzed in a previously determined statistical model, and any deviation from the previously established protocol may result in studies with low credibility. Retrospective and especially prospective studies must be carefully designed with rigorous sample size, proper randomization, and inclusion and exclusion criteria. Because the description of prospective and retrospective studies is beyond the scope of this chapter, the reader should refer to other sources where these types of studies are critically evaluated.[3,37–42]

## Implant retrieval analysis

The retrieval of previously functional endosseous implants (from a living tissue or obtained postmortem) is one of the most valuable tools for characterizing short- and long-term host-to-implant interactions as well potential failure mechanisms.[5,43] The information acquired through implant retrieval analysis is directly related to the amount of information available from patient, clinician, implant therapy modality, and implant system (ie, lot number); the lack of knowledge of any of these variables limits the amount of information that can be acquired from retrieved specimens, ultimately leading to erroneous conclusions. Therefore, protocol must be carefully designed prior to establishment of a retrieval program. If appropriately designed, implant retrieval analysis can be extremely useful in the reverse engineering of biomaterial and biomechanical designs, with investigators learning from both successes and failures.[5] Retrieval analyses of plateau root-form implants in clinical function for months and up to more than 10 years presented the variations in histomorphometric parameters as well as the bone microstructural evolution over time around loaded implants.[44,45] However, the limited number of currently active retrieval programs for which multidisciplinary expertise is available, added to the decreasing number of failure reports from both practitioners and implant manufacturers, is quickly decreasing the number of implant retrieval reports.

# Surface Modification of Dental Implants

The primary intention of further processing endosseous implant surfaces following device manufacturing is to positively modulate the host-implant tissue response. For this purpose, numerous surface engineering methods have been used to change endosseous dental implant surface topography and chemistry.

Although an exhaustive classification system with standardized chemical and physical parameters has been developed,[7] for the purposes of description, this chapter separates the surface modification methods into two categories. The first category, despite subtle to moderate differences in topographic and chemical composition between different designs, comprises primarily topographic surface changes. The second category includes the highly osseoconductive bioceramic coatings and novel approaches used to overcome processing limitations that result from surface modifications such as plasma-sprayed hydroxyapatite (PSHA).

## Topographic surface modifications

In order to describe some of the surface modifications currently used on a large scale in implant dentistry, it is important to describe the starting point of implant surface design. In the days of early implant dentistry, following machining (turning) of the implant bulk, the implant surface was cleaned, packaged, and sterilized prior to surgical placement. In general, after machining, the implant surface presents periodic grooves that vary based on specifications of the machining equipment, such as machining tool type and cutting angle (Fig 3-1). This procedure typically results in an implant with a clean, minimally rough surface (typically $R_a <$ 0.5 μm) that, according to classic protocols, requires several months for osseointegration. The machined implant surface was considered the gold standard of implant surface design for several decades and, to date, is the only surface design properly addressed from a statistical standpoint in the dental implant literature.[46] Thus, it is natural that most novel designs are compared with machined implant surfaces for in vitro, in vivo, and clinical investigations.

Despite the successful use of machined and sterilized implant surfaces for several decades, many studies have demonstrated that modification of the topographic pattern of the surface (especially if $R_a$ is 0.5 to 1.5 μm) tends to increase not only the BIC but also the resistance of the interface between the bone and implant.[2] Based on that, from the mid 1990s, experimental data obtained for rough surfaces ($R_a$ values around 1.5 μm) showed better bone response compared with machined or titanium plasma-sprayed (TPS) implant surfaces ($R_a >$ 2.0 μm). It should be noted that the majority of current commercial implant systems present $R_a$ ranging from 1 to 2 μm[2,8]; the effects of such characteristics on the osseoconductivity and bone apposition on the implant surface are still under investigation.

If further increases in surface roughness profiles are desired, TPS processing of the surface, which has been one of the methods commonly used for obtaining $R_a$ values higher than 2 μm and thus the highest surface area of all commercially available surfaces should be used. Based on that, TPS implants often have been recommended for use in regions with low bone density (Fig 3-2). The process is performed at high temperatures, and titanium powder is propelled toward the implant surface by a plasma (typically argon) to avoid the deleterious hydrogen contamination of the substrate.[6]

TPS processing may increase the surface area of dental implants up to approximately six times the initial surface area,[47] depending on implant geometry and processing variables, such as initial powder size, plasma temperature, and distance between the nozzle output and target. However, this significant increase in total area does not necessarily represent an effective increase in osseointegration area because spaces greater than 50 μm are typically required for bone formation and subsequent homeostasis.[48] Consequently, the real effective increase in functional area becomes 1.5 to 2.0 times the initial surface area[49] (see Fig 3-2). The increase of six times the original surface area may not be the sce-

# Surface Modification of Dental Implants

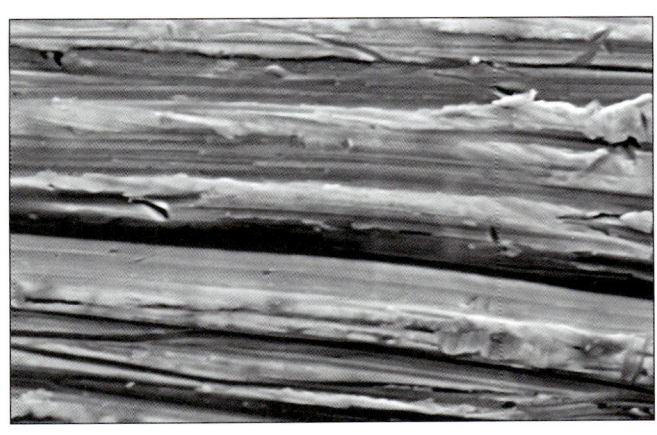

**Fig 3-1** Scanning electron micrograph (SEM) of a machined implant surface. Note the periodic grooves, which originate from the implant machining (original magnification ×1,500).

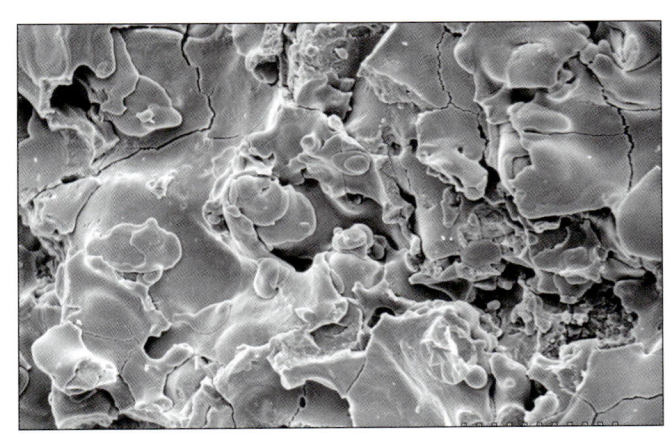

**Fig 3-2** SEM of a TPS implant surface. The micrograph also depicts the cracks that result from the rapid cooling that occurs during the TPS process (original magnification ×1,500).

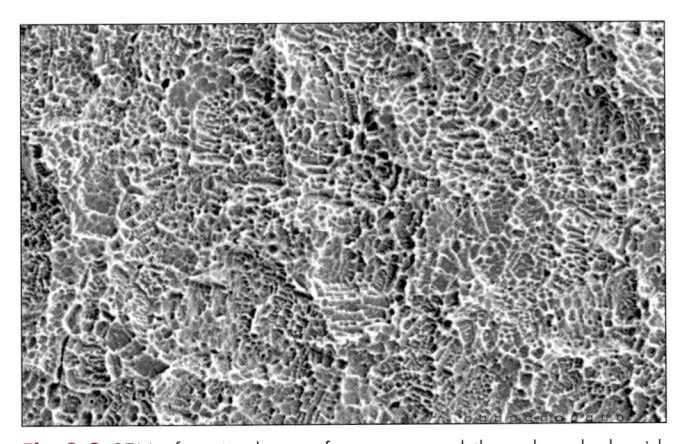

**Fig 3-3** SEM of an implant surface processed through a dual acid-etching procedure (original magnification ×1,500).

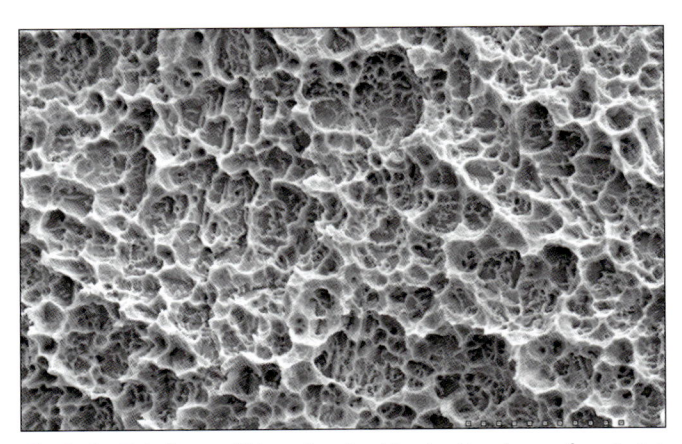

**Fig 3-4** SEM of a sand-blasted and acid-etched implant surface (original magnification ×1,500).

nario for bone growth and apposition but may become a factor when there is exposure of the implant surface to the oral fluids and bacteria. In addition, intercommunication between pores facilitates migration of pathogens to inner bone areas, potentially compromising the success of the implant therapy because of difficulties in controlling peri-implantitis.[50] Synergistically to bacteriologic contamination, autocatalytic chemical degradation may cause loss of metallic substrate and bone attachment.

Several in vivo studies have shown the importance of surface roughness for improvement and acceleration of osseointegration. Rough surfaces, such as those obtained by TPS, grit blasting, and acid etching have shown torque-to-failure values significantly higher than those of implants with machined profiles.[51] However, while favorable results have been achieved with the TPS surface in animal studies, its use has decreased because of the potential of coating debris in the surrounding tissues, leading biomaterials engineers to develop other techniques to change surface topography.

Over the last 5 to 10 years, implant surface roughness has been increased through a variety of methods in an attempt to increase surface area, cleanliness, and chemistry.[2,3] One of the earliest commercially available methods for increasing surface topography profiles was surface acid etching, either alone (Fig 3-3) or in combination with grit blasting (Figs 3-4 to 3-7). The majority of commercially available grit-blasted implant surfaces are subsequently acid etched. The acid-etching procedure aims to further enhance the topographic profile of the surface and remove processing byproducts. The grit-blasting procedure is generally performed via propulsion of variously sized particles of silica (sand) (see Fig 3-4), resorbable bioceramic (resorbable blast media [RBM]) (see Fig 3-5), alumina (see Fig 3-6), or titanium dioxide (see Fig 3-7) toward the metallic substrate.[6]

The most common acid-etching agents are hydrofluoric, nitric, sulfuric, or a combination of different solutions. The advantages of this method include an increase in the total surface area of the implant. This increase in surface area is due to the selective removal of the deeper parts of the topography, which degrade faster than the outer surface. However, this process should be carried out under controlled conditions because overetching decreases surface topography and creates mechanical properties that may be detrimental to osseointegration. In addition, it is important that the etching procedures following grit blasting remove any particle remnants (especially in the case of alumina or silica) because chemical analyses of failed implants have shown evidence that the presence of such particles could interfere with the titanium osseoconductivity regardless of their proven biocompatibility.[6] Alternatively, grit blasting the surface with bioceramic particles (RBM process) or titanium dioxide particles would not result in detrimental osseointegration kinetics because bioceramic particles are theoretically resorbed or dissolved over time.[6]

The most recent surface modifications presented to the market involve chemical changes to grit-blasted and acid-etched surfaces. The first modification comprises grit blasting and acid etching the surface with formulations that leave fluoride remnants on the surface to increase bone healing around the implant. The rationale for such modification is to gain the benefit of both optimal surface topography and chemical composition. However, the effect of this surface modification on bone formation around an implant is still unknown.

The second modification is submergence of implants in saline solution for sterilization and storage.[4] This method is used on sand-blasted, large-grit, acid-etched (SLA) implants (SLActive, Straumann). Topographically, this surface presents the same surface roughness pattern and chemical composition as the original SLA implant. A study has shown that the hydrophilic nature of the SLActive surface significantly increased the wound-healing kinetics compared to the previous SLA surface.[4] However, long-term clinical studies using the commercially available implant design with the SLActive surface are desirable because chamber models tend to favor intramembranous bone formation instead of appositional bone[16,52–55] (commonly observed in screw-type implants), and the effect of surface hydrophilicity may not be as evident in screw-type implants as it is in chamber models.

For better evaluation of the effects of such chemical modifications to rough substrates on the osseointegration process, more basic studies considering full surface characterization of experimental and control implants are desirable to elucidate the mechanisms by which these subtle surface chemistry changes speed up osseointegration.

Observations of the dual acid-etched as well as the grit-blasted and acid-etched surfaces showed that different roughness patterns are obtained depending on the processing condition and that higher surface areas are obtained compared with machined surfaces. It is also evident that different types of particles used for grit blasting result in surfaces with qualitatively different topographies. Based on the surface roughness, these different types of surface treatments typically result in $R_a$ values between 0.5 and 2.0 μm, which are associated with an increased early host-implant response in vivo.[2,3]

Considering three-dimensional parameters, it has been suggested that surfaces with an average roughness ($S_a$) of 1 to 2 μm may result in improved bone responses.[56,57] Another surface modification that increases the topography of the surface with potential surface chemistry changes and additions during processing is the anodization method (Fig 3-8). Studies have shown that this surface modification increases the early host-implant response.[58–60]

In general, moderately rough surfaces, such as those obtained through grit blasting with or without subsequent acid etching, anodization, or varied acid-etching procedures have presented higher torque values compared with machined surfaces. However, it should be noted that mechanical testing by means of torque, pull-out, or push-out tends to favor implants with rougher surface profiles because of mechanical interlocking of the bone and implant surface. Thus, whether rougher surface profiles favor the host-implant response, increasing bone mechanical properties at an earlier time point, or mechanical interlocking of rougher surfaces and bone is responsible for increased mechanical testing values needs further investigation. As previously mentioned, an increase in bone mechanical properties around rough surfaces (ie, dual acid etching, see Fig 3-3) has been demonstrated in a rat model,[17] and validation of this increase in humans through retrieval analysis is highly desirable.

Suzuki et al[34] compared various histomorphometric parameters between machined and TPS implants in rabbit tibiae for 6, 16, and 42 weeks. The histomorphometric results showed higher BIC for the rougher implant surfaces, and no differences in MAR were detected throughout the experiment. An investigation by Grizon et al[33] compared histomorphometric parameters between machined and rough cpTi implant surfaces in a goat model. The authors reported a positive relationship between bone volume and BIC around implants with rough implant surfaces. However, although trends were observed in the biologic response to machined and rough implant surfaces, the mechanism resulting in the increased bone response to rough surface is yet to be elucidated.

Studies comparing different implant surfaces are numerous, and it seems to be generally accepted that rough implant surfaces with $R_a$ values between 0.5 and 2.0 μm enhance the host-implant response.[2,3,29] However, direct comparison between different surgical sites, animal models, and the investigated time periods following implant placement cannot be made, which makes a concise evaluation concerning which rough surface better influences the host response to implants practically impossible.

In addition to contradictory findings concerning the performance of different implant surfaces in different animal models, most studies compare new rough surface designs with machined surfaces. The great majority of studies comparing moderately rough designs with machined implants usually assess a limited number of parameters (typically static parameters such as torque and BIC) and lack assessment of bone dynamics around different implant types as well as surface spatial and/or hybrid and chemistry implant surface characterization. This lack of bone dynamics assessment leads to unsubstantiated speculation with respect to the mechanism by which moderately rough surfaces may favor the host-implant response, making no contribution to further surface engineering development. If studies considering static

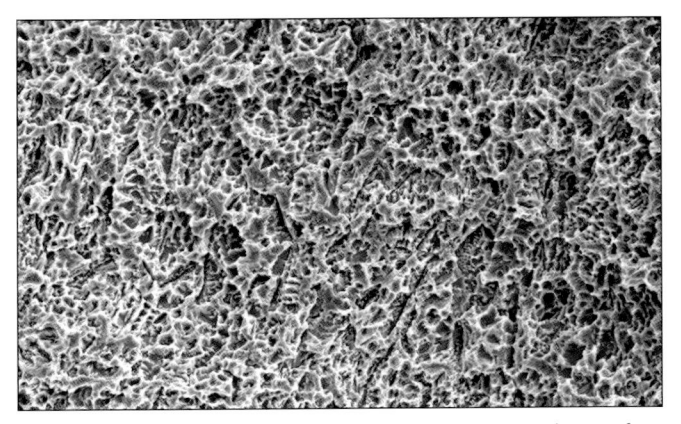

**Fig 3-5** SEM of an RBM-treated implant surface (original magnification ×1,500).

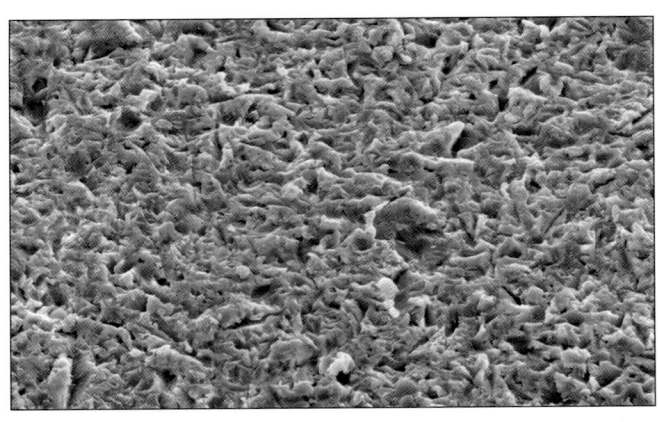

**Fig 3-6** SEM of an alumina-blasted and acid-etched implant surface (original magnification ×1,500).

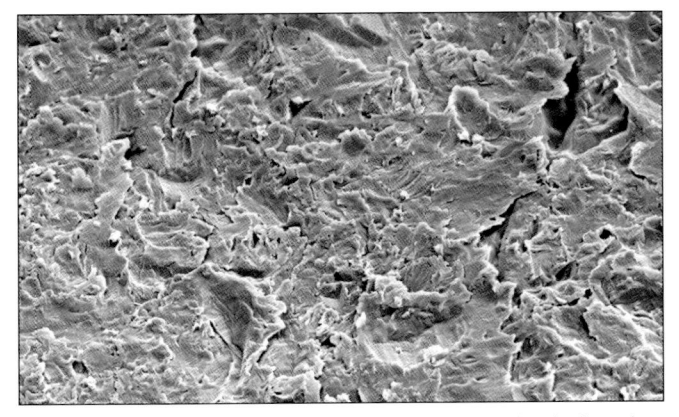

**Fig 3-7** SEM of a titanium oxide–blasted and acid-etched implant surface (original magnification ×1,500).

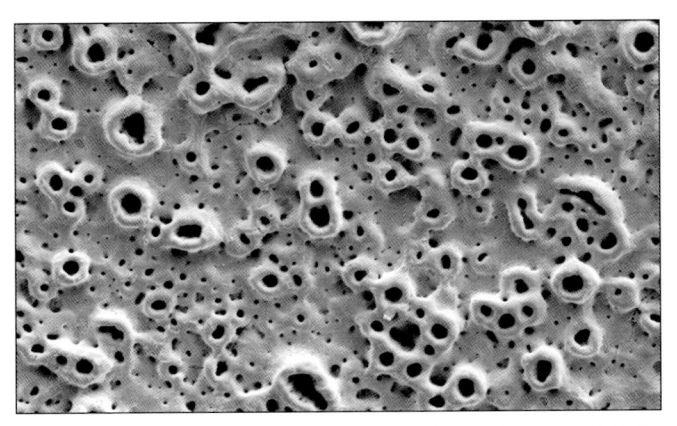

**Fig 3-8** SEM of an anodized surface (original magnification ×1,500).

and dynamic histomorphometric parameters compared various moderately rough surfaces with machined surfaces (as a control), biomaterials scientists would be able to determine the critical parameters necessary (the optimized oxide thickness, elemental chemistry, and texture) for enhanced host-implant response and use this information to design the next generation of implant systems.

## Bioceramic coating of dental implants

Among all engineering surface modifications for dental and orthopedic implants, the addition of calcium-and-phosphorus–based materials as coatings has received significant attention.[5,10,19,23,30,31,39] This interest has arisen in part because these elements are the same basic components of natural bone, and coatings can be applied along the implant surfaces using various industrial processing methods.[5,10]

Most commercially available bioceramic coatings are processed as 20- to 50-μm thick PSHA coatings[5,9,10,19,31,39] (Fig 3-9). Manufactured PSHA coatings normally rely on mechanical interlocking between grit-blasted or etched metallic surfaces and the ceramiclike PSHA material for physical integrity during implant placement and function.[6] While substantially enhanced in vivo bone-bioceramic bonding (bioactivity) and BIC magnitudes have been observed soon after PSHA implant placement,[5,9,10,19,23,31,39] PSHA implants have fallen out of favor in dental practice because studies have shown that such coatings do not uniformly dissolve or degrade after long periods in function, decreasing the mechanical properties of both the coating and the bone-coating interface.[19,23,31,39]

Retrieval analyses of PSHA implants have shown that the translational interface between the bulk metal, metal oxide, and bioceramic coating (Fig 3-10) may be regarded as a weak link where adhesive failure has been reported to occur.[5,9,10] Also, uniformity of coating composition and crystallinity has not always been achieved through the plasma-spray process, and a controversial literature database has developed with respect to coating composition and crystalline content and resultant in vivo performance.[24,61] Alterations of calcium-phosphorus atomic ratios throughout the coating surface and differences in relative thickness may change coating dissolution and degradation rates in vivo.[19,30,31,39] In addition to inherent process limitations and the unpredictable dissolution behavior of PSHA in vivo, the transmucosal nature of dental implants challenges PSHA coatings. These factors have contributed to the decreased use of PSHA coatings for implants in clinical dental practice. Despite the limitations, which may ultimately lead to implant failure, it has been well documented that PSHA-coated implants have elevated osseoconductive properties,[1,10,19,30,31,39,41-45] which may be a significant factor in implant survival under loading conditions, especially in areas where amount or quality of bone is compromised and generation of additional bone attachment is necessary.

## Nanotechnology in implant surface engineering

Evolution of engineering manufacturing processes has led to the controlled production of condensed matter domains with reduced dimensions. The production of reduced domains may strongly affect the electronic configuration of materials, supporting opportunities for a variety of applications, including biomedical engineering. In the case of biomaterials, the production of small domains may potentially change the host response at both cellular and tissue levels.[9]

Tissue engineering through nanobiomaterials is under active investigation. However, the benefits of nanobiomaterials compared with that of their bulk counterparts has not been fully characterized at either the cellular or the tissue level. On the other hand, manufacturing processes used for confined material dimensions production has been useful in overcoming limitations in biomedical device design and production, particularly in the case of bioceramic coatings of dental and orthopedic implants.[62]

In an attempt to improve on the limitations of the PSHA coating process, a thin film of bioceramic coatings has been developed for implant surfaces through processes like sol-gel deposition,[6] pulsed laser deposition (PLD),[61] sputtering coating techniques,[20,21] ion beam–assisted deposition (IBAD),[7,31,32,39] and electrophoretic deposition.[6] These techniques are often applied in substantially thinner coating thicknesses compared to PSHA coatings, typically ranging from 1 to 5 μm. As an alternative to thin coatings, discrete crystalline deposition (DCD)[63-65] and the development of a combination of RBM and modified acid-etching techniques have also been developed for the incorporation of calcium and phosphorus into implant surfaces.

### Ion beam–assisted deposition

Desirable features of thin-film coatings include controlled composition and thickness plus enhanced adhesion to the metallic substrate (40 MPa versus 7 to 9 MPa for PSHA implants).[5,7,19,30,31,39] Controlled composition and thickness achievable through any of these processes also influence coating dissolution in vivo,[31] thereby affecting osseoconductivity early postsurgery. Dissolution of thin films may also expose the metallic substrate after some time has elapsed following surgical placement. Therefore, the possibility of having close bone contact to the implant metallic substrate at the microscopic level after total dissolution of the coating may be an attractive feature of thin-film coatings. This close contact would avoid an interphase between bone, bioceramic, surface oxides, and implant metallic substrate, supporting favorable conditions for long-term anchorage of the implant.[24,49,66]

Animal studies including sputter-coated[20,21] and IBAD-coated[9,66,67] calcium-and-phosphorus–based thin films on titanium implants have demonstrated higher biomechanical fixation,[30,43,44,50] bioactivity,[50] and BIC[16,43,44] compared with noncoated implants soon after implant placement. Also, investigations comparing PSHA-coated implants to sputter-coated and IBAD-coated implants have shown favorable mechanical fixation 12 weeks after implant placement in dog femora.[68]

A potential drawback of the novel processing techniques for thin-film deposition is their high cost for large-scale production. Therefore, to decrease processing time and make the manufacture of thin coatings commercially viable, it is desirable to process the thinnest coating that would significantly increase the biologic response. A recent study[62] has shown that a coating thickness of 300 to 500 nm resulted in increased biologic response early postsurgery compared with a 20- to 50-nm coating thickness. The same study showed that the in vivo performance of the 300- to 500-nm coating thickness was somewhat comparable to that of PSHA.[62]

### Calcium phosphate DCD

Another engineering approach to incorporating calcium-and-phosphorus–based components into implant surfaces is the DCD method. This process incorporates nanometer-sized crystals of calcium phosphate in a previously treated surface (dual acid etching)[65] (Fig 3-11). While the DCD method yields a surface that is different in morphology and microstructure than that achieved with IBAD and other thin-film deposition methods, the rationale behind such surface treatment is also to attempt to provide an increased osseoconductive component to the surface while avoiding the potential long-term limitations of PSHA coatings.

The DCD surface has shown promising results in a controlled study in humans, in which higher BIC was found after 2 months in vivo.[65] Biomechanical testing comparing dual acid etching plus DCD versus dual acid etching alone showed higher values of hydroxyapatite nanocrystals for the surface with DCD.[64]

### Other nanotechnology techniques

In addition, the commercially available IBAD and DCD surface treatments for the incorporation of calcium and phosphorus into implant surfaces, other alternatives have been explored with the objective of chemically modifying implant surfaces to increase their biocompatibility and enhance wound healing.

The most common technique comprises a combination of surface treatments to increase implant surface roughness. This modification of grit blasting the sur-

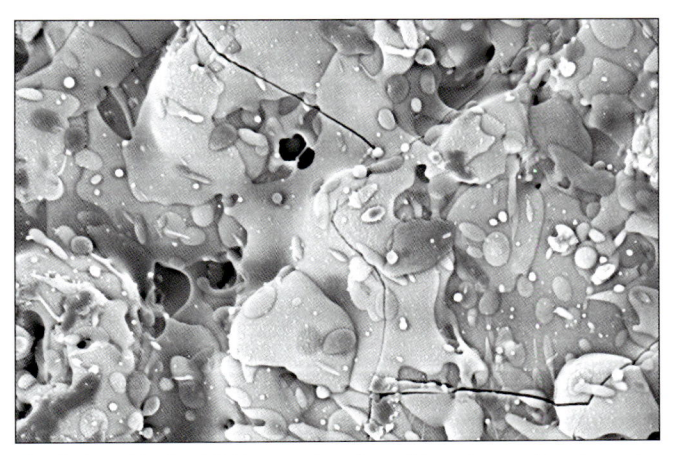

**Fig 3-9** SEM of a PSHA-coated surface. Note the resulting irregular surface due to hydroxyapatite particle propulsion toward the implant surface at high temperatures. The cooling cracks result from rapid cooling (original magnification ×1,500).

**Fig 3-10** Representative optical micrograph showing a ceramometal interface disruption after mechanical loading of a PSHA-coated implant retrieved after a 15-week period in beagle dog tibia. The fracture presented shows that the bone-bioceramic interface *(black arrows)* has increased mechanical properties compared to the bioceramic–metallic substrate interface *(white arrows)*, characterizing the weak link observed after osseointegration of PSHA-coated implants at longer terms in vivo.

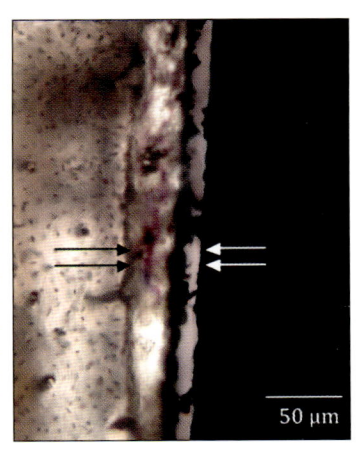

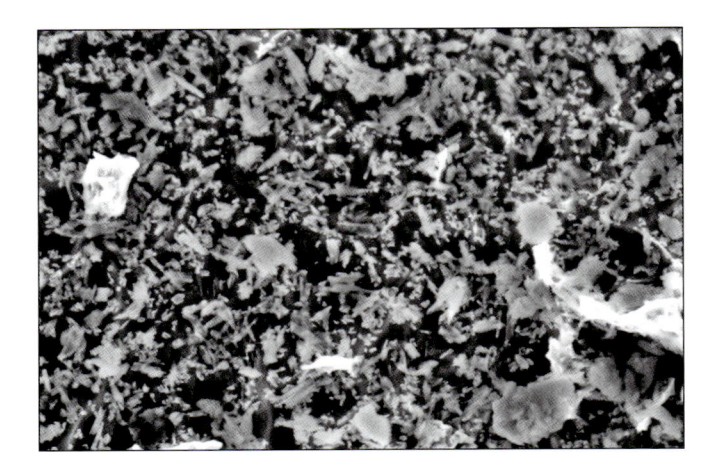

**Fig 3-11** Field emission SEM of a DCD implant surface. Note the nanoscale particles deposited in the dual acid-etched surface (original magnification ×30,000). (Courtesy of Biomet 3i.)

face with biocompatible bioceramics (ie, RBM) added to selective cleaning procedures (ie, modified acid-etch [MAE] procedures) leads to minimally to moderately rough surfaces with calcium and phosphorus remnants. The resulting RBM surface topography and chemistry are dependent on several variables, such as blasting media composition, particle size, and processing parameters, including blasting pressure and distance and subsequent acid-etching treatments.[69] To assess the effect of the calcium and phosphorus remnants on torque-to-interface failure and on BIC and BAFO, RBM surfaces have been tested in vivo in different evaluation periods against alumina-blasted/acid-etched (AB/AE) surfaces with either higher[70] or lower[71] $S_a$ and root mean square roughness ($S_q$) values. Interestingly, in both cited studies, torque-to-interface failure was not significantly different between AB/AE and the RBM surfaces presenting different surface roughness. Therefore, whether calcium and phosphorus amounts were too low to positively influence bone response or the resulting surface roughnesses were equally effective in resisting torque removal forces could not be elucidated from these studies.[70,71] In a sequel study, substantially higher amounts of calcium and phosphorus were tailored in an RBM surface by means of a nonwashing procedure, and in spite of its significantly lower $S_a$ and $S_q$ values compared to an AB/AE control surface, significantly higher removal torque was observed,[72] suggesting not only that surface chemistry improved bone response but also that there may be a yet-to-be investigated threshold for calcium and phosphorus amounts that positively modulates bone response.[56,69]

From a theoretical standpoint, all nanosurfaces presented in this chapter may benefit from both surface roughness and chemical modification to enhance the host response to implants. While promising results have been obtained in preliminary studies and short-term clinical trials, more laboratory in vivo and prospective clinical trials should be performed to better characterize the performance of these surfaces in vivo.

# Conclusion

The main purpose of surface modification of dental implants is to decrease the healing time required for osseointegration. This is a desirable feature for both clinicians and patients and, along with implant macrodesign evolution, may be another step toward minimizing healing times prior to implant restoration.

Because the surface is the first part of the implant to encounter the host, it is natural that surface engineering has become an extensively studied topic. Unfortunately, despite the extensive literature developed over the last decades on this topic, inconsistencies in methodologies have led to difficulties in isolating the topographic and chemical parameters that provide optimum bone healing around immediately and early loaded dental implants. Despite these inconsistencies, various laboratory in vivo and clinical studies have demonstrated that moderately rough surfaces accelerate wound healing and are potentially advantageous for early and immediate loading of implants.

The emerging technology comprising nanoscale bioceramic coatings attempts to use beneficial surface topographies and chemistry to increase surface osseoconductivity. This technology is under active basic and clinical investigation to determine which osseoconductive properties lead to favorable results.

Immediate loading is a modern and progressive treatment concept in implant dentistry. Because different implant surfaces have been associated with varying survival rates, modern surface technology is of great importance to the success of implants, especially in challenging clinical conditions, such as immediate loading in bone of poor quality and/or quantity. However, this area of study is in close relationship with selective implant design and is definitely in need of further research before specific implant surfaces are used in daily practice.

## References

1. Esposito M, Murray-Curtis L, Grusovin MG, Coulthard P, Worthington HV. Interventions for replacing missing teeth: Different types of dental implants. Cochrane Database Syst Rev 2007:CD003815.
2. Albrektsson T, Wennerberg A. Oral implant surfaces: Part 1—Review focusing on topographic and chemical properties of different surfaces and in vivo responses to them. Int J Prosthodont 2004;17:536–543.
3. Albrektsson T, Wennerberg A. Oral implant surfaces: Part 2—Review focusing on clinical knowledge of different surfaces. Int J Prosthodont 2004;17:544–564.
4. Buser D, Broggini N, Wieland M, et al. Enhanced bone apposition to a chemically modified SLA titanium surface. J Dent Res 2004;83:529–533.
5. Lemons JE. Biomaterials, biomechanics, tissue healing, and immediate-function dental implants. J Oral Implantol 2004;30:318–324.
6. Lacefield WR. Current status of ceramic coatings for dental implants. Implant Dent 1998;7:315–322.
7. Dohan Ehrenfest DM, Coelho PG, Kang BS, Sul YT, Albrektsson T. Classification of osseointegrated implant surfaces: Materials, chemistry and topography. Trends Biotechnol 2010;28:198–206.
8. Albrektsson T, Brånemark PI, Hansson HA, Lindström J. Osseointegrated titanium implants. Requirements for ensuring a long-lasting, direct bone-to-implant anchorage in man. Acta Orthop Scand 1981;52:155–170.
9. Coelho PG, Lemons JE. IBAD nanothick bioceramic incorporation on metallic implants for bone healing enhancement. From physico/chemical characterization to in-vivo performance evaluation. In: Nano Science & Technology Institute (ed). Technical Proceedings of the 2005 NSTI Nanotechnology Conference and Trade Show, vol 1. Anaheim, CA: Nanotech, 2005:316–319.
10. Damien E, Hing K, Saeed S, Revell PA. A preliminary study on the enhancement of the osteointegration of a novel synthetic hydroxyapatite scaffold in vivo. J Biomed Mater Res A 2003;66:241–246.
11. Kay J. Calcium phosphate coatings for dental implants. Dent Clin North Am 1992;36:1–18.
12. Lacefield WR. Hydroxyapatite coatings. Ann N Y Acad Sci 1988;523:72–80.
13. Pearce AI, Richards RG, Milz S, Schneider E, Pearce SG. Animal models for implant biomaterial research in bone: A review. Eur Cell Mater 2007;13:1–10.
14. Groth T, Falk P, Miethke RR. Cytotoxicity of biomaterials—Basic mechanisms and in-vitro test methods—A review. Altern Lab Anim 1995;23:790–799.
15. Richards RG, Stiffanic M, Owen GR, Riehle M, Ap Gwynn I, Curtis AS. Immunogold labelling of fibroblast focal adhesion sites visualised in fixed material using scanning electron microscopy, and living, using internal reflection microscopy. Cell Biol Int 2001;25:1237–1249.
16. Berglundh T, Abrahamsson I, Lang NP, Lindhe J. De novo alveolar bone formation adjacent to endosseous implants. Clin Oral Implants Res 2003;14:251–262.
17. Butz F, Aita H, Wang CJ, Ogawa T. Harder and stiffer bone osseointegrated to roughened titanium. J Dent Res 2006;85:560–565.
18. Coelho PG. Histomorphometric and Biomechanical Studies of a Surface Modified Ti-6Al-4V Implant [thesis]. Birmingham, AL: University of Alabama, 2002.
19. Garetto LP, Chen J, Parr JA, Roberts WE. Remodeling dynamics of bone supporting rigidly fixed titanium implants: A histomorphometric comparison in four species including humans. Implant Dent 1995;4:235–243.
20. Vercaigne S, Wolke JG, Naert I, Jansen JA. A mechanical evaluation of $TiO_2$-gritblasted and Ca-P magnetron sputter coated implants placed into the trabecular bone of the goat: Part 1. Clin Oral Implants Res 2000;11:305–313.
21. Vercaigne S, Wolke JG, Naert I, Jansen JA. A histological evaluation of $TiO_2$-gritblasted and Ca-P magnetron sputter coated implants placed into the trabecular bone of the goat: Part 2. Clin Oral Implants Res 2000;11:314–324.
22. Wolke JG, de Groot K, Jansen JA. In vivo dissolution behavior of various RF magnetron sputtered Ca-P coatings. J Biomed Mater Res 1998;39:524–530.
23. Wolke JG, van der Waerden JP, Schaeken HG, Jansen JA. In vivo dissolution behavior of various RF magnetron-sputtered Ca-P coatings on roughened titanium implants. Biomaterials 2003;24:2623–2629.
24. Yang Y, Kim KH, Ong JL. A review on calcium phosphate coatings produced using a sputtering process—An alternative to plasma spraying. Biomaterials 2005;26:327–337.
25. de Groot KKC, Wolke JGC, de Bieck-Hogervorst JM. Plasma-sprayed coating of calcium phosphate. In: Yamamuro T, Henck LL, Wilson J (eds). Handbook of Bioactive Ceramics, Vol II. Calcium Phosphate and Hydroxyapatite Ceramics. Boca Raton: CRC, 1990:17–25.
26. Jimbo R, Coelho PG, Vandeweghe S, et al. Histological and three-dimensional evaluation of osseointegration to nano-structured calcium phosphate-coated implants. Acta Biomater 2011;7:4229–4234.
27. Ogawa T, Ozawa S, Shih JH, et al. Biomechanical evaluation of osseous implants having different surface topographies in rats. J Dent Res 2000;79:1857–1863.
28. Seybold EA, Baker JA, Crisciitello AA, Ordway NR, Park CK, Connolly PJ. Characteristics of unicortical and bicortical lateral mass screws in the cervical spine. Spine (Phila Pa 1976) 1999;24:2397–2403.

# References

29. Klokkevold PR, Nishimura RD, Adachi M, Caputo A. Osseointegration enhanced by chemical etching of the titanium surface. A torque removal study in the rabbit. Clin Oral Implants Res 1997;8:442–447.
30. Baker MI, Eberhardt AW, Martin DM, McGwin G, Lemons JE. Bone properties surrounding hydroxyapatite-coated custom osseous integrated dental implants. J Biomed Mater Res B App Biomater 2010;95:218–224.
31. Recker R. Bone Histomorphometry: Techniques and Interpretation. Boca Raton: CRC, 1983.
32. de Bruijn JD, Bovell YP, van Blitterswijk CA. Structural arrangements at the interface between plasma sprayed calcium phosphates and bone. Biomaterials 1994;15:543–550.
33. Grizon F, Aguado E, Huré G, Baslé MF, Chappard D. Enhanced bone integration of implants with increased surface roughness: A long term study in the sheep. J Dent 2002;30:195–203.
34. Suzuki K, Aoki K, Ohya K. Effects of surface roughness of titanium implants on bone remodeling activity of femur in rabbits. Bone 1997;21:507–514.
35. Frost HM. Bone's mechanostat: A 2003 update. Anat Rec A Discov Mol Cell Evol Biol 2003;275:1081–1101.
36. Frost HM. A 2003 update of bone physiology and Wolff's Law for clinicians. Angle Orthod 2004;74:3–15.
37. Chuang SK, Hatch JP, Rugh J, Dodson TB. Multi-center randomized clinical trials in oral and maxillofacial surgery: Modeling of fixed and random effects. Int J Oral Maxillofac Surg 2005;34:341–344.
38. Chuang SK, Tian L, Wei LJ, Dodson TB. Kaplan-Meier analysis of dental implant survival: A strategy for estimating survival with clustered observations. J Dent Res 2001;80:2016–2020.
39. Chuang SK, Tian L, Wei LJ, Dodson TB. Predicting dental implant survival by use of the marginal approach of the semiparametric survival methods for clustered observations. J Dent Res 2002;81:851–855.
40. Chuang SK, Wei LJ, Douglass CW, Dodson TB. Risk factors for dental implant failure: A strategy for the analysis of clustered failure-time observations. J Dent Res 2002;81:572–577.
41. Clark GT, Mulligan R. Fifteen common mistakes encountered in clinical research. J Prosthodont Res 2011;55:1–6.
42. Pihlstrom BL, Barnett ML. Design, operation, and interpretation of clinical trials. J Dent Res 2010;89:759–772.
43. Lemons J, Brott B, Eberhardt A. Human postmortem device retrieval and analysis—Orthopaedic, cardiovascular, and dental systems. J Long Term Eff Med Implants 2010;20:81–85.
44. Coelho PG, Bonfante EA, Marin C, Granato R, Giro G, Suzuki M. A human retrieval study of plasma-sprayed hydroxyapatite-coated plateau root form implants after 2 months to 13 years in function. J Long Term Eff Med Implants 2010;20:335–342.
45. Coelho PG, Marin C, Granato R, Suzuki M. Histomorphologic analysis of 30 plateau root form implants retrieved after 8 to 13 years in function. A human retrieval study. J Biomed Mater Res B Appl Biomater 2009;91:975–979.
46. Albrektsson T, Jansson T, Lekholm U. Osseointegrated dental implants. Dent Clin North Am 1986;30:151–174.
47. Schroeder A, van der Zypen E, Stich H, Sutter F. The reactions of bone, connective tissue, and epithelium to endosteal implants with titanium-sprayed surfaces. J Maxillofac Surg 1981;9:15–25.
48. Bobyn JD, Pilliar RM, Cameron HU, Weatherly GC, Kent GM. The effect of porous surface configuration on the tensile strength of fixation of implants by bone ingrowth. Clin Orthop Relat Res 1980:291–298.
49. Lemons J, Dietch-Misch F. Biomaterials for dental implants. In: Misch CE (ed). Contemporary Implant Denstistry. St Louis: Mosby, 1999:271–302.
50. Mombelli A, Lang NP. The diagnosis and treatment of periimplantitis. Periodontol 2000 1998;17:63–76.
51. Gotfredsen K, Berglundh T, Lindhe J. Anchorage of titanium implants with different surface characteristics: An experimental study in rabbits. Clin Implant Dent Relat Res 2000;2:120–128.
52. Bonfante EA, Granato R, Marin C, et al. Early bone healing and biomechanical fixation of dual acid-etched and as-machined implants with healing chambers: An experimental study in dogs. Int J Oral Maxillofac Implants 2011;26:75–82.
53. Coelho PG, Suzuki M, Guimaraes MV, et al. Early bone healing around different implant bulk designs and surgical techniques: A study in dogs. Clin Implant Dent Relat Res 2010;12:202–208.
54. Leonard G, Coelho P, Polyzois I, Stassen L, Claffey N. A study of the bone healing kinetics of plateau versus screw root design titanium dental implants. Clin Oral Implants Res 2009;20:232–239.
55. Marin C, Granato R, Suzuki M, Gil JN, Janal MN, Coelho PG. Histomorphologic and histomorphometric evaluation of various endosseous implant healing chamber configurations at early implantation times: A study in dogs. Clin Oral Implants Res 2010;21:577–583.
56. Wennerberg A, Albrektsson T. Structural influence from calcium phosphate coatings and its possible effect on enhanced bone integration. Acta Odontol Scand 2009;31:1–8.
57. Wennerberg A, Albrektsson T. Effects of titanium surface topography on bone integration: A systematic review. Clin Oral Implants Res 2009;20(suppl 4):172–184.
58. Huang YH, Xiropaidis AV, Sorensen RG, Albandar JM, Hall J, Wikesjö UM. Bone formation at titanium porous oxide (TiUnite) oral implants in type IV bone. Clin Oral Implants Res 2005;16:105–111.
59. Jungner M, Lundqvist P, Lundgren S. Oxidized titanium implants (Nobel Biocare TiUnite) compared with turned titanium implants (Nobel Biocare mark III) with respect to implant failure in a group of consecutive patients treated with early functional loading and two-stage protocol. Clin Oral Implants Res 2005;16:308–312.
60. Xiropaidis AV, Qahash M, Lim WH, et al. Bone-implant contact at calcium phosphate-coated and porous titanium oxide (TiUnite)-modified oral implants. Clin Oral Implants Res 2005;16:532–539.
61. Kim H, Camata RP, Vohra YK, Lacefield WR. Control of phase composition in hydroxyapatite/tetracalcium phosphate biphasic thin coatings for biomedical applications. J Mater Sci Mater Med 2005;16:961–966.
62. Coelho PG, Freire JNO, Coelho AL, et al. Nanothickness bioceramic coatings: Improving the host response to surgical implants. In: Liepsch D (ed). 5th World Congress of Biomechanics. Munich: Medimont, 2006:253–258.
63. Davies JE. Bone bonding at natural and biomaterial surfaces. Biomaterials 2007;28:5058–5067.
64. Mendes VC, Moineddin R, Davies JE. The effect of discrete calcium phosphate nanocrystals on bone-bonding to titanium surfaces. Biomaterials 2007;28:4748–4755.
65. Orsini G, Piattelli M, Scarano A, et al. Randomized, controlled histologic and histomorphometric evaluation of implants with nanometer-scale calcium phosphate added to the dual acid-etched surface in the human posterior maxilla. J Periodontol 2007;78:209–218.
66. Park YS, Yi KY, Lee IS, Han CH, Jung YC. The effects of ion beam-assisted deposition of hydroxyapatite on the grit-blasted surface of endosseous implants in rabbit tibiae. Int J Oral Maxillofac Implants 2005;20:31–38.
67. Coelho PG, Suzuki M. Evaluation of an IBAD thin-film process as an alternative method for surface incorporation of bioceramics on dental implants. A study in dogs. J Appl Oral Science 2005;13:87–92.

68. Yang CY, Wang BC, Lee TM, Chang E, Chang GL. Intramedullary implant of plasma-sprayed hydroxyapatite coating: An interface study. J Biomed Mater Res 1997;36:39–48.
69. Coelho PG, Granjeiro JM, Romanos GE, et al. Basic research methods and current trends of dental implant surfaces. J Biomed Mater Res B Appl Biomater 2009;88:579–596.
70. Marin C, Granato R, Suzuki M, et al. Biomechanical and histomorphometric analysis of etched and non-etched resorbable blasting media processed implant surfaces: An experimental study in dogs. J Mech Behav Biomed Mater 2010;3:382–391.
71. Bonfante E, Marin C, Granato R, et al. Histologic and biomechanical evaluation of alumina-blasted/acid-etched and resorbable blasting media surfaces. J Oral Implantol doi:10.1563/AAID-JOI-D-10-00105 [Epub ahead of print 6 Oct 2010].
72. Coelho PG, Marin C, Granato R, Giro G, Suzuki M, Bonfante EA. Biomechanical and histologic evaluation of non-washed resorbable blasting media and alumina-blasted/acid-etched surfaces. Clin Oral Implants Res doi:10.1111/j.160-0501.2010.02147.x. [Epub ahead of print 24 March 2011].

# Role of Implant Design in Immediate Loading    4

As the field of implant dentistry has evolved over time, there have been different dental implant designs, such as blades, screws, and cylinders, each of which has various characteristics inherent to its macrodesign. For example, using cylindric implants, a press-fit technique in undersized osteotomies has been attempted. For screw-type implants, surgical steps with the use of specific-diameter drills allow an osteotomy preparation that enhances the mechanical stability of the implant body with the surrounding bone. The threads of the implant body support the increase of the mechanical implant stability and also allow bone adaptation to elevated shear forces.[1] Because of the shape of the osteotomy and the thread profile, there is sufficient space for bone in-growth. Screw-type implants have the advantage of adapting the bone to the surrounding compressive loads, especially when they are placed in cortical or cancellous bone. Some implant designs provide a thread profile with reduced height, increasing the number of threads per unit area of the implant surface.[2]

The external contour of an implant and the magnitude of occlusal loading can have significant effects on the load transfer characteristics and may result in different bone-failure rates for different implant systems. This is especially important in extreme occlusal load ranges (≥ 1,000 N), with the overload threshold of implants being dependent on their geometric shape.

During function, some implant designs present higher loads in the apical part of the implant and significant reduction of compression in the cervical part.[3,4] This advantage, offered by implant designs with a progressive thread profile, has been documented most often when small-diameter implants are placed in the molar region. Such studies showed no crestal bone loss over a period of 20 months of loading and no significant failures due to the narrow implant diameter in areas with highly demanding biomechanics.[5]

## Types of Implant Stability

### Primary stability

Primary stability is dependent on the correct use of surgical drills and the gentle preparation of the osteotomy. This stability is a mechanical interlocking between the implant body and the surrounding mature lamellar bone, which is characterized later by a series of biologic reactions, starting with bone turnover at the interface, followed by rapid repair.

### Secondary stability

After primary (mechanical) stability has been established, the wound-healing mechanisms lead to continuous tissue repair with cell differentiation to osteoblasts and bone formation. This phenomenon is known as *secondary* or *biologic stability*. Especially important to biologic stability is rapid remodeling under functional loading conditions. An annual remodeling rate of approximately 30% has been established at the bone-implant interface of functionally loaded implants,[6] with changes in mechanical properties occurring in this region.[7] However, even though functional loading has been shown to be important for the stimulation of bone remodeling, no studies have clearly answered the question as to which specific type of force—compressive versus tensile—is most beneficial. Some studies indicate that bone forms more quickly in areas exposed to severe compressive forces, while other studies point to tensile forces as the stimulating factor for osteogenesis.[8,9] Despite this controversy, there is no doubt that control of excessive loads is necessary for immediately loaded implants.

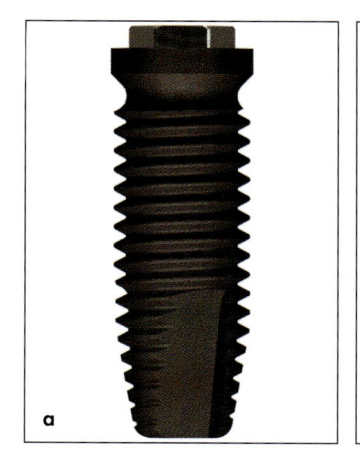

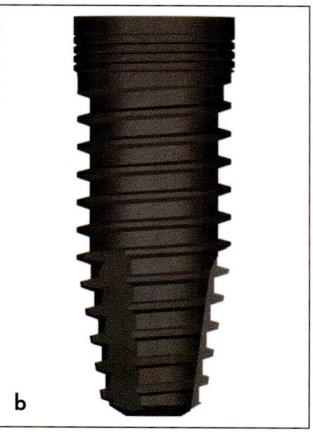

**Fig 4-1** Cylindric (a) and tapered (b) implants have different primary stability associated with the implant shape. Tapered implant designs are better for immediate loading in compromised bone qualities.

**Table 4-1** Stability measurements of various Straumann implant designs placed in vitro

| Test | Bone Level | Standard Plus | Tapered Effect |
|---|---|---|---|
| Periotest | −4.7 (± 1.18) | −6.07 (± 0.94) | −6.57 (± 0.7) |
| RFA | 75.02 (± 3.65) | 75.98 (± 3.00) | 79.83 (± 1.85) |

## Effect of implant design on primary stability

Osseointegration seems to be dependent on primary implant stability, which is determined by the implant design.[10,11] According to Meredith,[12] primary stability is influenced by the length, geometry, and surface area of the implant and by bone-implant contact (BIC) percentage at the histomorphometric level. Therefore, new implant designs have been developed for immediate function after implant placement (Fig 4-1). Glauser et al[13] stated that primary implant stability is determined by the bone density, the implant design, and the surgical technique. The clinical assessment of implant stability is empiric and subjective; however, it is important in achieving osseointegration.[14]

## Determining primary stability

Several methods to determine the primary stability and possible future prognosis of implants have been developed: peak insertion torque (cutting torque), Periotest (Medizintechnik Gulden) value, resonance frequency analysis (RFA), and removal torque.[15]

The geometric shape of implants (tapered versus nontapered) has been studied, with the primary stability assessed by RFA. Glauser et al[16] found significantly higher RFA values for tapered implants than nontapered implants in a comparative clinical study using RFA and insertion torques. In a human cadaver study, O'Sullivan et al[17] demonstrated higher primary stability (assessed by RFA values) for tapered implants compared to nontapered ones and found similar RFA values for tapered implants irrespective of bone quality.

After placement of Straumann implants with three different designs (Bone Level, Standard Plus, and Tapered Effect [Fig 4-2]), the RFA and Periotest values showed significantly higher implant stability for tapered implants[18] (Table 4-1).

The primary stability of self-tapping implants (Camlog, Camlog) was compared with that of non–self-tapping implants with a progressive thread design (Ankylos, Dentsply Friadent) using RFA and insertion torque measurements in a clinical study.[19] The insertion torque was significantly higher for the progressive thread design; however, there was no significant difference between the RFA values of the two implant designs.

Further in vitro studies showed an increased percentage of BIC histomorphometrically (more than 50%) after implant placement with a progressive thread design in cadaver jaws.[20] Similar results were found after in vitro placement of implants with different designs in cow ribs by experienced clinicians. The specimens were examined histomorphometrically as well as with microcomputed tomography immediately after implant insertion. The authors found that the design of the implant may be associated with different percentages of BIC because of the specific thread profile,[21,22] (Table 4-2) which seems to be an important parameter for successful osseointegration, especially in immediate loading concepts.

Implant designs that promote high stability because of the thread morphology at the middle and apical parts of the implant are important for placement in areas where alveolar bone is missing (ie, fresh extraction sockets or sites needing bone augmentation).

## Micromovement at the Bone-Implant Interface

A high percentage of primary bone contact with the implant body is important for decreasing micromovements at the interface. According to Brunski,[23] macromovements lead to fibrous encapsulation, but micromove-

**Fig 4-2** Different implant geometries for bone- or tissue-level placement have different primary stabilities. For example, Straumann system implants include Standard Plus *(a)*, Tapered Effect *(b)*, and Bone Level *(c)* implants.

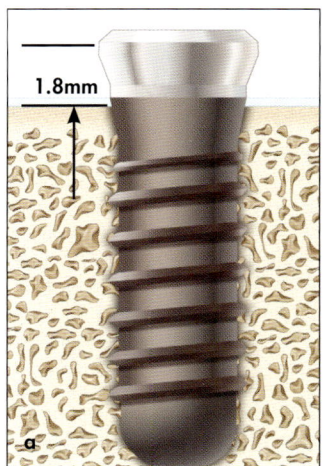

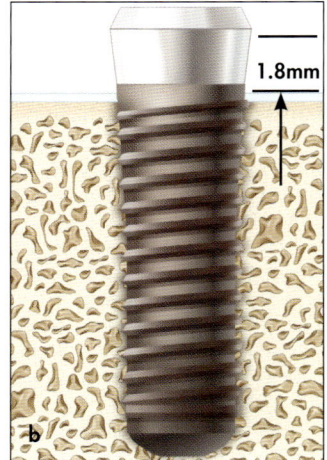

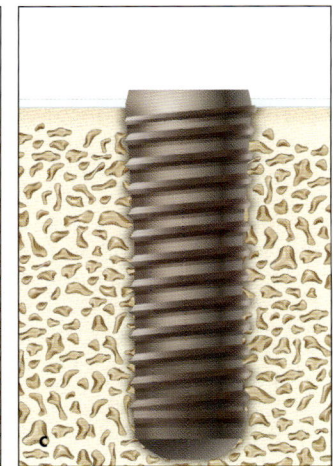

| Table 4-2 BIC percentages immediately after in vitro implant placement |||
|---|---|---|
| Implant design | Number of implants | Total BIC (%) |
| Progressive (Ankylos) | 11 | 65.13 ± 15.96 |
| Condensation, progressive (XiVE, Dentsply Friadent) | 10 | 58.25 ± 5.25 |
| Tapered screw-type (Frialit-2, Dentsply Friadent) | 11 | 55.86 ± 6.89 |
| Standard cylinder (Straumann) | 10 | 51.15 ± 17.85 |
| Tapered (Replace Select, Nobel Biocare) | 10 | 49.15 ± 15.99 |

ments to the threshold of 100 μm are not detrimental to osseointegration. Cameron et al[24] reported that motions of approximately 200 μm resulted in fibrous tissue integration rather than bone formation. When this micromotion occurs, bone formation is dependent on surface roughness; in its presence, micromotion does not necessarily lead to fibrous encapsulation. Other studies have also looked at the threshold of acceptable micromovements for bone formation as an important factor in implant design and surface characteristics.[25,26] The threshold level of micromotion was between 50 and 150 μm for bioinert materials.[27] To eliminate micromovement at the bone-implant interface, immobilization by rigid splinting of implants is necessary. A bar-retained, implant-supported restoration allows primary and immediate immobilization of implants.[28] Another suggestion is to provide a fixed, cross-arch prosthesis to control micromovements.[29] Biomechanical stability is increased by using a higher number of splinted implants. Skalak[30] recommended this as a biomechanical model to keep micromotions below the critical level.

Hashimoto et al[31] studied the effects of early loading of implants (after 4 weeks of healing) in monkeys and found no signs of connective tissue healing. Similar results were also observed by Deporter et al[32] in dogs with conical implants that had been loaded 6 weeks after surgery. Corigliano et al[33] confirmed osseointegration of single-tooth implants placed in monkeys when implants were loaded in the second week of healing. Piattelli et al[34] studied the healing of screw-type implants in monkeys using a split-mouth design in which one side was not loaded and the contralateral side was immediately loaded. They found significantly higher bone density around the immediately loaded (splinted) implants. In another monkey study, a significantly higher bone density within the threads of immediately loaded (splinted) implants compared with delayed loaded implants was found for implants with a progressive thread design.[35]

When rigid splinting is used to decrease micromovements immediately after surgery, the loading forces allow better healing and denser bone formation at the bone-implant interface. The exact mechanism of this observation at the molecular biologic level is not well understood; however, implant design and surface characteristics (see chapter 3) seem to be important factors in improving osseointegration.

# Conclusion

Tapered (or slightly tapered), screw-type implants are able to increase primary stability, especially in poor-quality bone, and should be used routinely for advanced immediate loading concepts. In such treatment concepts, where the bone quality is low and grafting techniques are necessary, the tapered implant design reduces dramatic shear forces and provides more stability at the bone-implant interface, allowing placement of fewer implants to restore grafted edentulous ridges. In addition, implant designs that provide high mechanical stability at the apical part because of the thread and pit morphology should be used in advanced surgical protocols with immediate functional loading.

# References

1. Brunski JB. The new millennium in biomaterials and biomechanics. Int J Oral Maxillofac Implants 2000;15:327–328.
2. Hansson S. The implant neck: Smooth or provided with retention elements. A biomechanical approach. Clin Oral Implants Res 1999;10:394–405.
3. Nentwig GH, Moser W, Knefel T, Ficker E. Dreidimensionale spannungsoptische Untersuchungen der NM-Implantatgewindeform im Vergleich mit herkömmlichen Implantatgewinden. Z Zahnärztl Implantol 1992;8:130–135.
4. Moser W, Nentwig GH. Finite-Element-Studien zur Optimierung von Implantatgewindeformen. Z Zahnärztl Implantol 1989;5:29–32.
5. Romanos GE, Nentwig GH. Single molar replacement with a progressive thread design implant system: A retrospective clinical report. Int J Oral Maxillofac Implants 2000;15:831–836.
6. Roberts WE, Marshall KJ, Mozsary PG. Rigid endosseous implant utilized as anchorage to protract molars and close an atrophic extraction site. Angle Orthod 1990;60:135–152.
7. Chen J, Lu X, Paydar N, Akay HU, Roberts WE. Mechanical simulation of the human mandible with and without an endosseous implant. Med Eng Phys 1994;16:53–61.
8. Frost HM. Skeletal structural adaptations to mechanical usage (SATMU): 1. Redefining Wolff's law: The bone modeling problem. Anat Rec 1990;226:403–413.
9. Oda J, Sakamoto J, Aoyama K, Sueyoshi Y, Tomita K, Sawaguchi T. Mechanical stresses and bone formation. In: Hayashi K, Kamiya A, Ono K (eds). Biomechanics: Functional Adaptation and Remodeling. Tokyo: Springer 1996:123–140.
10. Albrektsson T, Brånemark PI, Hansson HA, Lindström J. Osseointegrated titanium implants. Requirements for ensuring a long-lasting, direct bone anchorage in man. Acta Orthop Scand 1981;52:155–170.
11. Carlsson L. On the development of a New Concept for Orthopaedic Implant Fixation [thesis]. Göteborg: Göteborg University, 1989.
12. Meredith N. Assessment of implant stability as a prognostic determinant. Int J Prosthodont 1998;11:491–501.
13. Glauser R, Sennerby L, Meredith N, et al. Resonance analysis of implants subjected to immediate or early functional occlusal loading. Successful vs. failing implants. Clin Oral Implants Res 2004;15:428–434.
14. Meredith N, Book K, Friberg B, Jemt T, Sennerby L. Resonance frequency measurements of implant stability in vivo. A cross-sectional and longitudinal study of resonance frequency measurements on implants in the edentulous and partially dentate maxilla. Clin Oral Implants Res 1997;8:226–233.
15. Cehreli MC, Karasoy D, Akca K, Eckert SE. Meta-analysis of methods used to assess implant stability. Int J Oral Maxillofac Implants 2009;24:1015–1032.
16. Glauser R, Portmann M, Ruhstaller P, Gottlow J, Schaerer P. Initial implant stability using different implant designs and surgical techniques. A comparative clinical study using insertion torque and resonance frequency analysis. Appl Osseointegration Res 2001;2:6–8.
17. O'Sullivan D, Sennerby L, Meredith N. Measurements comparing the initial stability of five designs of dental implants: A human cadaver study. Clin Implant Dent Relat Res 2000;2:85–92.
18. Ciornei G, Jucan A, Feng C, Caton J, Romanos GE. In vivo assessment of primary stability of different implant designs. Presented at the 25th Anniversary Meeting of the Academy of Osseointegration, Orlando, FL, 4–6 March 2010.
19. Rabel A, Köhler SG, Schmidt-Westhausen AM. Clinical study on the primary stability of two dental implant systems with resonance frequency analysis. Clin Oral Invest 2007;11:257–265.
20. Bade H, Günes Y, Koebke J. Untersuchungen zur Primärstabilität von Dentalimplantaten. Z Zahnärztl Implantol 2000;16:33–39.
21. Romanos GE, Damouras M, Veis A, Schwarz F, Parisis N. Oral implants with different thread designs. A histometrical evaluation. Presented at the Annual Meeting of the International Association for Dental Research, New Orleans, 21–24 March 2007.
22. Romanos GE, Damouras M, Veis A, Schwarz F, Parisis N. Dental implants and their different thread designs. A radiological and histological evaluation. Presented at the 42nd Annual Meeting of the International Association for Dental Research Continental European and Israeli Divisions, Thessaloniki, Greece, 26–29 Sept 2007.
23. Brunski JB. Avoid pitfalls of overloading and micromotion of intraosseous implants. Dent Implantol Update 1993;4(10):77–81.
24. Cameron HU, Pilliar RM, MacNab I. The effect of movement on the bonding of porous metal to bone. J Biomed Mater Res 1973;7:301–311.
25. Pilliar RM, Lee JM, Maniatopoulos C. Observations on the effect of movement on bone in-growth into porous-surfaced implants. Clin Orthop Relat Res 1986;208:108–113.
26. Szmukler-Moncler S, Salama H, Reingewirtz Y, Dubruille JH. Time of loading and effect of micromotion on bone-dental implant interface: Review of experimental literature. J Biomed Mater Res 1998;43:192–203.
27. Søballe K, Hansen ES, Brockstedt-Rasmussen H, Bünger C. Tissue ingrowth into titanium and hydroxyapatite coated implants during stable and unstable mechanical conditions. J Orthopaedic Res 1992;10:285–299.
28. Ledermann PD. Über 20jährige Erfahrung mit der sofortigen funktionellen Belastung von Implantatstegen in der Regio interforaminalis. Z Zahnärztl Implantol 1996;12:123–136.
29. Schnitman PA, Wöhrle PS, Rubenstein JE, DaSilva JD, Wang NH. Ten years results for Brånemark implants immediately loaded with fixed prostheses at implant placement. Int J Oral Maxillofac Implants 1997;12:495–503.
30. Skalak R. Biomechanical considerations in osseointegrated prostheses. J Prosthet Dent 1983;49:843–848.
31. Hashimoto M, Akagawa Y, Nikai H, Tsuru H. Single-crystal sapphire endosseous dental implant loaded with functional stress—Clinical and histological evaluation of periimplant tissues. J Oral Rehabil 1988;15:65–76.
32. Deporter DA, Watson PA, Pilliar RM, Chipman ML, Valiquette N. A histological comparison in the dog of porous-coated vs. threaded dental implants. J Dent Res 1990;69:1138–1145.
33. Corigliano M, Quaranta M, Scarano A, Piattelli A. Bone reaction to early loaded plasma-sprayed titanium implants [abstract 275]. J Dent Res 1995;74(special issue):435.
34. Piattelli A, Corigliano M, Scarano A, Quaranta M. Bone reactions to early occlusal loading of two-stage titanium plasma-sprayed implants: A pilot study in monkeys. Int J Periodontics Restorative Dent 1997;17:162–169.
35. Romanos GE, Toh CG, Siar CH, Wicht, H, Yacoob H, Nentwig GH. Bone-implant interface around implants under different loading conditions. A histomorphometrical analysis in the Macaca fascicularis monkey. J Periodontol 2003;74:1483–1490.

# Histologic Evaluation of Immediately Loaded Implants

## 5

Biologic and endogenous components influence bone metabolism and structure during loading. Bone metabolism can be significantly increased with a resulting increase in bone-implant contact (BIC) if the implant surface is sand-blasted, acid etched, etched and sand-blasted, titanium plasma sprayed (TPS), or coated with hydroxyapatite (HA). Furthermore, macrointerlocking properties (ie, implant design) are important for achieving improved osseointegration.

Biomechanical factors around endosseous implants are known to influence the modeling and remodeling processes in bone and thus play an important role in the quality of anchorage between implant and surrounding bone tissue. The bone response depends on the direction, magnitude, and repetition rate of loading forces. Bone can better resist rapidly applied loads than slowly applied forces. Repetitive forces increase bone volume, whereas markedly reduced loading forces decrease the bone volume.

There is no doubt that immediate loading with excessive loading forces after implant placement may cause excessive micromotion at the implant-bone interface and lead to fibrous tissue formation (encapsulation), which may cause implant failure.[1] Immediate loading of implants can be successful if certain conditions are met. Two factors are (1) excellent primary stability of the implants and (2) adequate splinting between implants to tolerate the loading forces. Appropriate microinterlocking and macrointerlocking properties are also important because they are beneficial in improving implant stability.

Histology is the best way to study implant healing, assess micromovement, and evaluate the degree of osseointegration that can be achieved using various techniques and materials. Studies evaluating histologic and histomorphometric parameters both in animals and in humans have produced quantitative and qualitative data regarding the efficacy of immediately loaded implants, independent of their design.

## Animal Studies

### Bone response to immediately loaded implants

Animal studies have demonstrated that osseointegration of immediately loaded implants is influenced by the surface roughness and thread design of implants.[2–7] For instance, in a nonhuman primate model, immediately loaded HA-coated blade implants were shown to have undergone superior osseointegration in comparison with titanium blade implants, which engendered fibrous connective tissue growth.[2] Likewise, osseointegration occurred with bilaterally splinted, immediately loaded, one-stage titanium threaded implants placed in dogs. The BIC of immediately loaded implants did not differ from that of implants loaded after healing, and only marginal bone resorption was found.[3] Additionally, Piattelli et al[5] have found histologic and histomorphometric evidence that bone density is higher around immediately loaded screw-shaped TPS implants in comparison with unloaded implants in the maxilla and mandible of *Macaca fascicularis*. The histomorphometric analysis in this study demonstrated that the BIC percentage in immediately loaded implants was 67.3% in the maxilla and 73.2% in the mandible; these percentages in the unloaded implants were 54.5% in the maxilla and 55.8% in the mandible. Moreover, bone around the immediately loaded implants had a more compact appearance.

Histomorphometric analysis of the bone-implant interface also shows no statistical difference in the BIC percentages between immediately loaded and delayed loaded implants.[7] Several studies using *Macaca fascicularis* have indicated that, in the posterior mandible, osseointegration of immediately loaded splinted implants occurs with a hard and soft tissue peri-implant response that is similar to that of delayed loaded implants[6–8]; however, the bone volume (density) within the implant threads was characteristically higher with immediately loaded versus delayed loaded implants.[7,9] The immediately loaded implants evaluated in these studies were osseointegrated with no gaps or fibrous connective tissue observed between the titanium surface and the surrounding alveolar bone. Bone lamellae parallel to the implant surface were found within the implant threads, with the greater formation of new bone characterized by numerous lacunae with osteocytes observed in the crestal and middle parts of the implants.[7,10] There was no statistically significant difference in the BIC percentages between the two implant loading groups (delayed versus immediate loading). In contrast, implants had higher BIC percentages under both loading conditions (delayed and immediate) compared with the unloaded situations.[10]

The following histologic and histomorphometric observations were made during a study in which nonloaded, delayed loaded, and immediately loaded implants with a progressive thread design and a Morse taper implant-abutment connection were placed in the posterior mandible of monkeys.[9,10] All implants healed uneventfully and integrated with the bone. No gaps or soft tissue formation were found between the implant and the abutment (conical seal) during loading. No obvious bone resorption around the implants could be observed. The abutments were maintained in place during the entire observation period without removal, which may have been the reason for the crestal bone stability.

## Histologic observations

### Nonloaded implants
The bone surrounding the nonloaded implants with different geometries had a loose structure with a high number of spaces filled with fat tissue and marrow. Some areas of the implants were covered by thin trabecular bone (Fig 5-1).

### Delayed loaded implants
Serial sectioning of the delayed loaded implants showed that all implants were osseointegrated and interfaced with healthy-looking bone. In general, the bone response was excellent, and no resorption or infrabony pockets were observed. Close apposition of haversian systems was evident within the newly apposed woven bone (Fig 5-2).

### Immediately loaded implants
The histologic examination of immediately loaded implants showed excellent bone response with compact, cortical bone and small bone trabeculae in contact with the implant surface, especially in the coronal portion of the implants. The bone trabeculae around the immediately loaded implants were thickened and appeared as fingerlike (or carpetlike) projections oriented parallel to all of the implant surfaces as well as within the implant threads. Some distance from the implant surface, the bone contained numerous marrow spaces. In areas with increased loading force (according to the direction of the force), greater and denser bone formation was observed. No gaps or connective tissue formation was found between the bone and the metal surface. The peri-implant hard tissues did not show any signs of resorption. Some bone resorption and connective tissue proliferation were found in the crestal region of the alveolar bone of a few implants (Fig 5-3). This resorption was not accompanied by inflammatory cellular reactions, but in some areas macrophages were found.

Healthy-looking haversian systems were clearly identified close to the implant surface, especially within the grooves of the implant. A characteristic demarcation between old and new bone was apparent. Numerous viable osteocytes in their lacunae were seen in the newly formed woven bone, and in some areas, giant cells in close contact with the titanium implant surface were present. In some cases, the new bone also covered the top of the implant (Fig 5-4a).

In general, there were no significant histologic differences between immediately and delayed loaded implants. Mineralized tissue was found to be in close approximation with the titanium implant surface with increased density around the middle and cervical parts of the implants.

Newly formed lamellar bone, stained and differentiated from the surrounding bony tissue, presented parallel lamellae in close contact with the titanium surface (Fig 5-4b).

It is significant that a sealing between the abutment and the inner part of the implant was observed without any migration of the epithelium at the implant-abutment interface, which characterizes the stability of the peri-implant soft tissues in the sulcular area (Fig 5-5a). The stability of the Morse taper connection at the implant-abutment interface under occlusal loading was observed histologically. This proves the complete sealing of such mechanical connections (Fig 5-5b).

## Histomorphometric observations

The histomorphometric findings at the interface of nonloaded, delayed loaded, and immediately loaded implants are presented in Table 5-1. BIC percentages were lower in the nonloaded implants and increased significantly ($P < .05$) during loading. Although these values were higher in the delayed loaded implants, they were not statistically different ($P > .05$) from those obtained with the immediately loaded implants. Bone volume (density of the mineralized bone) was greater in the loaded implants compared with the nonloaded implants ($P < .05$) in all of the measured implant areas. The immediately loaded implants presented a statistically significant ($P < .05$) higher quantity of mineralized bone tissue in the areas within the threads. Bone areas (density) in the distant regions of the bone (ie, not at the interface) showed no statistically significant difference ($P > .05$) around the delayed loaded as compared with the immediately loaded implants.

Animal Studies

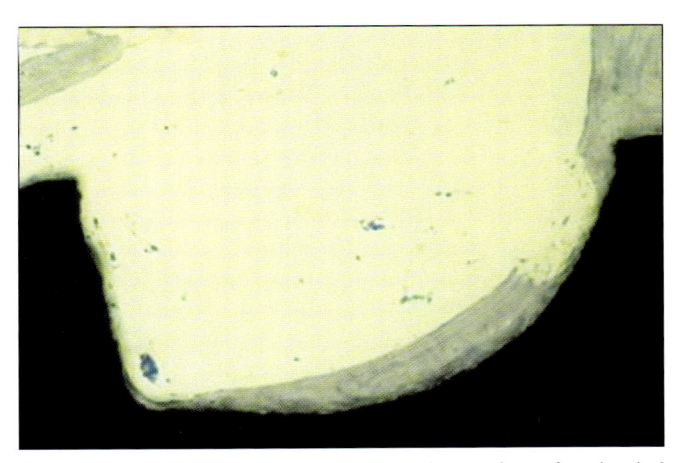

**Fig 5-1** Carpetlike (thin) bone formation at the interface of nonloaded implants 3 months after healing.

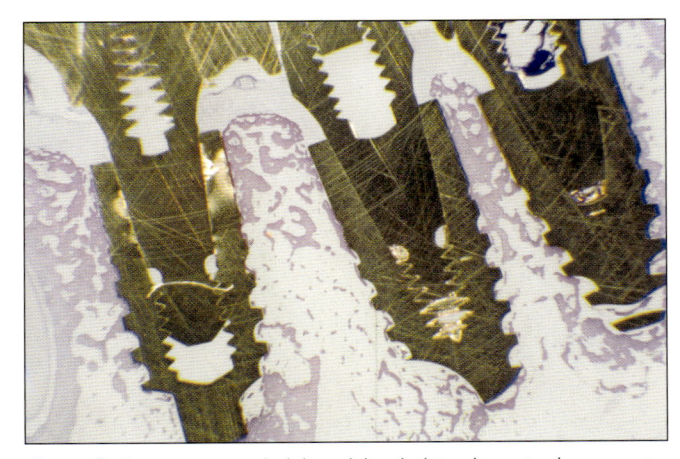

**Fig 5-2** Osseointegrated delayed loaded implants in the posterior mandible presenting vital lamellar bone at the interface similar to the bone around healthy teeth.

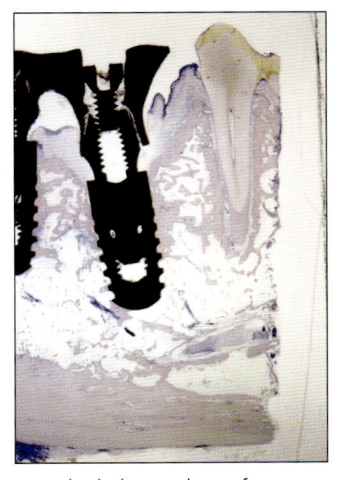

**Fig 5-3** New high-density bone formation around immediately loaded implants in the posterior mandible.

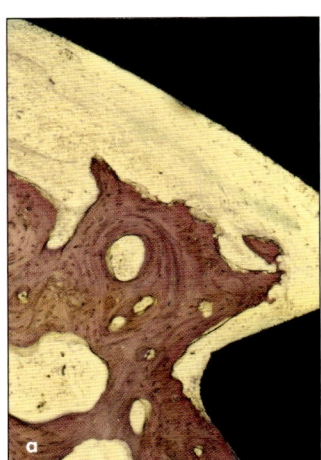

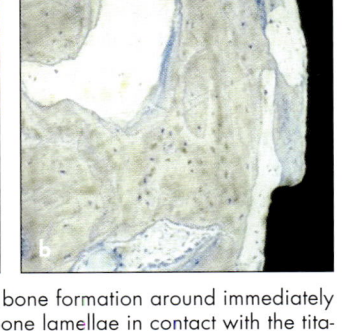

**Fig 5-4** *(a and b)* Characteristic bone formation around immediately loaded implants presenting vital bone lamellae in contact with the titanium surface. Observe the new bone formation over the implant top in an implant with platform switching without abutment removal. A high number of osteocytes localized in lacunae are presented in the new woven bone formation within the implant threads.

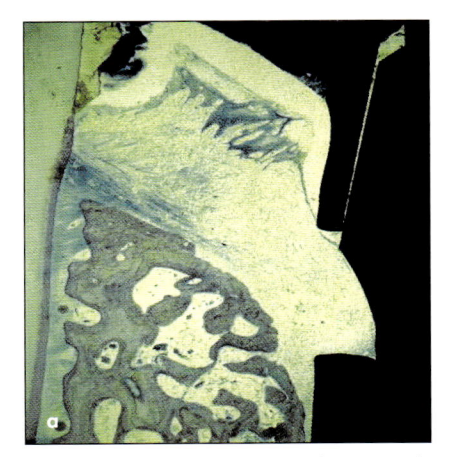

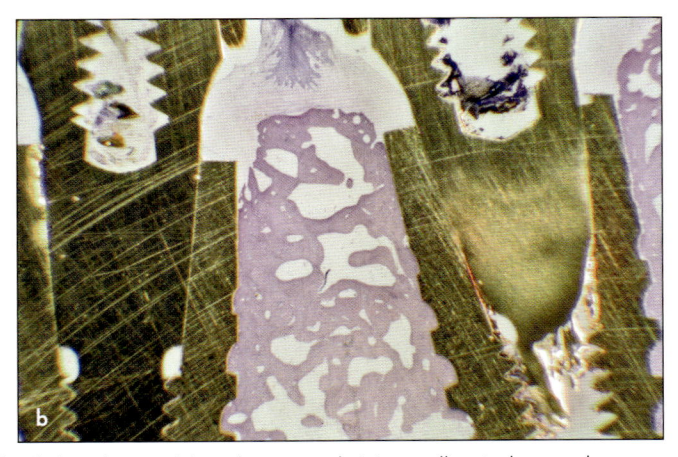

**Fig 5-5** Bone formation around an immediately loaded implant and the adjacent tooth *(a)* as well as in the area between two implants *(b)* demonstrates excellent formation of dense lamellar bone.

**Table 5-1** Histomorphometric findings at the interface of implants (3.5 mm in diameter, 8 mm in length) placed in the posterior mandible under different loading conditions*

| Loading condition | N | BIC (%) | BA-t (%) | BA-a (%) | BA-c (%) |
|---|---|---|---|---|---|
| No loading | 6 | 50.20 ± 9.06 | 27.02 ± 12.28 | 37.59 ± 18.04 | 31.71 ± 18.01 |
| Delayed loading | 24 | 67.93 ± 1.60 | 65.42 ± 19.88 | 73.97 ± 23.59 | 44.99 ± 20.02 |
| Immediate loading | 24 | 64.25 ± 0.65 | 76.95 ± 11.35 | 54.34 ± 17.13 | 47.79 ± 27.20 |

BA, bone area (density); t, within the threads; a, at the apical part of the implant; c, at the cervical part of the implant.
*Based on data from Romanos.[9]

## Peri-implant soft tissue response

### Immediately loaded implants

The stability of soft tissue surrounding immediately loaded implants is a critical topic of research because soft tissue sealing and integration around the abutment is essential in achieving successful long-term biofunctionality of the implant.[11,12] The soft tissue mucosal barrier serves complex functions in preventing bacterial invasion and food impaction.[13,14] The underlying mechanisms of attachment, which influence the integrity of this biologic seal between implant and soft tissues, are not well understood.[15]

Compared with the standard two-stage protocol, a major advantage of the one-stage protocol to place dental implants with immediate loading is the immediate restoration of esthetics and function.[16,17] The increasing application of this one-stage technique has led to the need for concurrent clinical and experimental investigations to evaluate the effects of immediate loading on the soft tissue–implant interface. A search of the existing literature reveals that the structure and dimensions of this interface in immediately loaded implants has not been well investigated.[4,5]

#### Histologic observations
The definitive microscopic examination of the soft tissues around immediately loaded implants was published in the study described above by Siar et al.[8] The authors found that the peri-implant soft tissue was histologically similar to the mucosa around natural teeth. The coronal mucosa was covered by a keratinized stratified squamous epithelium (SSE) with a thickness of several cell layers and rete pegs formation, supported by fibrous connective tissue with minimal inflammation (in monkeys, excellent plaque control is not possible). The mucosal epithelium continued apically to form the sulcular epithelium, which consisted of nonkeratinized SSE that also had rete ridges. Toward the apical region, the sulcular epithelium became contiguous with the junctional epithelium (JE). The latter occurred as a thin, nonkeratinized epithelium that was a few cell layers thick and had a flat epithelia–connective tissue interface. A mild, diffuse, mononuclear inflammatory infiltrate was observed in the adjacent connective tissue. Separating the apical JE and the first BIC was a narrow zone of relatively avascular and acellular hyalinized connective tissue. This connective tissue layer contained fine short collagen fibers running parallel to the smooth surface of the transmucosal collar of the implant abutment (see also Fig 5-5a).

#### Histomorphometric observations
All sections in the Siar et al[8] study were analyzed under several magnifications of light microscopy to identify specific anatomical landmarks. Areas of histologic artifacts were avoided. Six peri-implant soft tissue parameters were quantified:

1. Sulcus depth (SD): Distance between the gingival margin (GM) and the most coronal point of the JE (cJE)
2. JE: Distance between the cJE and the most apical point of the JE (aJE)
3. Connective tissue contact (CTC): Distance between the aJE and the first point of BIC
4. DIM: Distance between the GM and the top of the implant
5. DIB: Distance between the top of the implant and the first point of BIC
6. Biologic width (BW): SD + JE + CTC

### Delayed loaded implants

#### Histologic observations
In the Siar et al[8] study, histologic examination of the soft tissues around delayed loaded implants revealed peri-implant mucosa structurally similar to that around natural teeth. The coronal keratinized SSE, sulcular nonkeratinized SSE, and attenuated JE were likewise identified. In the underlying connective tissue, a mild inflammatory cell infiltrate was present. The CTC also occurred as a zone of scarlike connective tissue, poor in cells and blood vessels, that was devoid of any inflammatory reaction.

#### Histomorphometric observations
Comparison of the overall mean values obtained by Siar et al[8] showed no significant difference between the delayed loaded and immediately loaded implants ($P > .01$). For the BW, no significant difference between the two loading groups was found ($P > 0.01$). The mean vertical dimensions of the components of BW (ie, SD, JE, and CTC) were comparable with those of the natural teeth (Table 5-2).

**Table 5-2** Mean values of soft tissue parameters for immediately loaded and delayed loaded implants*

| Parameter | Immediate loading N | Immediate loading Mean score (mm) | Delayed loading N | Delayed loading Mean score (mm) | P values |
|---|---|---|---|---|---|
| SD | 48 | 0.68 ± 0.63 | 47 | 0.88 ± 0.57 | 0.099 |
| JE | 51 | 1.71 ± 1.04 | 50 | 1.66 ± 0.77 | 0.809 |
| CTC | 52 | 1.51 ± 1.14 | 49 | 1.24 ± 0.92 | 0.877 |
| DIM | 48 | 2.27 ± 1.18 | 50 | 2.38 ± 0.81 | 0.516 |
| DIB | 54 | 1.32 ± 1.21 | 52 | 1.19 ± 0.91 | 0.540 |

*Based on data from Siar et al.[8]

## Influence of implant system

Soft tissue integration in relation to different implant systems[18,19] has been studied previously based on clinical observations.[19,20] Histologic[21,22] and histomorphometric analyses[19,21] also have been used to report on soft tissue integration in relation to different implant systems[18,19] following abutment disconnection and reconnection,[23] different abutment types[24] in implants with different surface topography,[11] in submerged versus nonsubmerged implants,[14,18] and in one-piece versus two-piece implants.[12,25] Most of these experimental studies used the dog model,[14,18] which permitted only a hinge jaw movement. In contrast, the monkey model has anatomical similarities with the human in terms of dentition and jaw movements.

## Soft tissue thickness

According to histomorphometric soft tissue data, the DIM is an important parameter in providing information on the morphology of the outer implant epithelium. Plaque accumulation in the abutment area as well as the marginal part of the prosthetic suprastructure has been shown to cause reactive hyperplasia of the outer mucosa, resulting in soft tissue morphology alteration in this area.[22] Such changes in turn affect the vertical dimension of the DIM. In studies[8,9] that used implants with platform shifting (Ankylos, Dentsply Friadent), a mild degree of peri-implant inflammation was observed clinically (monkey specimens). The DIM scores for immediately loaded and delayed loaded implants showed no significant differences, indicating that factors relating to oral hygiene control, implant design, and soft tissue levels relative to the implant posts and their superstructures were comparable in both groups and were not influenced by the different loading protocols after healing. This characteristic soft tissue finding is probably associated with the shape of the abutment and the implant-abutment connection (conical seal). In their study on healed tissues around implants in beagle dogs, Weber et al[14] observed that there was no significant difference in the DIM between submerged implants (uncovered 3 months after implant placement by stage-two surgery) and nonsubmerged implants.

## Biologic width

The BW is the sum of the vertical dimensions of SD, JE, and CTC.[12,25–27] Gargiulo et al[26] demonstrated that, in the natural teeth, the BW is a physiologically formed and stable dimension whose level is dependent on the location of the crest of the alveolar bone. Recent studies on endosseous dental implants confirmed that the same phenomenon of a dimensionally stable BW was recapitulated by the peri-implant soft tissues.[12,25,27] Dynamic changes[25] were shown to occur within the components of this stable structure, and their dimensions were found to be dependent on (1) the presence or absence of a microgap (interface) between the implant and abutment and (2) the location of the microgap in relation to the crest of the bone.[12]

Siar et al[8] demonstrated that the vertical dimensions constituting the BW were not significantly different ($P > .01$) between the immediately loaded implant group (3.9 mm) and the delayed loaded implant group (3.78 mm). These results suggest that the parameters were not influenced by differences in the loading protocol, surgical treatments, or anatomical location of the implants. Successful soft tissue integration was achieved because of the smooth transmucosal collar and the absence of microgaps (Morse taper connection) between the implant and the abutment in the implant system used.[6] A long JE was observed and can be attributed to epithelial downgrowth alongside the surface of the abutment and the machined collar of the implants.

## Junctional epithelium and connective tissue contact

The JE and CTC are important parameters, providing information related to the location of the apical extension of junctional epithelial cells, the crestal bone height, and the extent of BIC. Berglundh et al[13] found that, at both tooth and implant sites, the apical cells of the epithelium terminated approximately 1.0 to 1.5 mm coronal to the alveolar bone crest. Studies evaluating the healing patterns of soft tissues in submerged versus nonsubmerged implants disclosed that apical extension of peri-implant epithelium is significantly greater and the attachment level significantly more apical adjacent to submerged implants with stage-two transmucosal abutments than in nonsubmerged one-stage implants.[14,27] The histomorphometric analysis showed that the mean JE and CTC between the test and control groups disclosed no significant differences.[27] This finding implies that the crestal bone height adjacent to implants was not influenced by the different loading protocols in the two groups, specifically for implants with platform shifting and a conical implant-abutment connection. These findings correlated well with experimental and clinical studies demonstrating that immediate loading did not compromise soft and hard tissue integration.[6,9,28,29]

The abutments used were not removed in the entire loading period. This is important to achieve peri-implant soft and hard tissue stability.

## Discussion and conclusions

It is still not clear what changes occur in the mechanical environment around the implant and what mechanical parameters are dominant in initiating bone activity. Some researchers have reported that bone formation occurs in areas with compression.[30,31] Other studies have shown that both tensile and compressive stresses promote the amount and maturation of bone and that the promotion of bone formation depends on the quantity of the stress forces.[32]

According to histologic and histomorphometric observations, it may be concluded that loading influences new bone formation. Gentle occlusal stresses may increase blood circulation in bone, thus enhancing bone metabolism and consequently promoting bone remodeling. Moreover, immediate loading seems to increase ossification within the threads of the alveolar bone around endosseous implants. The findings presented in this study[32] suggest that the interface reacts according to Wolff's law on loading, which states that bone can change or adapt its shape and microstructure to changes in the mechanical environment (ie, form follows function).[33]

The histologic and histomorphometric observations gathered from studies of implants placed in monkeys under different loading conditions demonstrate the quality and quantity of peri-implant bone and soft tissues. They further show that the bone next to an immediately loaded implant surface can be remodeled without fibrous tissue formation when excellent primary stability (with appropriate implant design selection and careful osteotomy preparation) and adequate splinting (immobilization of the implants immediately after placement with rigid provisional restorations) are achieved. Immediate loading seems to increase the quantity of the mineralized bone within the implant threads in monkeys when the implants are immediately loaded with composite resin provisional prostheses in the first month of healing and later restored with the definitive restorations. Experimental studies in rabbits have provided histomorphometric evidence that the apposition of neocortical bone after implant placement is achieved very quickly, does not increase after the first month of healing, and remains unchanged between 3 and 6 months.[34] Similar observations also have been reported in sheep.[35]

# Human Studies

## Bone response to immediately loaded implants

The immediate loading treatment concept can be successfully used in implant dentistry independent of the geometry of the implant used. Based on histologic observations from different animal studies, immediately loaded implants form a direct bone-implant interface without any fibrous tissue formation. Bone cells migrate onto the implant surface and establish a stable anchorage of the titanium surface into the bone. Mature bone formation is dependent on the loading period. Experiments on animals can be consulted, but the results cannot be directly transferred to humans because of different loading conditions between the different species. Therefore, data from retrieved implants placed in humans are necessary. There are limited data from human biopsies presenting bone integration of immediately loaded implants after functional loading of several years. There are limited data showing direct BIC in patients with well-defined immediate loading protocols in association with the clinical and radiologic parameters of the examined implants.[36]

Moreover, there is a paucity of information about wound healing at the bone-implant interface in heavy smokers and other immunocompromised patients with immediately loaded implants. Data regarding implants removed because of fracture or other (eg, orthodontic, psychologic) reasons are extremely important from the scientific point of view because they present the bone response at the interface during different periods of healing. Furthermore, such histologic data demonstrate different kinds of implant systems with various surface patterns placed in different bone qualities in the maxilla and the mandible. The biomechanical response of the bone during loading is dependent on the implant shape (eg, cylindric, tapered) as well as the thread geometry interfacing with different bone qualities. A necessary requirement for long-term success after immediate functional loading is the primary stability and immobilization of the implant during and after surgery. It is important that the clinician understand the bone response at the interface of immediately loaded implants placed in humans before undertaking the use of this treatment concept in routine daily practice.

Histologic and histomorphometric evaluations of immediately loaded implants of various shapes and thread designs retrieved from humans yielded the following results:

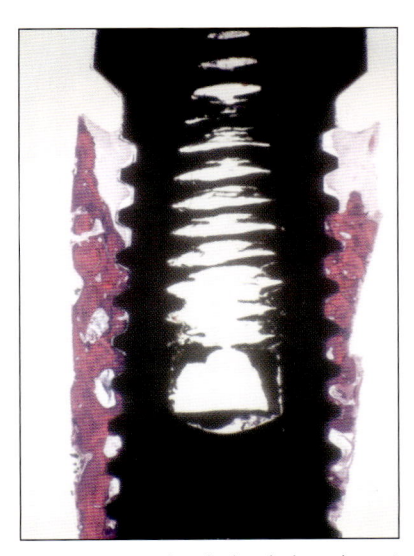

**Fig 5-6** Immediately loaded implant 4 months after placement presenting excellent bone formation at the interface (original magnification ×1.5).

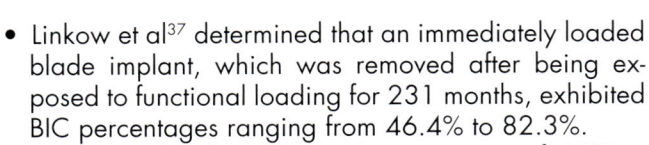

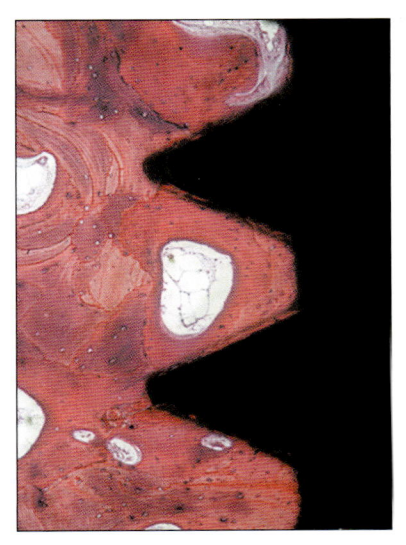

**Fig 5-7** Immediately loaded implant 4 months after placement demonstrating thick lamellar bone formation (original magnification ×25).

- Linkow et al[37] determined that an immediately loaded blade implant, which was removed after being exposed to functional loading for 231 months, exhibited BIC percentages ranging from 46.4% to 82.3%.
- Froum et al[38] showed a BIC percentage of 40% to 72% in humans after retrieval of immediately loaded implants.
- Ledermann et al[39] reported high percentages of BIC (70% to 80%) after histologically examining four retrieved immediately loaded mandibular implants in a human after 12 years of function.

In general, examinations of histologic nondecalcified sections revealed mostly cancellous-type bone (with large marrow spaces) around the apical two-thirds of the implant surface. Soft tissue pockets were frequently observed around the cervical nonthreaded part, where the bone surfaces were undergoing some resorption.

Parallel to the qualitative evaluation, histomorphometric data demonstrated similar BIC percentages in maxillary and mandibular implants—44% and 48%, respectively. Whether or not these values indicate good or poor integration of the implants is unknown. Bone-anchored implants are referred to as *clinically stable implants*. However, there is no consensus about the amount of BIC needed for a clinically stable implant, although it has been demonstrated that bone tissue density around implants will increase with time of observation.[40] Other quantitative parameters investigated in this autopsy report[36] were bone areas formed both inside and outside the threads. Comparisons between bone areas formed within the implant threads placed in the maxilla and mandible demonstrated no differences (about 52%), while generally there was a bit more bone formed immediately outside the inner threads in the maxilla compared to the mandible. Less bone within the threads compared with outside the threads may indicate that the bone area inside the threads was not fully remodeled. One can only speculate as to whether this is related to a short healing time or host tissue factors, the latter being influenced by smoking, the execution of the immediate loading concept of implants in poor-quality bone, or a combination of these parameters.

# Histologic information from retrieved implants: Case reports

## Nontapered implants

### Case 1

Two Osseotite (Biomet 3i) implants were immediately loaded and in function for 4 months in the mandible of a healthy, nonsmoking 61-year-old man. All immediately loaded implants were placed in normal bone quality and achieved clinical osseointegration. Subsequently, they were loaded using a definitive fixed prosthesis. The sites of the retrieved implants healed without complications, as confirmed by radiologic evaluation at 24 months.

At the mandibular right lateral incisor site, osseointegration was achieved with close bone apposition as observed under the light microscope; histomorphometrically, the BIC percentage was 80%. The implant-bone interface consisted of a combination of newly formed and old bone. Bone was in contact with the entire implant surface. Occasionally, bone was not present at the tip of some threads. On the buccal side, the bone crest was localized above the first thread level, while on the lingual side it was slightly above the second thread (Fig 5-6). Epithelium downgrowth was not found contacting the implant surface at the supracrestal level.

At the mandibular left second premolar site, all slides showed osseointegration, and the mean BIC percentage was 81.5% (78% to 85%). Old and new bone was found at the interface. The new bone was undergoing remodeling (Fig 5-7); the implant surface was covered by bone and did not lack bone patterns at the tip of the threads. Again, epithelium downgrowth was not found at the interface.

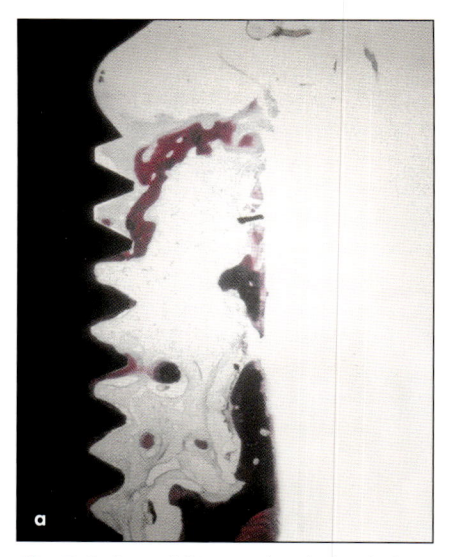

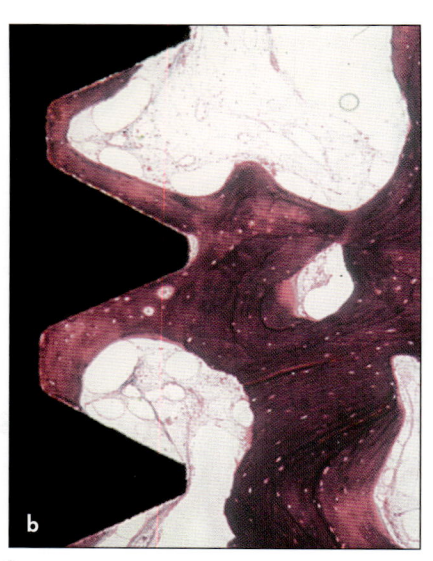

**Fig 5-8** *(a and b)* Immediately loaded implants 2 months after placement in soft bone ([a] original magnification ×5; [b] original magnification ×15).

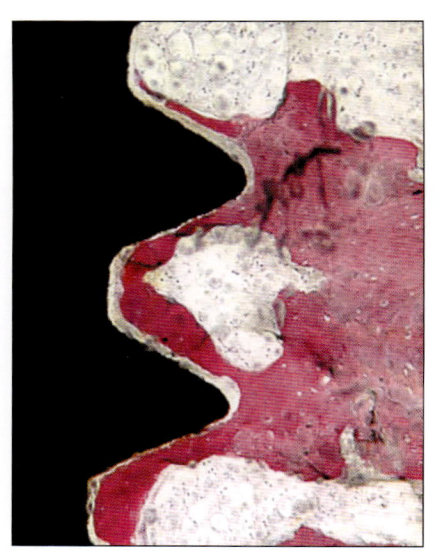

**Fig 5-9** In most areas of the bone-implant interface, bone appeared to be separated from the titanium surface of the immediately loaded implant (2-μm gap). No gaps or fibrous tissue was present at the interface. Inflammatory cells were absent (original magnification ×40).

### Case 2

An immediate loading protocol was used in the edentulous mandible of a healthy, nonsmoking 52-year-old man. All immediately loaded implants achieved clinical osseointegration and were included in the definitive fixed prosthesis. A panoramic radiograph taken at 24 months confirmed that the sites had healed uneventfully and were filled with bone.

At the mandibular right canine site, healing took place under occlusal function for 2 months. One section from this immediately loaded implant, which was placed in soft bone quality, was available for evaluation. Only the labial side was evaluated. Osseointegration was achieved, the measured BIC was 64.2%, and fibrous encapsulation was not seen. Bone marrow occupied most of the crestal and cancellous areas. The bone crest was level with the first implant thread (Fig 5-8a), but the first point of BIC occurred more apically, at the level of the third thread. The adjacent cortical bone was composed of newly formed bone, and remnants of old bone were found embedded in this bone. Under the cortical bone, a single marrow space extended to the ninth thread. In this cancellous area, the implant textured surface was covered by a quasi-continuous thin shell of newly formed bone in continuation with the crestal cortex (see Fig 5-8a). More apically, bone was denser with large marrow spaces (Fig 5-8b). New bone covered the titanium surface, interposing between the old bone (more purple aspect, on the right side) and the interface. Epithelial downgrowth was not observed.

### Case 3

Implants were placed and loaded the same day of surgery in the maxilla of a 60-year-old man who was a heavy smoker (approximately 60 cigarettes per day). The most distal implant, located in the left tuberosity, was retrieved with a trephine for psychologic reasons after 6 months of loading. Before retrieval, the implant appeared to be clinically stable, and a periapical radiograph showed there was minimal resorption around the most coronal portion of the implant.

In most areas, bone appeared to be separated from the implant surface by a 2-μm gap. At higher magnification, the bone was trabecular with wide marrow spaces (Fig 5-9). In the areas where the bone was in close contact with the implant surface, bone tended to grow down to the bottom of the threads. The mean BIC percentage was 60% ± 3.8%. Bone remodeling areas were present around the implant, and no gaps or fibrous tissue was present at the interface. Inflammatory cells were absent, and no foreign body reaction or bone loss was found at the bone-implant interface. No epithelial downgrowth was present.

### Case 4

A total of four implants, two IMZ-TwinPlus (Dentsply Friadent) screw-type implants and two cylindric implants, were placed and immediately loaded in the posterior maxilla and the mandible. These implants were distal abutments of fixed implant-supported provisional restorations. After 10 months of loading, the implants were retrieved and examined histologically.

A mean vertical bone loss of 1.5 ± 0.1 mm was present. In the area of bone loss, fibrous connective tissue with no inflammatory infiltrate could be observed. Direct contact between lamellar bone and the implant surface was present without gaps or fibrous connective tissue at the interface in both samples (Fig 5-10). In most areas

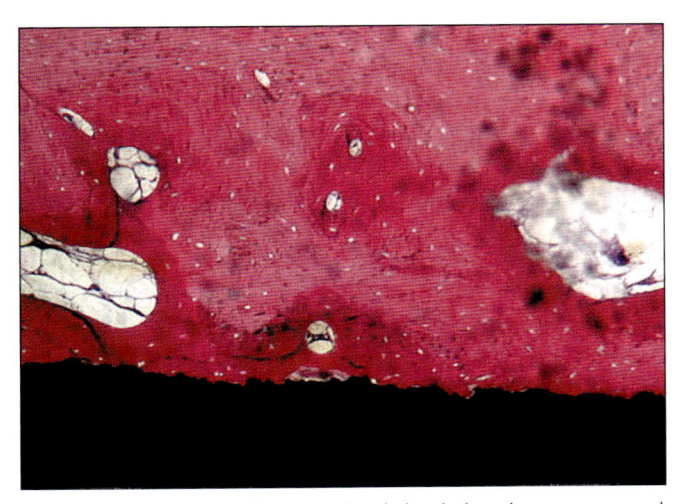

**Fig 5-10** The surface of the immediately loaded implant was covered with mature compact lamellar bone. Direct contact between bone and implant surface was present without gaps or fibrous connective tissue at the interface (original magnification ×100).

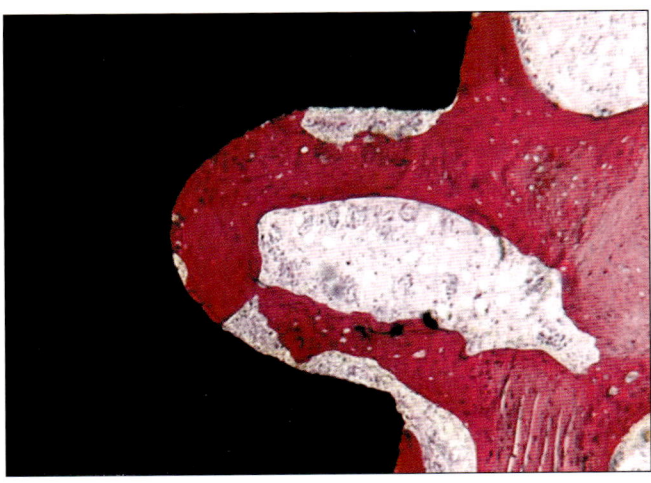

**Fig 5-11** Only newly formed bone was found at the interface with the implant, while old preexisting bone (weaker staining) was found at a distance from the interface, embedded in newly formed bone. No gaps or fibrous tissue was present at the interface of any of the implants (original magnification ×50).

of the interface, it was possible to see the presence of newly formed bone. Preexisting bone was occasionally seen embedded in the newly formed bone. None of the specimens contained inflammatory or multinucleated giant cells at the interface or in the peri-implant tissues. No gaps were present at the interface, even at higher magnification. A limited number of marrow spaces were present at the bone-implant interface. The histomorphometric analysis showed the mean BIC percentage to be 64.5% ± 4.7%.

## Case 5

Three (two HA-coated and one sand-blasted) immediately loaded Maestro implants (BioHorizons) were retrieved after a 6-month loading period in two patients. All three implants appeared to be osseointegrated. Periapical radiographs showed a mean vertical bone resorption of 0.5 ± 0.1 mm. The implants were treated to obtain thin sections for histologic examination of the bone at the interface.

On the surface of the abutment and on the first cervical 0.5 mm of the implant, it was possible to observe the presence of mild bacterial invasion. At low-power magnification, bone was present around all three implants, starting from the concavity of the first thread. Only newly formed bone was found at the interface with the implant, while old preexisting bone was found at a distance from the interface embedded in newly formed bone (Fig 5-11). Intense remodeling activity was found at a distance of about 3 mm from the implant surface, where Howship lacunae and active rims of osteoblasts were present. Bone was present in all three concavities of every thread in the three implants. Bone trabeculae, with a thickness of about 150 to 200 μm, were also present in the thread concavities at the interface with large marrow spaces and supracrestal connective tissues. In the HA-coated implants, the HA that was located in the central portion of the concavities was not resorbed, while resorption was present in the most external portion of the concavities. In the areas where the coating had been resorbed, it was possible to see multinucleated giant cells with HA particles in their cytoplasm. The bone near the HA coating presented wide osteocyte lacunae; this bone showed a partially organized lamellar structure. No gaps or fibrous tissue was present at the interface of any of the three implants. In the sand-blasted mandibular implant, bone was in close and direct contact with the titanium surface.

The mean BIC percentage was 80.6% ± 4.7%, excluding the nonthreaded portion. The mean SD in all examined implants was 0.9 ± 0.1 mm, while the mean length of the JE was 0.9 ± 0.05 mm, and the mean length of the CTC was 1.1 ± 0.05 mm. Epithelial downgrowth was not present in any of the examined implant specimens.

### Tapered (root-form) implants

## Case 1

Twelve Ankylos implants were placed and immediately loaded in a woman who was a heavy smoker. Six implants were placed in each arch on the same day, connected and loaded using provisional resin prostheses. A soft diet was advised for the first stages (4 to 6 weeks) of healing, after which the definitive restorations were placed in situ and the masticatory function reestablished. The patient died after 7 months of loading because of a bronchial carcinoma. The implants were retrieved postmortem.[36]

The implants were osseointegrated to some extent and surrounded by mostly cancellous bone, although a great part of the bone was resorbed, especially around the cervical nonthreaded part of the implants. In this region, fibrous connective tissue was in close contact with the titanium surface, and nonepithelial migration was found (Fig 5-12). All implants in the maxilla were osseointegrated to some extent. Incomplete mineralized bone filled some of the implant threads. In some areas, soft connective tissue covered the peri-implant crestal section without any epithelial proliferation or migration, and very small pocket formation was observed. Only small, single blood vessels and single macrophages were found. Fibrous connective and fat tissue also covered some of the apical part of the implants. Single remnants of vital bone were found in the cervical peri-implant areas; the collagen fibers were oriented parallel to the titanium surface. A high number of blood vessels were located in the bone marrow spaces.

All implants in the mandible had direct bone contact to some extent. The peri-implant bone had a lamellar structure and was less mineralized or not remodelled. Some peri-implant bony pockets and resorptive areas were found without epithelial proliferation and were completely filled by soft connective tissue. The peri-implant soft tissue was not inflamed, and the connective tissue adjacent to the implant surface was collagen rich. Parallel-oriented fibers and bundles as well as blood vessels were found. The epithelium was proliferated only on the abutment surface and did not reach the coronal portion of the implants.

The mean percentage of BIC inside and outside the threads for the maxillary specimens was 53% compared to 48% for the mandibular specimens. The mean bone area measurement within the threads was 53% for maxillary specimens compared to 50% for the samples in the mandible.

**Case 2**
Seven Frialit-2 implants (Dentsply Friadent) with 8-mm length and 3.8-mm diameter were inserted in the posterior maxilla (two implants) and the mandible (five implants) and loaded immediately after surgery. After 10 months of loading, the implants were retrieved with a trephine and examined histologically.

All seven implants were surrounded by bone. A mean vertical bone loss of 1.02 ± 0.3 mm was observed. Newly formed, strongly stained, compact, mature cortical bone with few marrow spaces was observed around all implants. Active remodeling was observed in some areas. In the maxilla, the bone presented a higher percentage of marrow spaces, whereas in the mandible it was possible to observe well-organized haversian systems. Few marrow spaces were observed directly on the implant surface. Osteoblasts were found around the implant, or in the marrow spaces. Osteoclasts were shown in only a few areas, and no inflammatory infiltrate was present around the implants. No dense, fibrous connective tissue was found at the bone-titanium interface (Fig 5-13). Histomorphometric evaluation showed that the mean BIC percentage was 66.8% ± 3.8%.

**Case 3**
Eight XiVE implants (Dentsply Friadent) were inserted in the edentulous mandible of a 53-year-old man and immediately loaded. After a healing period of 6 months, two implants were removed with the surrounding tissues. The implants were osseointegrated and showed no clinical signs of mobility. No bone resorption was found in the radiologic evaluation that was performed before the implants were retrieved.

At the mandibular right second molar site, higher magnification of the bone presented wide marrow spaces, with a few of these abutting the implant surface. In some areas, newly formed bone was present at the interface. On one side of the implant, there was no evidence of vertical bone resorption at the level of the crestal bone; on the other side, 1.3 ± 0.2 mm of crestal bone resorption was present. Signs of bone loss were present in the most coronal bone, while no resorption was seen in the bone at its interface with the implant. Newly formed bone tended to grow down into the bottom of the threads of the implant. The mean BIC percentage was 72% ± 2.9%. No gaps or fibrous tissues were present at the interface, nor were there any inflammatory cells, a foreign body reaction, or epithelial downgrowth. Bone lamellae parallel to the threads were found between the threads. In the crestal and middle part of the implant, a higher deposition of new bone was found (Fig 5-14).

At the mandibular left second molar site, the implant showed more trabecular bone with large marrow spaces at the interface. The BIC percentage was 61% ± 4.2%. A mean vertical bone resorption of 2.3 ± 0.3 mm was present on both sides of the retrieved implant. No inflammatory cells or fibrous gaps were present at the interface. At the apical portion of the implants, only a few very thin bone trabeculae covered the titanium surface.

# Conclusion

Based on the evaluation of human retrieved implants, there is histologic evidence of osseointegration of immediately loaded implants in the maxilla and mandible using different implant systems. The histomorphometric data of the analysis of the retrieved implants presented in the international literature show a mean BIC percentage of 66.83% ± 8.96% (Table 5-3; see also Romanos et al[41]).

# Acknowledgment

The data presented in this chapter are derived from previously published studies performed with Prof C. G. Toh and Prof C. H. Siar (University of Malaya, Kuala Lumpur, Malaysia) as well as Prof A. Piattelli and Dr T. Traini (University of Chieti, Italy), Dr T. Testori (University of Milano, Italy), Dr M. Degidi (Bologna, Italy), Prof Dr mult K. Donath (University of Hamburg, Germany [deceased]), and Prof C. Johansson (University of Gothenburg, Sweden). The author would like to extend his appreciation for the long-term collaboration of this internationally recognized research team.

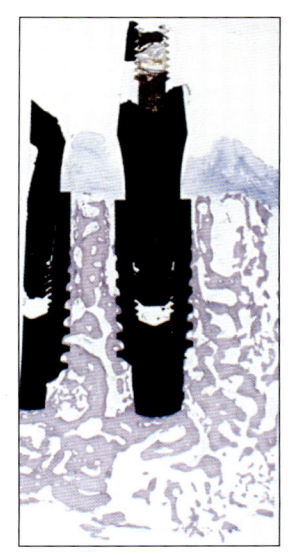

**Fig 5-12** Immediately loaded implants placed in the mandible 7 months after loading in a heavy smoker. Excellent bone integration was observed between the implants in the poor-quality posterior mandibular bone.

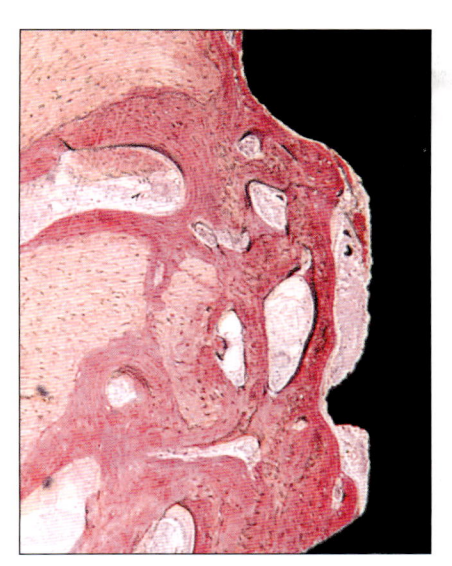

**Fig 5-13** Newly formed, strongly stained, compact, mature cortical bone with few marrow spaces was observed around the immediately loaded implant. No inflammatory infiltrate was present around the whole implant surface. No fibrous connective tissue was found at the bone-implant interface (original magnification ×40).

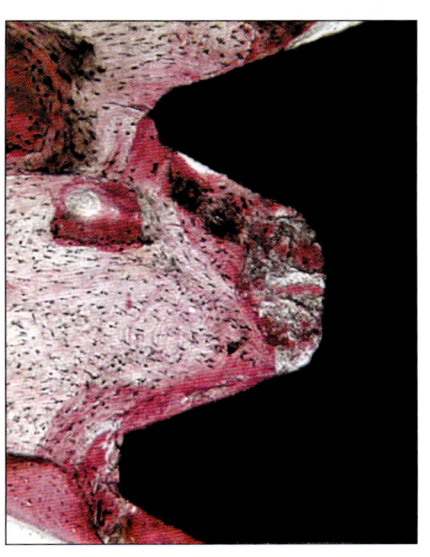

**Fig 5-14** Mature, compact bone was present around the immediately loaded implant. Newly formed bone tended to grow down into the bottom of the threads of the implant. No gaps or fibrous tissues were present at the interface, nor were there any inflammatory cells, a foreign body reaction, or epithelial downgrowth (original magnification ×40).

**Table 5-3** Histomorphometric findings of immediately loaded implants in humans

| Implant type | Loading (mo) | Implants (n) | Area | BIC (%) |
| --- | --- | --- | --- | --- |
| 3i Osseotite | 4 | 1 | Maxillary second molar | 80 |
| 3i Osseotite | 2 | 1 | Maxillary second molar | 64.2 |
| Nobel TiUnite | 6 | 1 | Maxilla | 60 |
| IMZ-TwinPlus (sand-blasted) | 10 | 2 | Mandible | 54.2–64.5 |
| Maestro (HA-coated, (sand-blasted) | 6 | 3 | Mandible | 80.6 |
| Ankylos (sand-blasted) | 7* | 6 | Maxilla | 65 |
| Ankylos (sand-blasted) | 7* | 6 | Mandible | 59 |
| Frialit-2 (sand-blasted) | 10 | 7 | Maxilla (2); mandible (5) | 66.8 |
| XiVE (sand-blasted) | 6 | 2 | Mandibular second molar | 61–72 |
| **TOTAL** | | | | 66.83 ± 8.96 |

*Heavy smoker receiving chemotherapy.

# References

1. Zubery Y, Bichacho N, Moses O, Tal H. Immediate loading of modular transitional implants: A histologic and histomorphometric analysis in dogs. Int J Periodontics Restorative Dent 1999;19:343–353.
2. Lum LB, Beirne OR, Curtis DA. Histologic evaluation of hydroxylapatite-coated versus uncoated titanium blade implants in delayed and immediately loaded applications. Int J Oral Maxillofac Implants 1991;6:456–462.
3. Sagara M, Akagawa Y, Nikai H, Tsuru H. The effects of early occlusal loading on one-stage titanium alloy implants in beagle dogs: A pilot study. J Prosthet Dent 1993;69:281–288.
4. Piattelli A, Paolantonio M, Corigliano M, Scarano A. Immediate loading of titanium plasma-sprayed screw-shaped implants in man: A clinical and histological report of two cases. J Periodontol 1997;68:591–597.
5. Piattelli A, Corigliano M, Scarano A, Costigliola G, Paolantonio M. Immediate loading of titanium plasma-sprayed implants: A histologic analysis in monkeys. J Periodontol 1998;69:321–327.

6. Romanos GE, Toh CG, Siar CH, et al. Peri-implant bone reactions to immediately loaded implants. An experimental study in monkeys. J Periodontol 2001;72:506–511.
7. Romanos GE, Toh CG, Siar CH, Swaminathan D. Histologic and histomorphometric evaluation of peri-implant bone subjected to immediate loading: An experimental study with *Macaca fascicularis*. Int J Oral Maxillofac Implants 2002;17;44–51.
8. Siar CH, Toh CH, Romanos GE, et al. Peri-implant soft tissue integration of immediately loaded implants in the posterior macaque mandible: A histomorphometric study. J Periodontol 2003;74;571–578.
9. Romanos GE. Immediate Loading in the Posterior Area of the Mandible. Animal and Clinical Studies. Berlin: Quintessence, 2005.
10. Romanos GE, Toh CG, Siar CH, Wicht, H, Yaacob H, Nentwig GH. Bone-implant interface around implants under different loading conditions. A histomorphometrical analysis in the *Macaca fascicularis* monkey. J Periodontol 2003;74:1483–1490.
11. Abrahamsson I, Zitzmann NU, Berglundh T, Wennerberg A, Lindhe J. Bone and soft tissue integration to titanium implants with different surface topography: An experimental study in the dog. Int J Oral Maxillofac Implants 2001;16:323–332.
12. Hermann JS, Buser D, Schenk RK, Schoolfield JD, Cochran DL. Biologic width around one- and two-piece titanium implants. A histometric evaluation of unloaded nonsubmerged and submerged implants in the canine mandible. Clin Oral Implants Res 2001;12:559–571.
13. Berglundh T, Lindhe J, Ericsson I, Marinello CP, Liljenberg B, Thomsen P. The soft tissue barrier at implants and teeth. Clin Oral Implants Res 1991;2:81–90.
14. Weber HP, Buser D, Donath K, et al. Comparison of healed tissues adjacent to submerged and nonsubmerged unloaded titanium dental implants. A histometric study in beagle dogs. Clin Oral Implants Res 1996;7:11–19.
15. Donley TG, Gillette WB. Titanium endosseous implant–soft tissue interface: A literature review. J Periodontol 1991;62:153–160.
16. Chiapasco M, Gatti C, Rossi E, Haefliger W, Markwalder TH. Implant-retained mandibular overdentures with immediate loading. A retrospective multicenter study on 226 consecutive cases. Clin Oral Implants Res 1997;8:48–57.
17. Grunder U, Polizzi G, Goené R, et al. A 3-year prospective multicenter follow-up report on the immediate and delayed-immediate placement of implants. Int J Oral Maxillofac Implants 1999;14:210–216.
18. Abrahamsson I, Berglundh T, Wennström J, Lindhe J. The peri-implant hard and soft tissues at different implant systems. A comparative study in the dog. Clin Oral Implants Res 1996;7:212–219.
19. Arvidson K, Fartash B, Hilliges M, Köndell PA. Histological characteristics of peri-implant mucosa around Brånemark and single-crystal sapphire implants. Clin Oral Implants Res 1996;7:1–10.
20. Adell R, Lekholm U, Rockler B, et al. Marginal tissue reactions at osseointegrated titanium fixtures. (I) A 3-year longitudinal prospective study. Int J Oral Maxillofac Surg 1986;15:39–52.
21. Gotfredsen K, Rostrup E, Hjørting-Hansen E, Stoltze K, Budtz-Jørgensen E. Histological and histomorphometrical evaluation of tissue reactions adjacent to endosteal implants in monkeys. Clin Oral Implants Res 1991;2:30–37.
22. Berglundh T, Lindhe J, Marinello C, Ericsson I, Liljenberg B. Soft tissue reaction to de novo plaque formation on implants and teeth. An experimental study in the dog. Clin Oral Implants Res 1992;3:1–8.
23. Abrahamsson I, Berglundh T, Lindhe J. The mucosal barrier following abutment dis/reconnection. An experimental study in dogs. J Clin Periodontol 1997;24:568–572.
24. Abrahamsson I, Berglundh T, Glantz PO, Lindhe J. The mucosal attachment at different abutments. An experimental study in dogs. J Clin Periodontol 1998;25:721–727.
25. Hermann JS, Buser D, Schenk RK, Higginbottom FL, Cochran DL. Biologic width around titanium implants. A physiologically formed and stable dimension over time. Clin Oral Implants Res 2000;11:1–11.
26. Gargiulo AW, Wentz FM, Orban B. Dimensions and relations of the dentogingival junction in humans. J Periodontal 1961;32:261–267.
27. Cochran DL, Hermann JS, Schenk RK, Higginbottom FL, Buser D. Biologic width around titanium implants. A histometric analysis of the implanto-gingival junction around unloaded and loaded nonsubmerged implants in the canine mandible. J Periodontol 1997;68:186–197.
28. Romanos GE, Nentwig GH. Immediate versus delayed functional loading of implants in the posterior mandible: A 2-year prospective clinical study of 12 consecutive cases. Int J Periodontics Restorative Dent 2006;26:459–469.
29. Romanos GE, Nentwig GH. Immediate functional loading in the maxilla using implants with platform switching. Five-year results. Int J Oral Maxillofac Implants 2009;24:1106–1112.
30. Nakabayashi Y, Shiba R. An experimental study of bone remodeling influenced by mechanical stress [in Japanese]. Nippon Seikeigeka Gakkai Zasshi 1987;61:1429–1436.
31. Sakai K, Tomita K, Sawaguchi T, Akagawa S, Oda J. An experimental study on quantitative relation between the mechanical stimuli and the bone formation. Orthop Biomech 1990;12:99–103.
32. Oda J, Sakamoto J, Aoyama K, Sueyoshi Y, Tomita K, Sawaguchi T. Mechanical stresses and bone formation. In: Hayashi K, Kamiya A, Ono K (eds). Biomechanics. Functional Adaptation and Remodeling. Tokyo: Springer, 1996:123–140.
33. Wolff J. Das Gesetz der Transformation der Knochen. Berlin: Hirschwald Verlag, 1892:1–126.
34. Chappard D, Grizon F, Brechet I, Baslé M, Rebel A. Evolution of the bone-titanium interface on implants coated/noncoated with xenogeneic bone particles: Quantitative microscopic analysis. J Biomed Mater Res 1996;32:175–180.
35. Chappard D, Aguado E, Huré G, Grizon F, Baslé MF. The early remodeling phases around titanium implants: A histomorphometric assessment of bone quality in a 3- and 6-month study in sheep. Int J Oral Maxillofac Implants 1999;14:189–196.
36. Romanos GE, Johansson C. Immediate loading with complete implant-supported restorations in an edentulous heavy smoker: Histologic and histomorphometric analyses. Int J Oral Maxillofac Implants 2005;20:282–290.
37. Linkow LI, Donath K, Lemons JE. Retrieval analyses of a blade implant after 231 months of clinical function. Implant Dent 1992;1:37–43.
38. Froum S, Emtiaz S, Bloom MJ, Scolnick J, Tarnow DP. The use of transitional implants for immediate fixed temporary prostheses in cases of impant restorations. Pract Periodontics Aesthet Dent 1998;10:737–746.
39. Ledermann PD, Schenk RK, Buser D. Long-lasting osseointegration of immediately loaded, bar-connected TPS screws after 12 years of function: A histologic case report of a 95-year-old patient. Int J Periodontics Restorative Dent 1998;18:552–563.
40. Garetto LP, Chen J, Parr JA, Roberts WE. Remodeling dynamics of bone supporting rigidly fixed titanium implants: A histomorphometric comparison in four species including humans. Implant Dent 1995;4:235–243.
41. Romanos GE, Testori T, Degidi D, Piattelli A. Histological and histomorphometric findings from retrieved, immediately occlusally loaded implants in humans. J Periodontol 2005;76:1823–1832.

Georgios E. Romanos and Dittmar May

# Immediate Loading in the Anterior Mandible Using Overdentures

6

## Immediate Loading in the Edentulous Patient

In the edentulous mandible, it is possible to load implants immediately after surgery if certain requirements are met (Box 6-1). Maintaining primary stability and ensuring rigid immobilization are the two main factors required to successfully load four intraforaminal implants using an overdenture.[1–4]

### Implant-supported bar overdentures

Treatment in the anterior mandible with an immediately loaded bar overdenture supported on four Ledermann threaded (one-piece) implants has been proven scientifically and clinically successful in more than 20 years of use.[3] For instance, Ledermann[1,4] placed four implants in the interforaminal areas of the mandible and loaded them immediately after surgery using a bar-retained restoration. This treatment enabled patients to be provided with a restoration immediately after implant placement without having to wait for the osseointegration period to elapse. In a clinical study of 1,523 immediately loaded implants in 411 patients, a cumulative success rate of 92% was found after a mean observation period of 7.23 years[3] (Fig 6-1).

Babbush et al[2] employed a similar treatment using four screw-type implants with a success rate of 88%. Their results indicate that the success of immediate loading is due to the protective effects of the splinted implant–bone interface against masticatory forces. Between 2 and 3 days after implant placement, the implants were splinted

**Box 6-1** Requirements for successful treatment with immediately loaded, implant-supported, bar-retained overdentures

- High primary stability of the implants
- Rigid immobilization of the implants immediately after surgery
- Good bone quality and quantity at the implant site
- Simple clinical and laboratory steps and chairside techniques that make use of prefabricated components
- Good patient compliance

with a Dolder bar, and the denture base was cut back to accommodate the bar and then lined with soft material. Bone quality in the anterior part of the mandible was relatively dense. In a clinical study performed by Dietrich et al,[5] two different implant systems were used: (1) IMZ-TwinPlus (Dentsply Friadent) for submerged healing and later conventional loading and (2) bar-supported titanium plasma-sprayed (TPS) implants for immediate loading. Five years after the surgery, 94.6% of the conventionally loaded implants and 83.6% of the immediately loaded implants were in function.

Even higher success rates have been reported in other studies. In a multicenter study carried out by Chiapasco et al[6] among 226 patients with 776 immediately loaded implants splinted with a bar, the survival rate over a mean period of 6.4 years was about 96.9%. Similarly, Spiekermann et al[7] documented cases of mandibular overdentures fixed to three implants splinted with a Dolder bar and loaded immediately. The 5-year survival rate in this study was 97.3%.

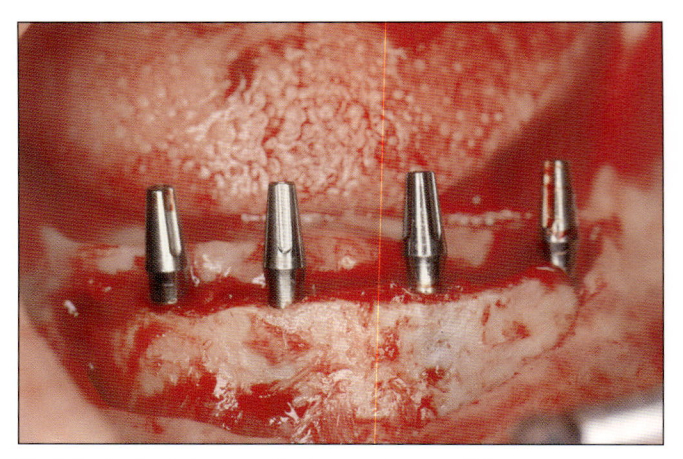

**Fig 6-1a** Implant placement in the anterior mandible.

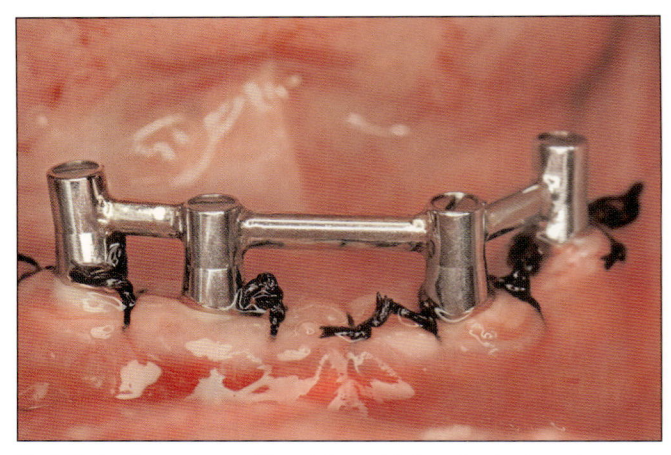

**Fig 6-1b** Implant-supported bar delivered 1 day after implant placement.

A drawback of immediately loaded implants supporting a bar overdenture is the considerable laboratory procedures and costs. In addition, a 12- to 24-hour delay between the surgical appointment and delivery of the overdenture should occur in most cases. Furthermore, some peri-implant mucosal irritation, gingival hyperplasia, and difficulty in plaque control associated with bar overdentures have also been reported.[8]

One early loading (not immediate loading) treatment approach uses the Brånemark (Nobel Biocare) implant system and the healing abutments as a restorative component for loading. In a study conducted by Becker et al,[9] implants were functionally loaded 5 days after surgery. After 2 years of loading, a cumulative survival rate of 96.3% was observed.

## Telescopic abutment–retained overdentures

Some studies have presented the possibility of using telescopic abutments in the mandible as an alternative to the bar-supported technique. For example, May and Romanos[10] placed four implants (Ankylos, Dentsply Friadent) with a progressive thread design and high primary stability in the anterior region of the mandible and immobilized them indirectly using an overdenture. According to this treatment protocol, the implants were not splinted with a bar but were connected with prefabricated conical abutments (Ankylos SynCone, Dentsply Friadent) having a 4-, 5-, or 6-degree angulation. Angulation of the abutments along the long axis of the implants (0, 7.5, 15, 22.5, and 30 degrees) allows parallelization using special alignment guides (Fig 6-2a). The prefabricated abutments (Ankylos SynCone) fit very precisely with the secondary copings, which were inserted into the overdenture without cementation (Fig 6-2b). The copings were placed over the abutments (Fig 6-2c), the undercuts were closed using rubber dam or elastic retraction rings, and the final relining was performed chairside (Fig 6-2d). The denture was then polished and placed immediately after surgery without removal for 10 days. Patients were encouraged to follow a soft or liquid diet during the initial healing stages, which is an important part of this protocol. In addition, an antibiotic was administered to control infection due to food debris. Typically after healing, the peri-implant soft tissues are in excellent condition and plaque control is good (Fig 6-2e). This treatment protocol has been used in a total of 204 implants for a mean observation period of 2 years and has presented a cumulative survival rate of 97.54%.[10]

In a recent clinical study,[11] the same concept was used but over a longer loading period of 79 ± 29.8 months (range: 17 to 129 months) and with 488 implants placed in the anterior mandible of 122 patients using prefabricated telescopic abutments (with an angulation of 4, 5, or 6 degrees). The survival rate was 94.06%.

In both studies, the peri-implant crestal bone levels were stable and did not present any bone loss because of the special implant design as well as the conical (tight) implant-abutment connection, in which the abutment collar is narrower than the head of the implant (called *platform switching* in other implant systems).

When using this technique, it is important to avoid disturbing the sensitive area between the head of the implant and surrounding alveolar bone because frequent removal of the prosthetic components (ie, healing abutments) is associated with an apical migration of the junctional epithelium in the sulcus, resulting in pocket formation and bone loss.[12] It is not necessary to remove abutments when implants are placed and connected with their definitive abutments using full torque immediately following surgery.

The use of Ankylos SynCone prefabricated telescopic abutments has many benefits for the clinician (Box 6-2).

Immediate Loading in the Edentulous Patient

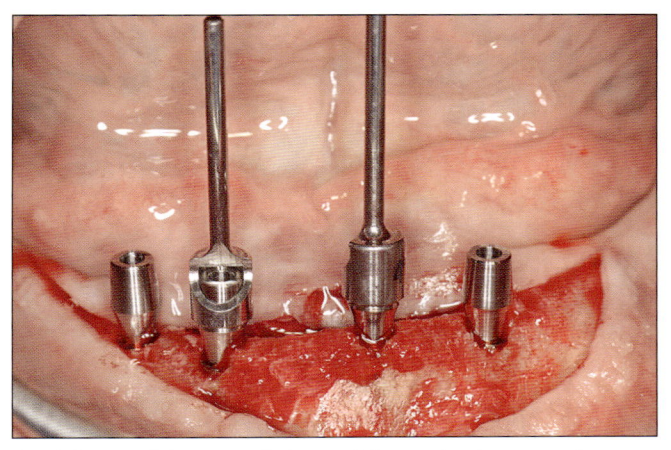

**Fig 6-2a** Parallelization of the prefabricated telescopic abutments (Ankylos SynCone) using alignment guides.

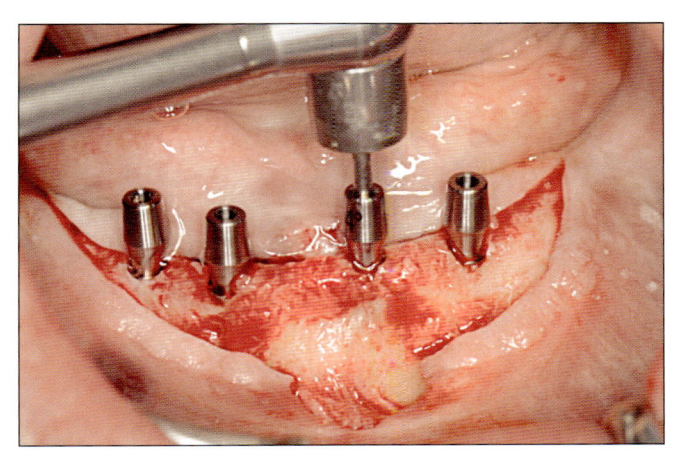

**Fig 6-2b** Placement of prefabricated telescopic abutments (Ankylos SynCone) using 15-Ncm final torque for a telescopic abutment–retained overdenture and immediate loading.

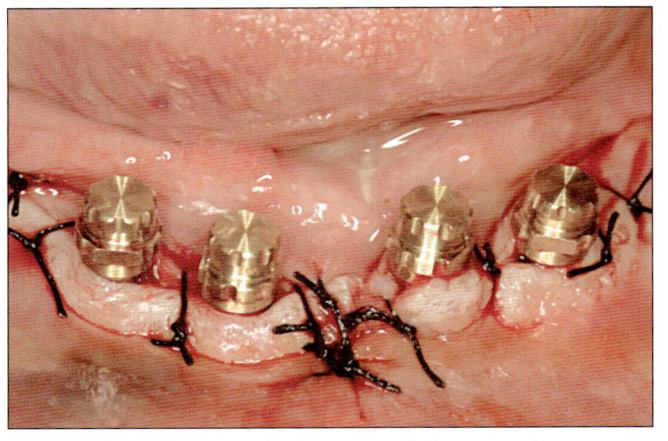

**Fig 6-2c** Flap closure and placement of the secondary copings (without any cementation material) for immediate loading. Rubber dam is placed to avoid undercuts.

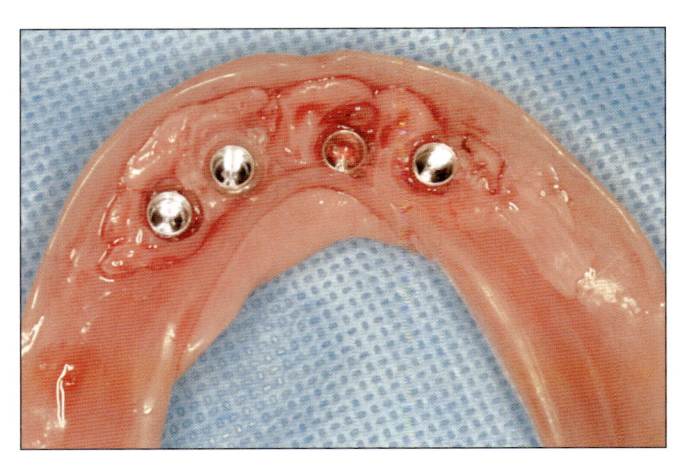

**Fig 6-2d** Base of the denture after relining with cold resin.

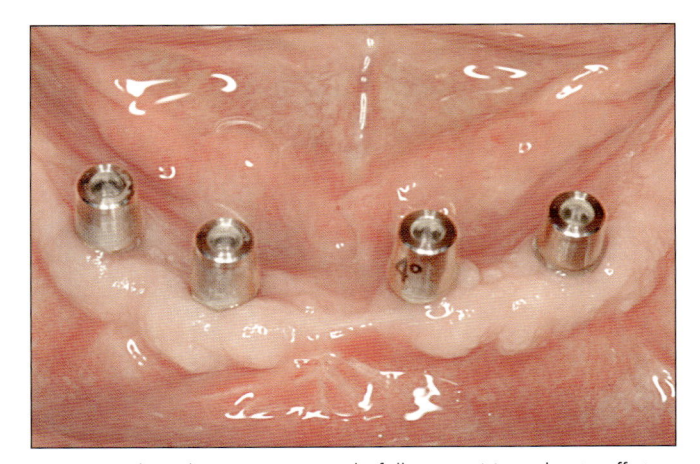

**Fig 6-2e** Clinical view at 6-month follow-up. Note the insufficient plaque control, but excellent peri-implant soft tissues.

**Box 6-2** Advantages of using telescopic abutment–retained, implant-supported overdentures

- Excellent three-dimensional immobilization of the restoration
- Defined release force
- Flexibility of design
- Optimum access for oral hygiene

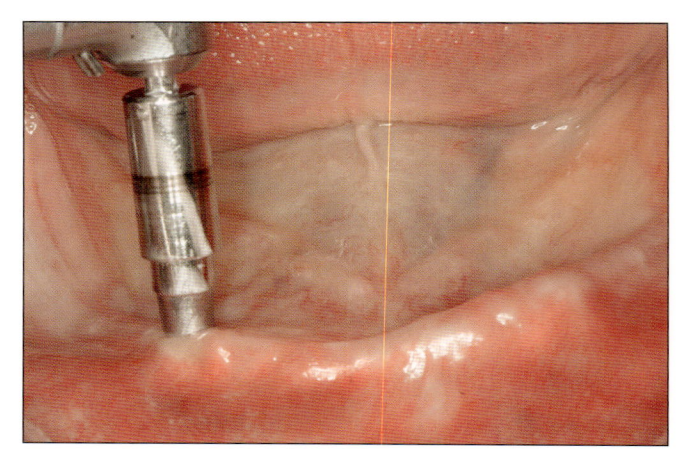

# Immediate Loading in the Anterior Mandible Using Overdentures

**Fig 6-3a** Flapless implant placement after soft tissue removal with a tissue punch.

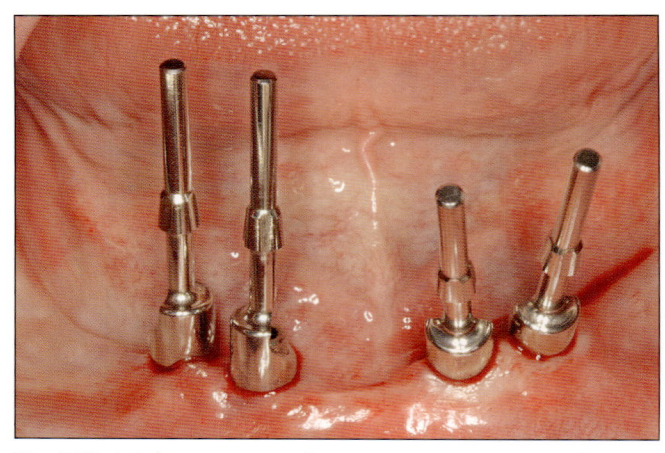

**Fig 6-3b** Ankylos SynCone abutment connection using alignment guides to align nonparallel abutment positions.

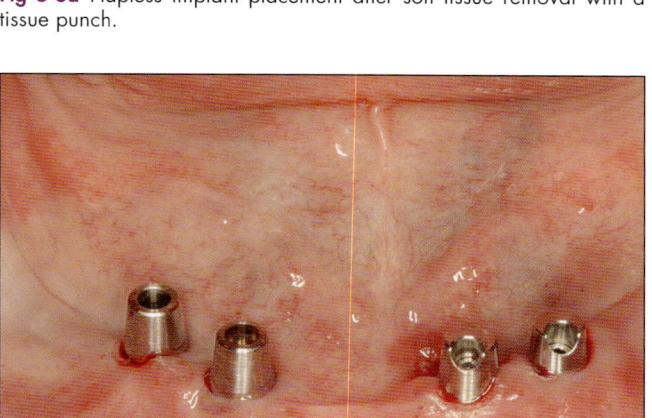

**Fig 6-3c** Following correct placement and angulation of the Ankylos SynCone abutments, final torque was used.

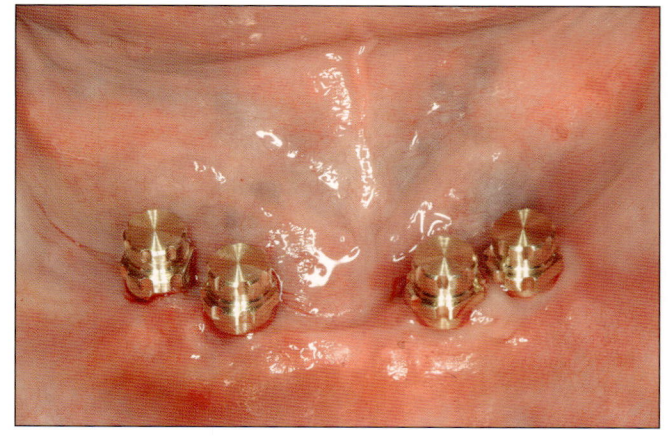

**Fig 6-3d** Placement of the secondary copings immediately prior to denture relining.

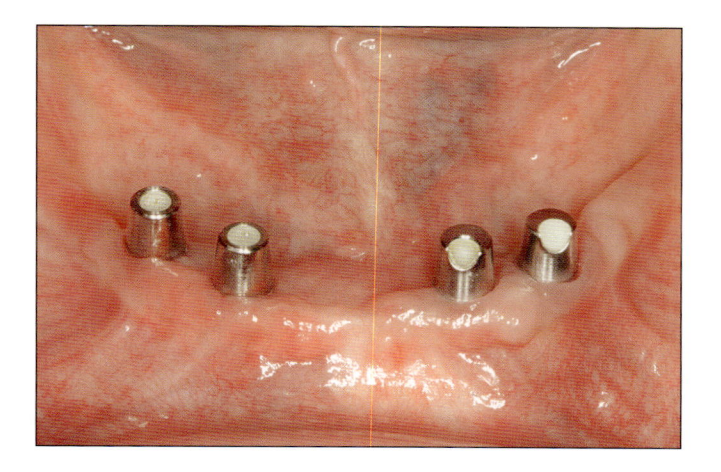

**Fig 6-3e** Peri-implant soft tissues in excellent condition 6 months after surgery.

They significantly reduce costs associated with the fabrication of customized abutments (no casting and milling), and they allow for better plaque control compared with implant-supported, bar-retained overdentures. This treatment protocol also may be used without raising a flap when the surgeon has a very high level of surgical skill and the bone quantity is sufficient to avoid complications such as perforations and exposure of the implant threads (Fig 6-3).

The concept of immediate loading can be used successfully in the maxilla using four or more implants (Fig 6-4). With the use of prefabricated telescopic abutments, edentulous jaws can be restored with removable prostheses, which provide excellent patient comfort and plaque control. Excellence in implant maintenance can be a significant factor in long-term success in implant dentistry.

Immediate Loading in the Edentulous Patient

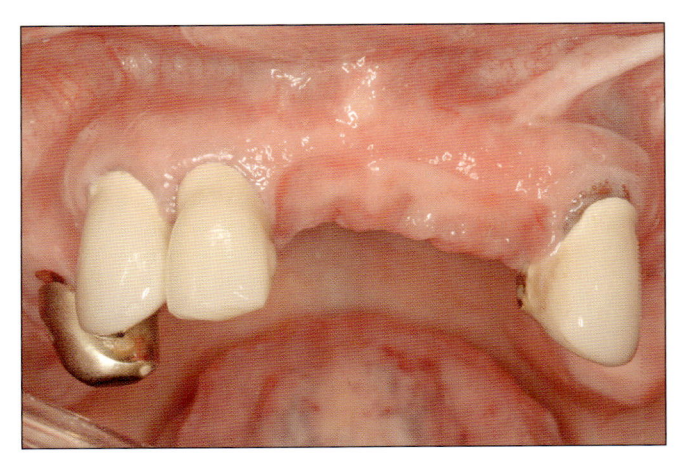

Fig 6-4a Maxillary teeth with a hopeless prognosis.

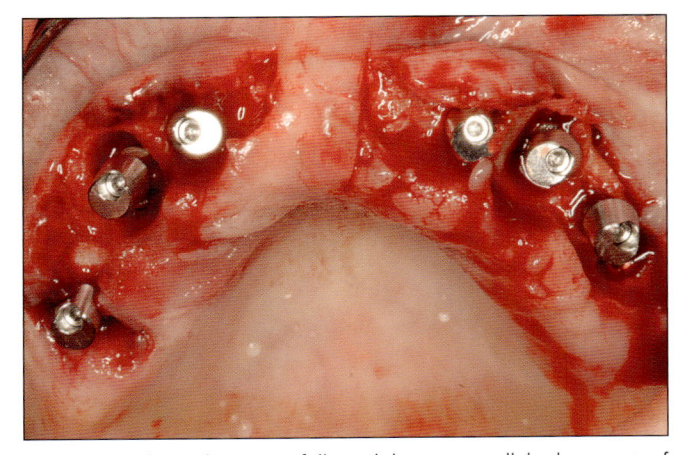

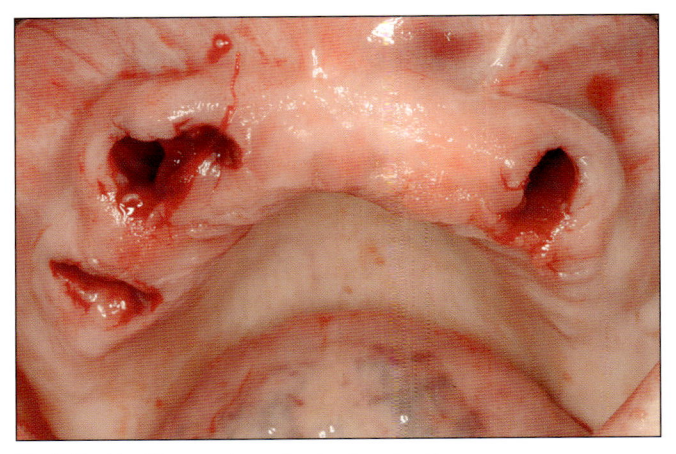

Fig 6-4b Maxillary sockets after tooth extraction.

Fig 6-4c Implant placement followed by nonparallel placement of Ankylos SynCone telescopic abutments.

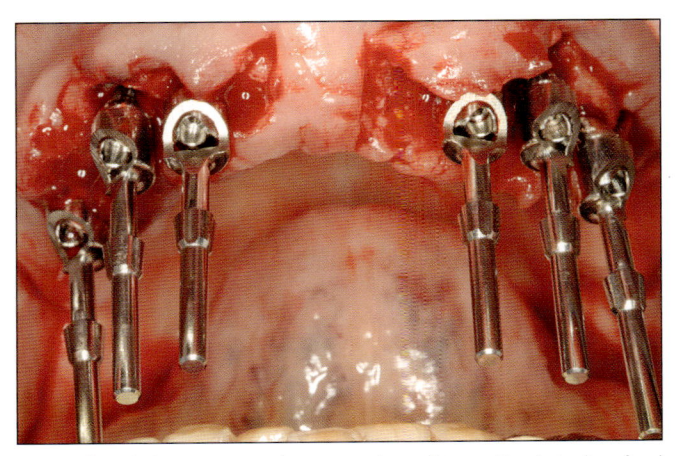

Fig 6-4d Ankylos SynCone abutments aligned immediately before final torque.

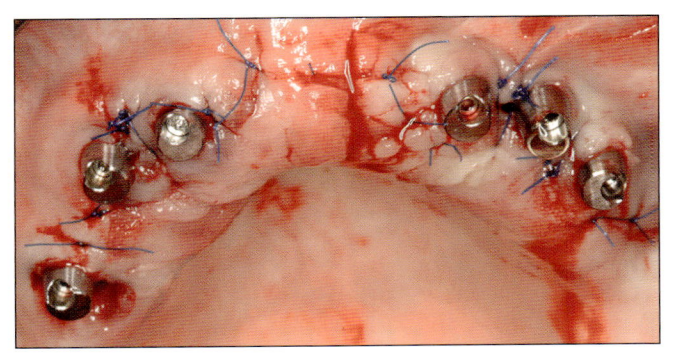

Fig 6-4e Final torque (15 Ncm) of the abutments and flap closure.

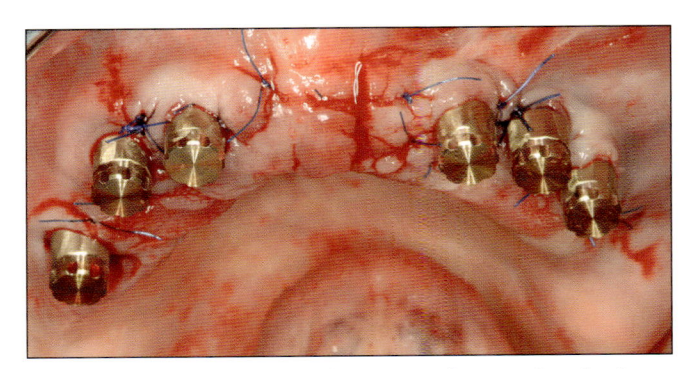

Fig 6-4f Placement of the secondary copings for immediate loading.

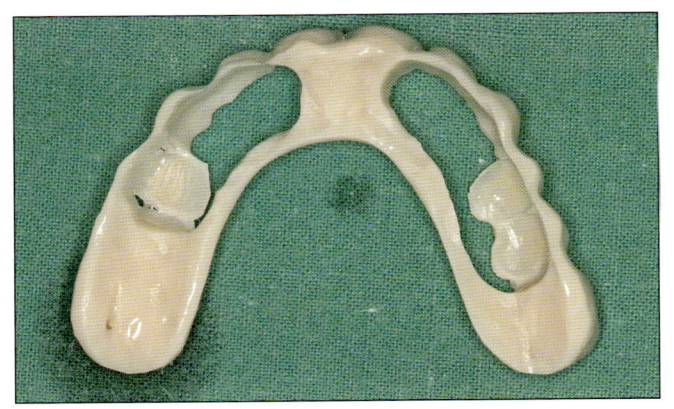

Fig 6-4g Provisional template prior to relining.

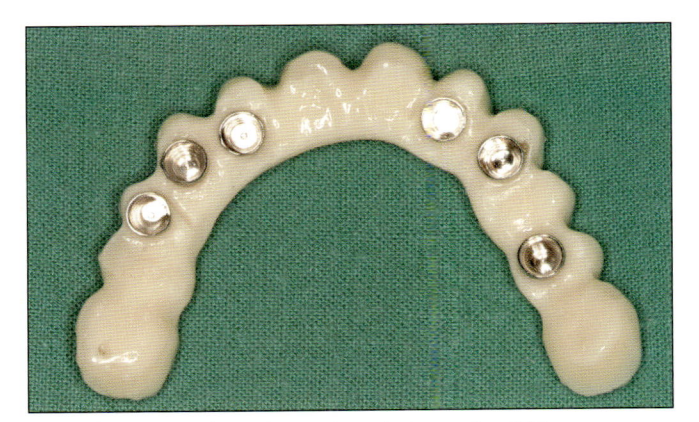

Fig 6-4h Provisional prosthesis after relining and polishing

59

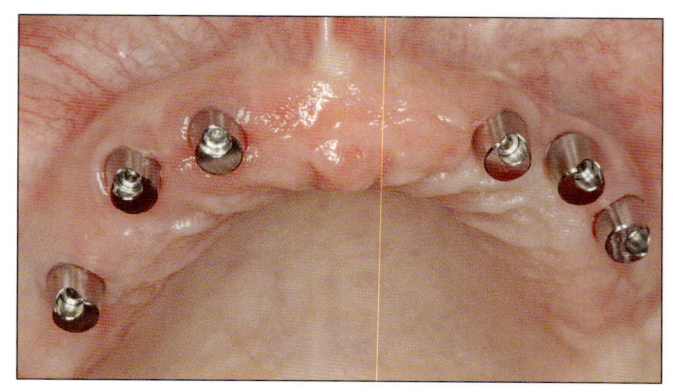

## 6 Immediate Loading in the Anterior Mandible Using Overdentures

**Fig 6-4i** Five months after immediate loading, the peri-implant soft tissue is in excellent condition and the implants have high stability.

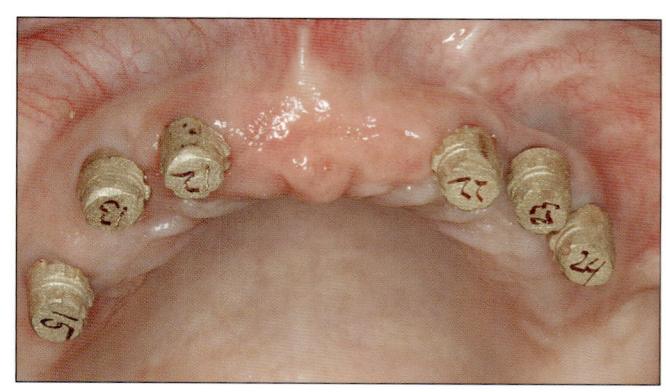

**Fig 6-4j** Five months after immediate loading, secondary copings (sand-blasted) are prepared for fabrication of the final prosthesis. In the transitional stage, the patient had standard temporary abutments. The framework of the final prosthesis was prepared using Ankylos SynCone telescopic abutments.

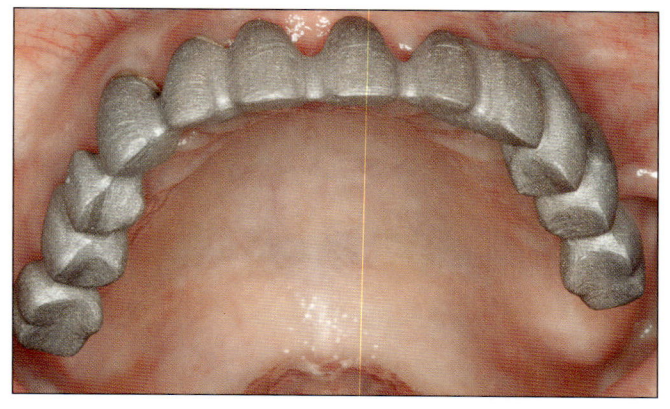

**Fig 6-4k** Framework try-in with passive fit for cementation over the secondary copings using Nimetic Cem (Espe).

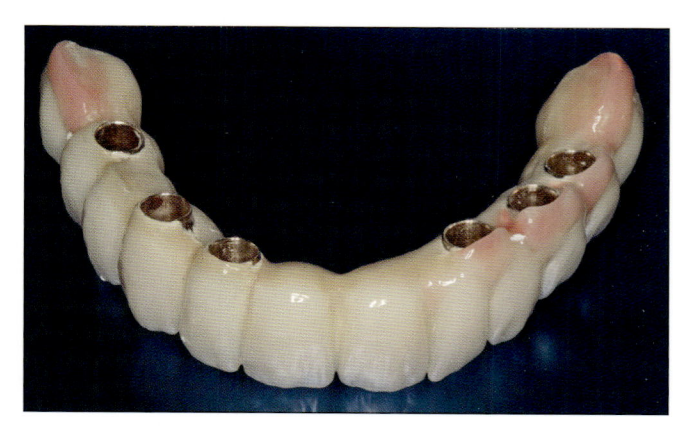

**Fig 6-4l** Final prosthesis before delivery.

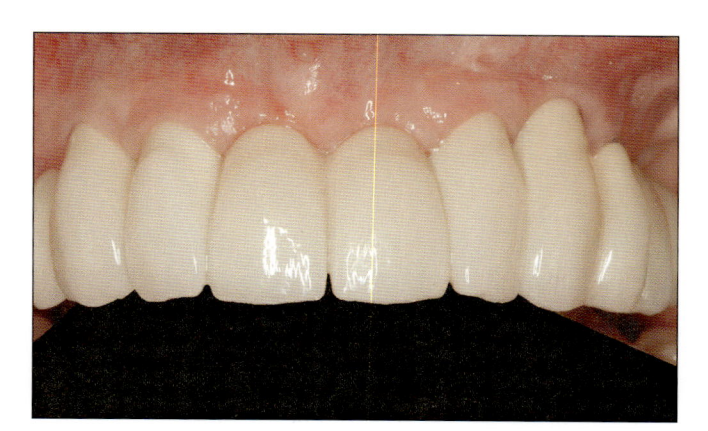

**Fig 6-4m** Final prosthesis in place.

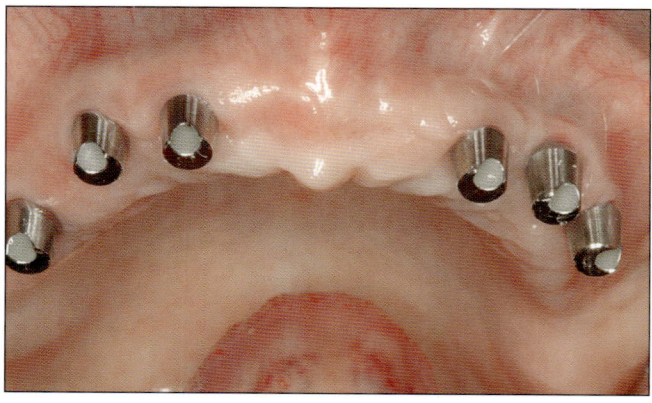

**Fig 6-4n** Excellent peri-implant soft tissues 2 months after delivery of the final prosthesis.

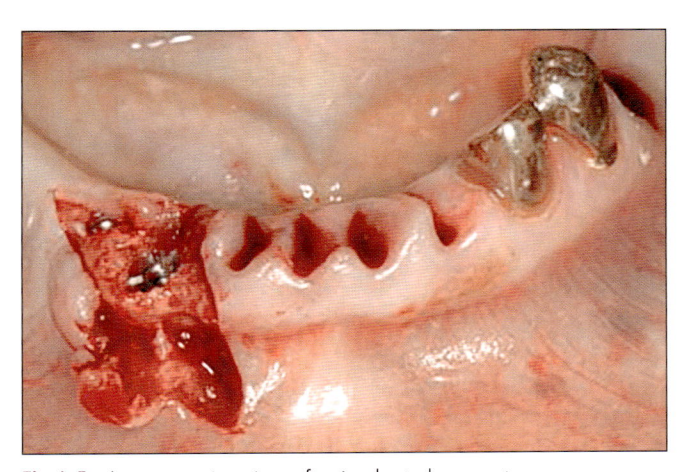

**Fig 6-5a** Intraoperative view after implant placement.

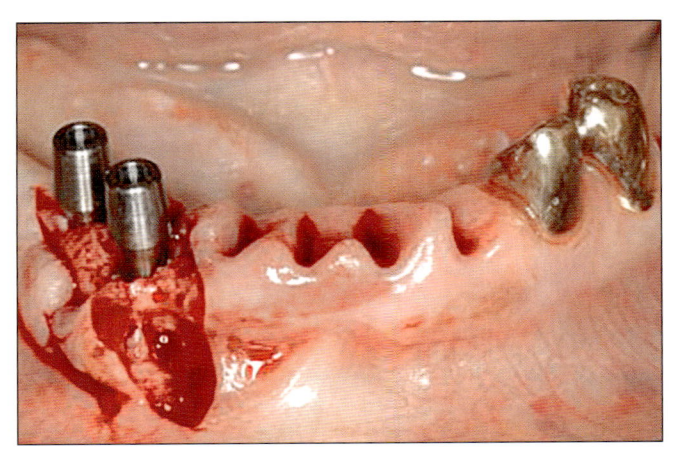

**Fig 6-5b** Abutments in place and parallel to residual teeth.

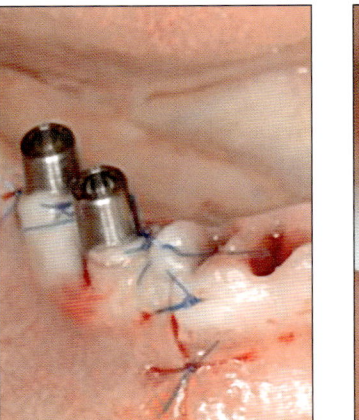

**Fig 6-5c** Flap closure.

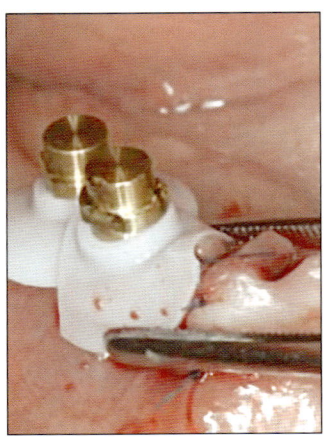

**Fig 6-5d** Rubber dam in place to avoid undercuts during relining.

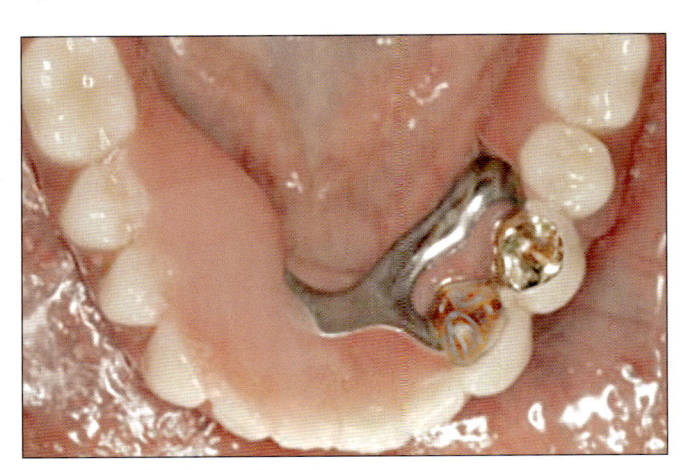

**Fig 6-5e** Occlusal view of prosthesis in place.

# Immediate Loading with Telescopic Abutments in the Partially Edentulous Patient

Additional benefits of the telescopic abutment method are observed when patients have a partially edentulous mandible and need implants for retention of a restoration. With the use of prefabricated abutments (Ankylos SynCone), it is possible to use a combination of residual teeth and implants to support a restoration when teeth have telescopic crowns (Fig 6-5). This concept can be used immediately after implant placement (immediate loading).

Our initial pilot study[13] showed that the implant survival is very high 2 years after loading. In this study, 62 Ankylos implants were placed in 31 patients (mean age: 68.45 ± 10.77 years). At the same visit, the implants were connected to teeth using the original telescopic abutment–retained restorations. The dentures were relined chairside with cold resin and left in place for 10 days, which provided secondary splinting of the implants and teeth. Administration of a systemic antibiotic was recommended for the first 10 postoperative days, and a soft or liquid diet was advised for the initial stages of healing. The peri-implant clinical indices (ie, plaque index, sulcus bleeding index, probing pocket depth, keratinized mucosa width, and Periotest values using the Periotest device [Medizintechnik Gulden]) and radiologic parameters were evaluated after a total loading period of 24.53 ± 20.04 months. Vertical as well as horizontal bone loss were also evaluated on radiographs. At the end of this loading period, no implants were lost, which represented a survival rate of 100%. All implants showed parameters demonstrating healthy soft and hard tissue peri-implant conditions. Horizontal and vertical bone loss were not found in most areas. No tooth failure due to splinting and no periodontal destruction or tooth intrusion during loading were observed. In fact, bone gain (higher bone density) was found in some areas. Better ossification of the bone due to loading processes was also demonstrated. These preliminary data show that immediate implant loading using prefabricated telescopic abutments may be successful when implants are splinted with teeth, an approach that minimizes costs for the patient (because it is a chairside treatment) and that allows beneficial treatment options for general practitioners.

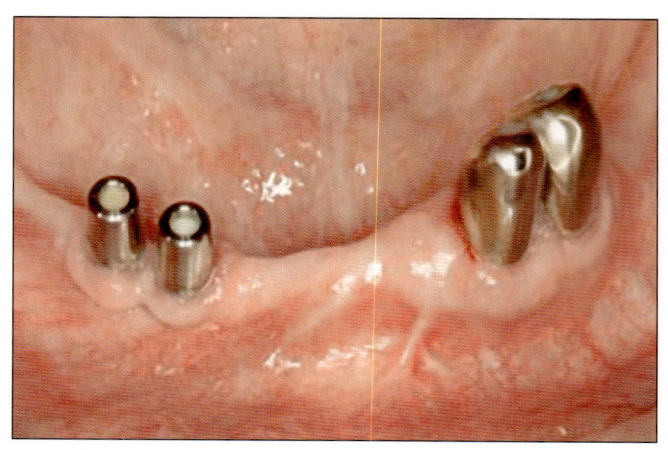

**Fig 6-5f** Clinical view 2 years after surgery presenting excellent peri-implant soft tissues.

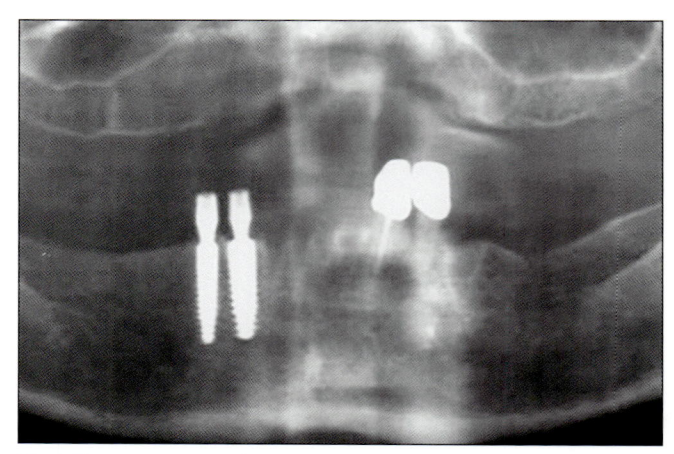

**Fig 6-5g** Panoramic radiograph 2 years after loading presenting no crestal bone loss. Given the close proximity (less than 3 mm) of the implants, the intact crestal bone is due to platform switching.

## Conclusion

The use of immediately loaded implants with telescopic abutment–retained overdentures in the mandible or maxilla has many advantages. Biologic benefits include prevention of crestal bone loss, avoidance of two-stage surgery with advanced periosteal elevation and bone exposure, and no disruption of the implant-abutment connection. Reduction of the total treatment period, the number of dental visits, and patient stress and anxiety due to dental treatment are among the psychologic benefits. The requirements and advantages of this treatment protocol have also have been presented in prosthodontic books with significant clinical interest.[14]

## References

1. Ledermann PD. Stegprothetische Versorgung des zahnlosen Unterkiefers mit Hilfe von plasmabeschichteten Titanschrauben-implantaten. Dtsch Zahnärztl Z 1979;34:907–911.
2. Babbush CA, Kent JN, Misiek DJ. Titanium plasma-sprayed (TPS) screw implants for the reconstruction of the edentulous mandible. J Oral Maxillofac Surg 1986;44:274–282.
3. Ledermann PD. Über 20jährige Erfahrung mit der sofortigen funktionellen Belastung von Implantatstegen in der Regio interforaminalis. Z Zahnärztl Implantol 1996;12:123–136.
4. Ledermann PD. 6-year clinical trial with titanium plasma-coated ITI (Internationales Team für Implantologie) screw implants in the mandibular interforaminal region [in German]. SSO Schweiz Monatsschr Zahnheilkd 1983;93:1070–1089.
5. Dietrich U, Lippold K, Dirmeier T, Behneke W, Wagner W. Statistical 13-year results for implant prognosis based on 2,017 IMZ implants in different indications [in German]. Z Zahnärztl Implantol 1993;9:9–18.
6. Chiapasco M, Gatti C, Rossi E, Haefliger W, Markwalder TH. Implant-retained mandibular overdentures with immediate loading. A retrospective multicenter study on 226 consecutive cases. Clin Oral Implants Res 1997;8:48–57.
7. Spiekermann H, Jansen VK, Richter EJ. A 10-year follow-up study of IMZ and TPS implants in the edentulous mandible using bar-retained overdentures. Int J Oral Maxillofac Implants 1995;10:231–243.
8. den Dunnen AC, Slagter AP, de Baat C, Kalk W. Professional hygiene care, adjustments and complications of mandibular implant-retained overdentures: A three-year retrospective study. J Prosthet Dent 1997;78:387–390.
9. Becker W, Becker BE, Huffstetlert S. Early functional loading at 5 days for Brånemark implants placed into edentulous mandibles: A prospective, open-ended, longitudinal study. J Periodontol 2003;74:695–702.
10. May D, Romanos GE. Immediate implant-supported mandibular overdentures retained by conical crowns: A new treatment concept. Quintessence Int 2002;33:5–12.
11. Romanos GE, May S, May D. Treatment concept of the edentulous mandible with prefabricated telescopic abutments and immediate functional loading. Int J Oral Maxillofac Implants 2011;26:593–597.
12. Abrahamsson I, Berglundh T, Lindhe J. The mucosal barrier following abutment dis/reconnection. An experimental study in dogs. J Clin Periodontol 1997;24:568–572.
13. Erker J, May D, Romanos GE. Immediately loaded implants with prefabricated telescopic abutments in tooth-implant telescopic-retained overdentures: A pilot study [abstract]. Int J Oral Maxillofac Implants 2005;20:475–476.
14. May D, Romanos GE, Shafie H. Loading approaches for mandibular implant overdentures. In: Shafie HR (ed). Clinical and Laboratory Manual of Implant Overdentures. Ames, Iowa: Blackwell, 2007:192–205.

# Immediate Loading in Edentulous Jaws

There are some general considerations for using the immediate loading technique when the maxilla and/or the mandible have to be restored with fixed, full-mouth restorations. Correct implant selection, which includes such factors as design, surface, diameter, and length, is significant in getting high primary stability at the time of implant placement. It is important to avoid tapping in the osteotomy site when the bone quality is very poor and to splint the implants with the provisional restorations as early as possible using resin materials. Use of metal reinforcement with metal wires or resin bonding materials such as Ribbond (Ribbond) limits fracture of the provisional restoration, thereby increasing implant prognosis due to secured immobilization. Other factors critical to the successful use of this treatment protocol include patient selection criteria (eg, good compliance and the absence of bruxism history) and implementation of a soft or liquid diet that significantly reduces loading forces in the initial stages of healing and controls overloading, especially in areas of compromised bone quality.

The following clinical examples provide step-by-step case presentations of the full-mouth treatment concept using six Ankylos (Dentsply Friadent) implants. High primary stability is achieved because of the characteristic tapered and progressive thread design of this implant system. The following clinical cases demonstrate that peri-implant bone dehiscences and simultaneous augmentations are not contraindications for immediate occlusal loading. Furthermore, the definitive long-term results demonstrate the importance of primary implant stability, immobilization (splinting), and patient adherence to a soft or liquid diet during the initial stages of healing.

## Case Reports

### Case 1: Immediate loading in conjunction with bone grafting in the mandible with fixed distal cantilever restorations

A 55-year-old woman presented with increased mobility of her teeth associated with advanced periodontal disease. The patient had partial dentures to replace the mandibular left first premolar through the third molar and the right first premolar through the second molar. All of the remaining teeth—the maxillary dentition and the mandibular anterior dentition from right canine to left canine—had to be removed because of increased mobility from advanced periodontal bone destruction. The preoperative radiologic examination showed advanced periodontal destruction around all teeth in both jaws (Fig 7-1a). All residual teeth were extracted, and after 3 to 4 months, when the soft and hard tissues were completely healed, implant placement was planned.

Before surgery, a prosthetic guide was fabricated based on the new full dentures. Radiologic examination of the patient was performed to determine the exact position of the implants. Implant placement was achieved after making a midcrestal incision, raising an envelope flap, and preparing the osteotomy sites according to the prosthetic guide (Figs 7-1b and 7-1c).

The implants were placed with high primary stability in accordance with the protocol of the implant system used. Immediately after implant placement, the parallelism of the abutments was verified before seating them with a final torque of 15 Ncm. All maxillary implants had primary stability and were covered by bone. Because of the poor bone quality in the maxilla, osteotomy tapping was not performed.

# 7  Immediate Loading in Edentulous Jaws

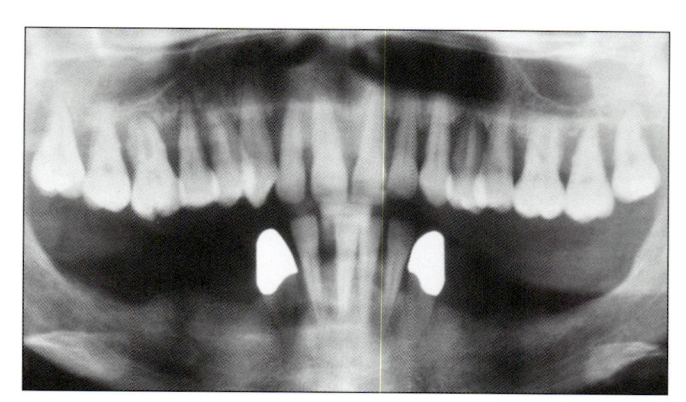

**Fig 7-1a** Radiologic evaluation of hopeless dentition due to advanced periodontal destruction.

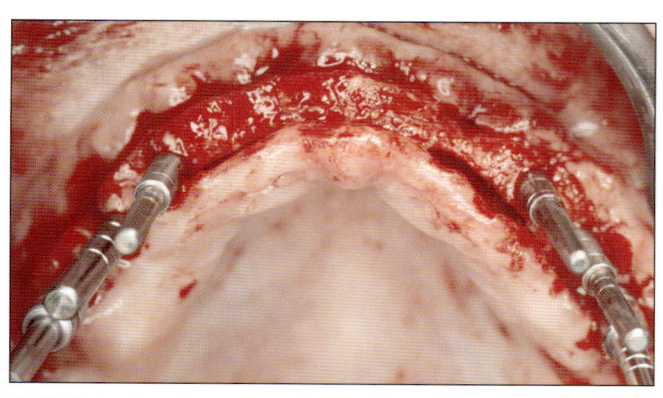

**Fig 7-1b** Implant placement in the maxilla presenting the need for angulation of the osteotomies.

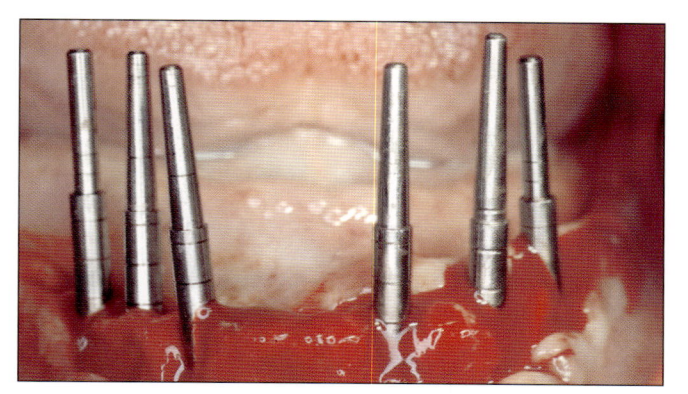

**Fig 7-1c** Parallelization of the osteotomies in the mandible during implant placement.

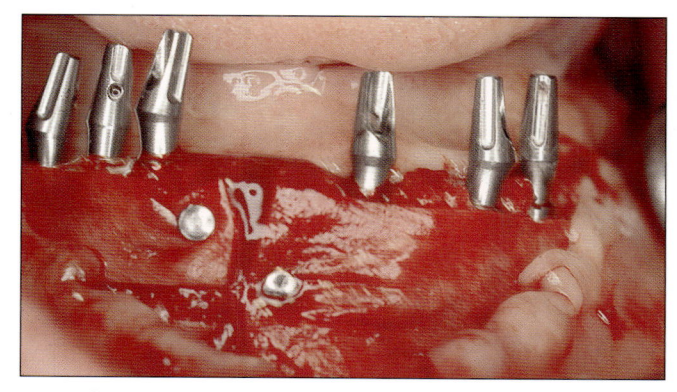

**Fig 7-1d** Correctly angled abutments seated on the implants. Note the autogenous bone graft covered with a collagen membrane.

The mandibular implants were placed in positions analogous to those of the maxilla, with the exception of the osteotomy at the left lateral incisor site that could not be performed because of the extremely soft bone. Instead, the adjacent central incisor site was selected for implant placement. Because of the exposed threads at the buccal aspect of the placed implants, autogenous bone was harvested from the mandible (adjacent donor sites) and used to cover the implant threads. An additional collagen membrane (Bio-Gide, Geistlich) was fixed in place with titanium tacks (Frios, Dentsply Friadent). After removal of the cover screws (incorporated in the implant body immediately after the implant placement), abutments with the correct angulations were used (Fig 7-1d).

Temporary healing caps were seated, and the flap was closed using 4-0 silk suture material in both the maxilla (Fig 7-1e) and the mandible (Fig 7-1f). In accordance with the prosthetic guide, provisional prostheses were fabricated from ProTemp (Espe) resin material, and the vertical dimension was kept in centric relation (Figs 7-1g and 7-1h). Open space was maintained between the soft tissues and the margins of the provisional restorations to optimize plaque control. The provisional bridges were cemented with TempBond (Kerr) and were not removed for the next 2 to 3 weeks. The occlusion was checked to avoid excessive contacts in the lateral movements of the mandible, and the patient was instructed to maintain a soft or liquid diet for the next 6 to 8 weeks to avoid overloading the implants in the critical initial stages of healing. The patient was also advised to use chlorhexidine digluconate (0.12%) mouthrinse for 10 days prior to suture removal, and clindamycin (300 mg) was prescribed 3 times per day for the first 10 postoperative days.

Figures 7-1i and 7-1j present the pre- and postoperative radiographs, respectively. All implants in the maxilla and mandible were placed on the same day under local anesthesia. To avoid sinus perforation during sinus floor elevation with simultaneous implant placement and immediate occlusal loading, an Ankylos implant with a diameter of 3.5 mm and a length of 8.0 mm was placed at the site of the maxillary left second premolar. The other implants had diameters of 3.5 mm and lengths of 11 or 14 mm.

## Case Reports

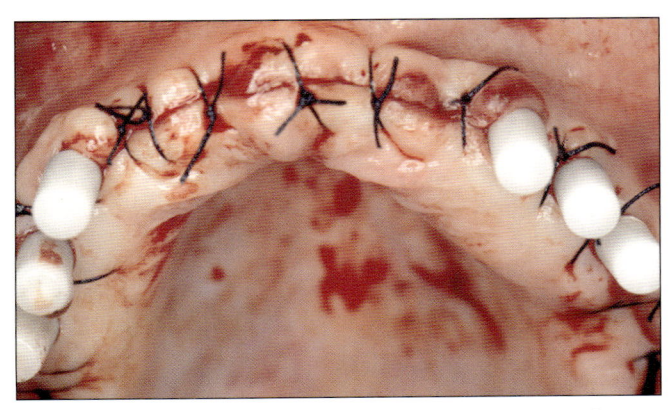

**Fig 7-1e** Plastic caps placed over the final abutments preserve the margins of the provisional prostheses immediately after surgery.

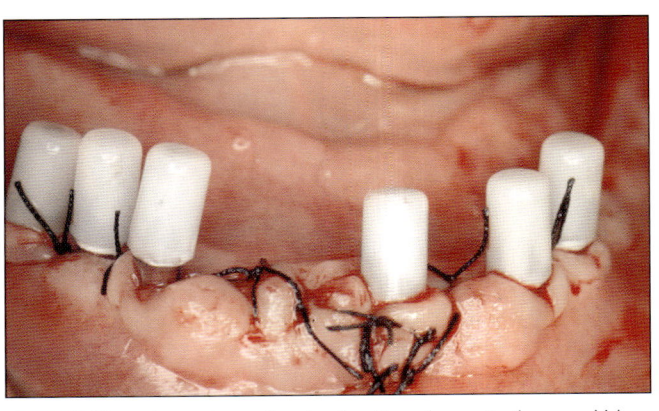

**Fig 7-1f** Clinical sites immediately after flap closure in the mandible.

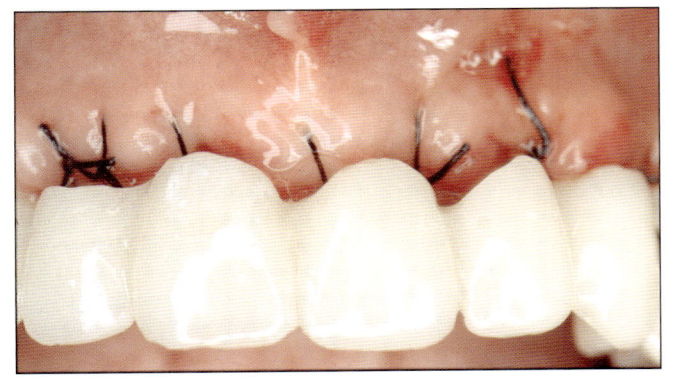

**Fig 7-1g** Provisionalization of the maxilla maintains space at the margins for sufficient plaque control after surgery.

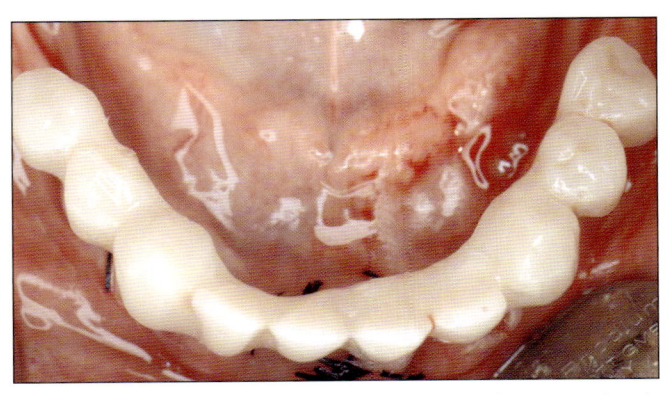

**Fig 7-1h** Design of the mandibular provisional prosthesis immediately after surgery. Note the relatively flat cusps of the teeth.

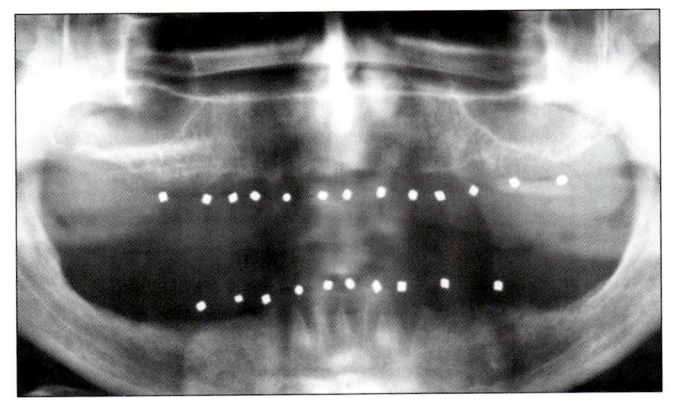

**Fig 7-1i** Preoperative radiograph.

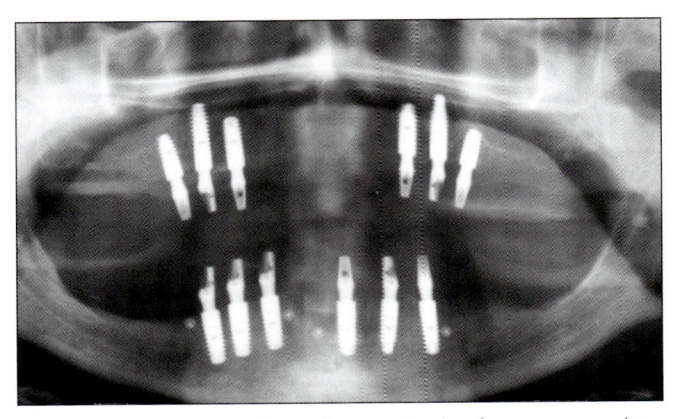

**Fig 7-1j** Postoperative radiograph immediately after surgery and immediate loading.

# 7 Immediate Loading in Edentulous Jaws

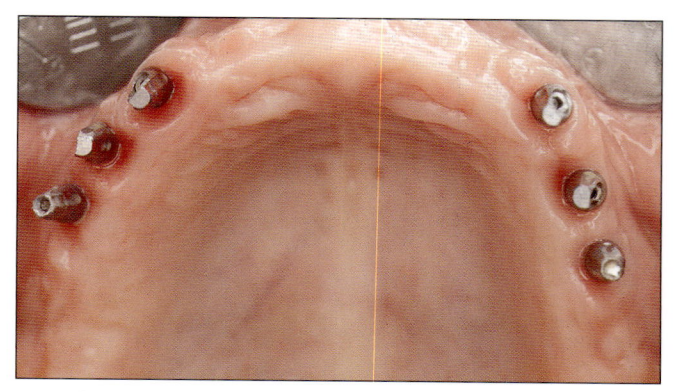

**Fig 7-1k** Peri-implant soft tissues in an excellent condition in the maxilla 3 weeks after surgery.

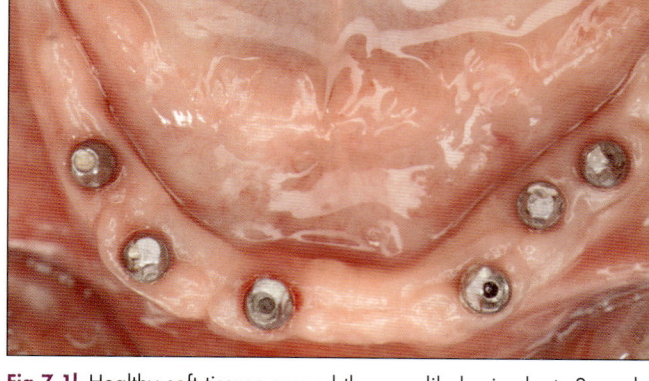

**Fig 7-1l** Healthy soft tissues around the mandibular implants 3 weeks after surgery.

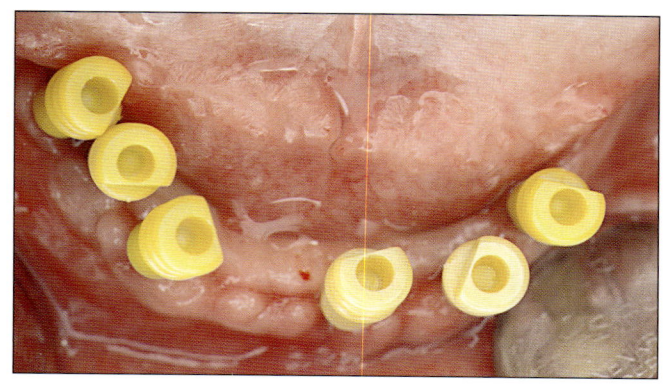

**Fig 7-1m** Impression copings in place for an abutment-level impression. The abutments were not removed from the implants.

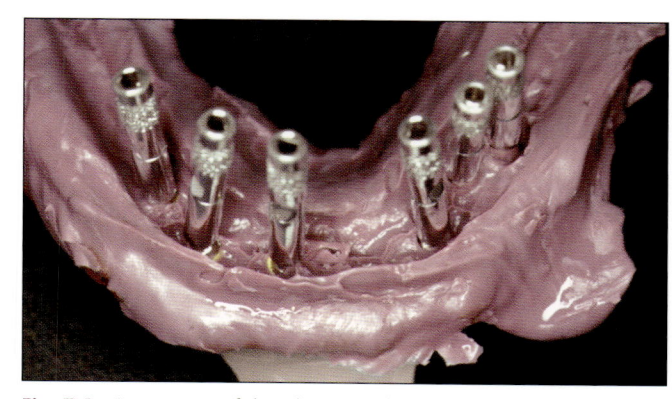

**Fig. 7-1n** Impression of the abutments for final prosthesis delivery using customized trays.

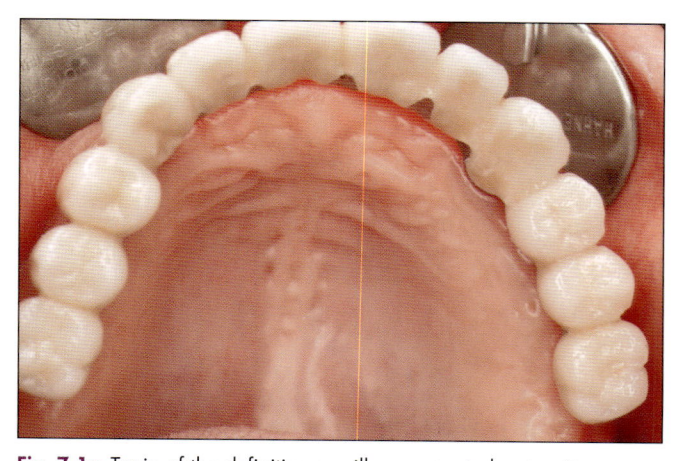

**Fig. 7-1o** Try-in of the definitive maxillary cemented restoration.

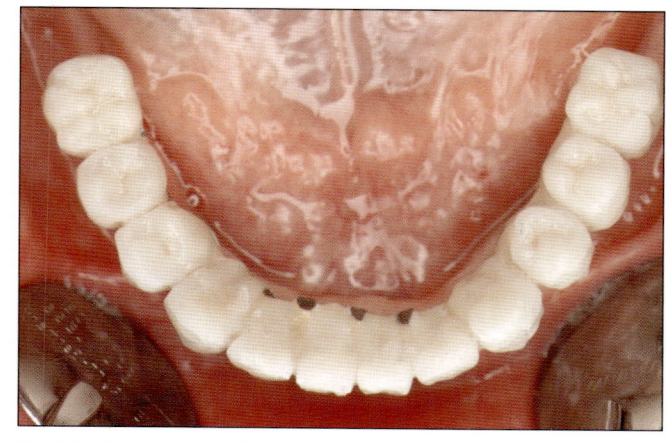

**Fig 7-1p** Try-in of the definitive mandibular prosthesis.

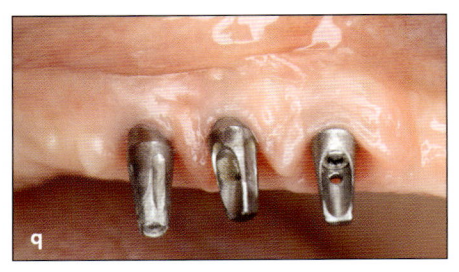

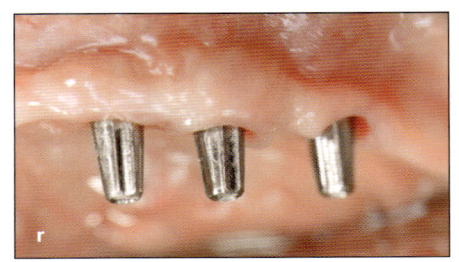

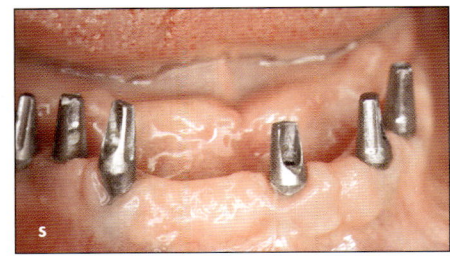

**Figs 7-1q to 7-1s** Excellent peri-implant soft tissues 2 years after immediate loading in the maxilla *(q and r)* and mandible *(s)*.

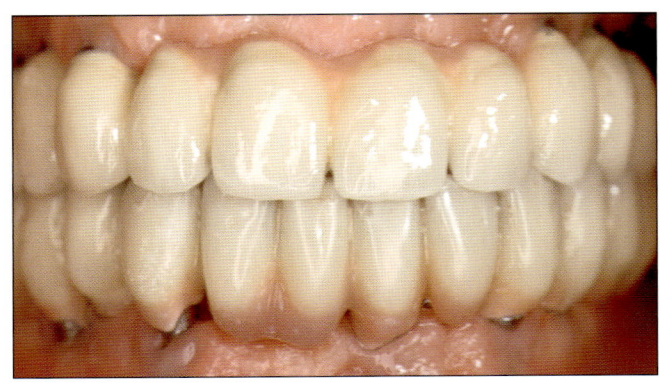

**Fig 7-1t** Definitive restorations 2 years after immediate loading.

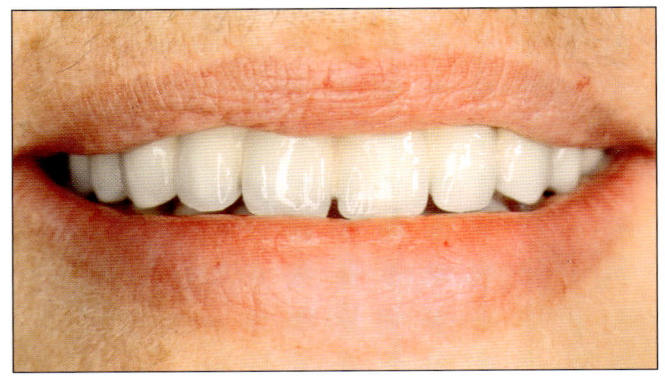

**Fig 7-1u** Esthetic result after 2 years. (Dental technician: Marion Biaesch, Frankfurt, Germany.)

Three weeks after implant placement and immediate loading, the soft tissue presented healthy color and condition (Figs 7-1k and 7-1l). The provisional prostheses were removed and impressions of the maxilla and mandible were taken (Fig 7-1m) using impression copings (abutments were not removed) with the use of Impregum impression material (Espe) in custom trays (Fig 7-1n).

Implant-supported metal-ceramic restorations were fabricated, and prior to their cementation, all clinical peri-implant indices were evaluated. The prostheses were cemented in place 6 weeks after implant placement using temporary cement (TempBond) (Figs 7-1o and 7-1p). Distal cantilevers were used in the maxilla and mandible to establish the molar occlusion.

*Note: The abutments were placed on the day of the implant placement and were never removed from their final position during the entire observation period.*

Two years after loading, the implants presented excellent peri-implant soft tissue in both jaws (Figs 7-1q to 7-1t). The esthetic result was good (Fig 7-1u), and the patient was very happy with the function, esthetics, and phonetics. Radiographs revealed that the peri-implant bone was stable without any bone loss. Five years after loading, the peri-implant soft tissue condition was healthy (Fig 7-1v), and the radiographic examination showed stability of the bone levels (Fig 7-1w). Even in the posterior implants connected to distal cantilevers, there were no fractures at the implant-abutment connection, in the implant body, or at the connection with the cantilevers. These results can be explained by the high stability and precision of the implant system used (implant body of pure titanium grade II and abutment of titanium alloy) and the excellent casting in the dental laboratory. Periotest (Medizintechnik Gulden) measurements were performed immediately after surgery and at 3 months, 6 months, 10 months, and 18 months after loading. The measurements are listed in Table 7-1. It was not possible to evaluate the Periotest values of the individual implants after 5 years because of permanent cementation of the prosthesis.

The final follow-up examination 11 years after immediate loading showed stable peri-implant conditions. At that time, the mandibular prosthesis was replaced with a new one (Fig 7-1x).

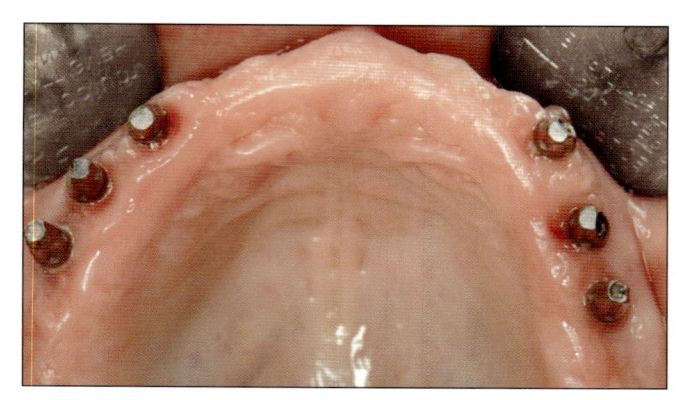

**Fig 7-1v** Healthy peri-implant soft tissues after 5 years.

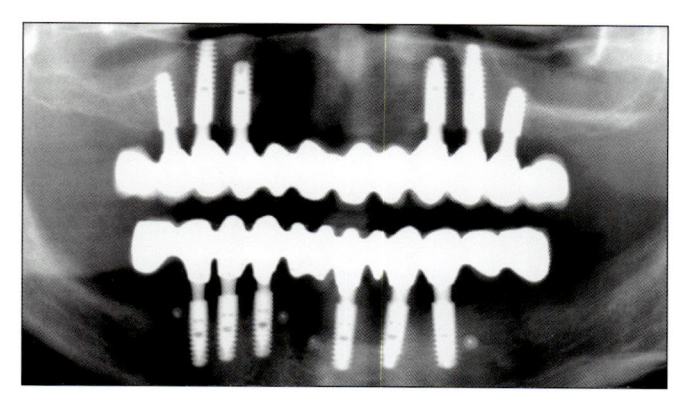

**Fig 7-1w** Postoperative radiograph showing stability of all implant bone levels 5 years after immediate loading.

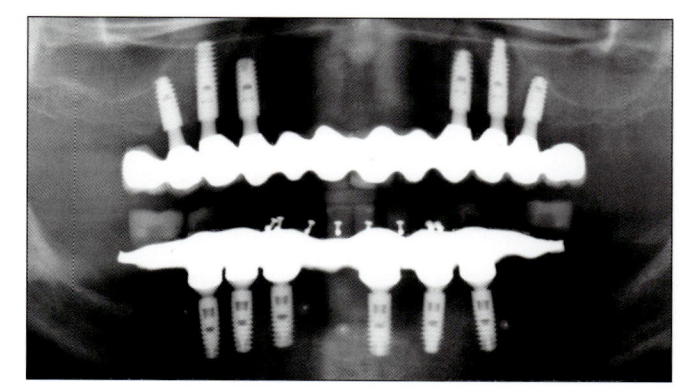

**Fig 7-1x** Panoramic radiograph of the same case 11 years after immediate loading. Note the crestal bone stability in the maxilla and mandible.

**Table 7-1** Periotest values in case 1 at different postsurgical time points

| Implant area | T0 | T1 | T2 | T3 | T4 |
|---|---|---|---|---|---|
| Maxillary right second premolar | 5 | 5 | 3 | 1 | 0 |
| Maxillary right first premolar | 4 | 4 | 6 | 1 | −1 |
| Maxillary right canine | 5 | 5 | 5 | 2 | 1 |
| Maxillary left canine | 6 | 6 | 3 | 1 | −1 |
| Maxillary left first premolar | 5 | 5 | 2 | −2 | −3 |
| Maxillary left second premolar | 5 | 6 | 5 | 0 | −1 |
| Mandibular left first premolar | 1 | −2 | −3 | −3 | −4 |
| Mandibular left canine | 2 | −2 | −4 | −2 | −3 |
| Mandibular left central incisor | 1 | −2 | −3 | −2 | −3 |
| Mandibular right canine | 0 | −1 | 0 | −2 | −3 |
| Mandibular right first premolar | −2 | −2 | −2 | −2 | −3 |
| Mandibular right second premolar | −3 | −3 | −4 | −4 | −4 |
| Mean | 2.3 | 1.5 | 0.6 | −1.0 | −2.0 |

T0, immediately after surgery; T1, 3 months; T2, 6 months; T3, 10 months; T4, 18 months after loading.

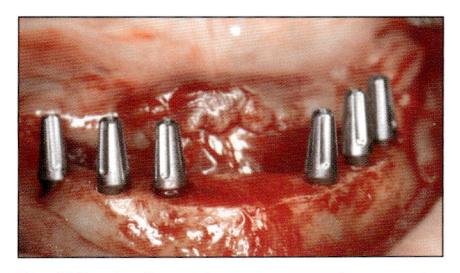

**Fig 7-2a** Implant placement in the anterior mandible with final abutment connection for immediate functional loading.

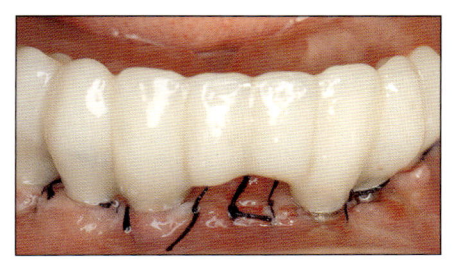

**Fig 7-2b** Provisional prosthesis in place immediately after surgery.

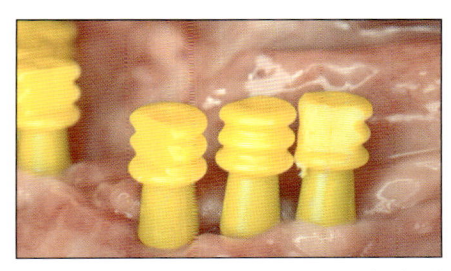

**Fig 7-2c** Impression copings in place for final impression. The abutments were not removed.

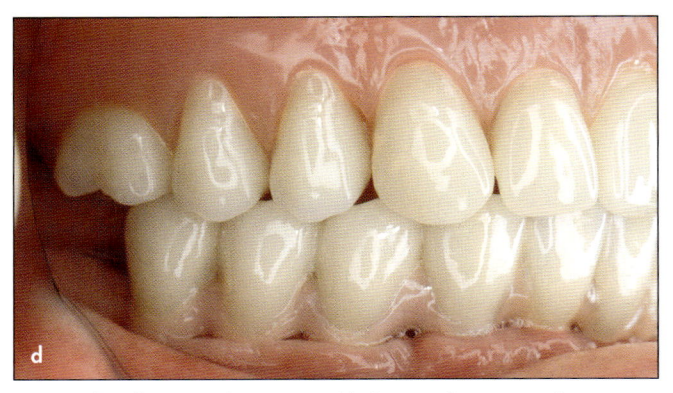

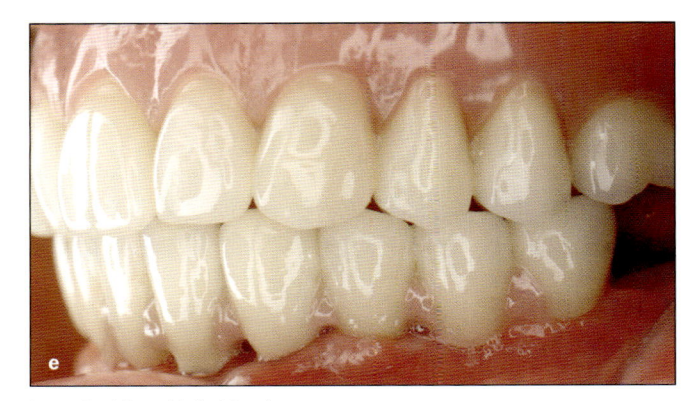

**Figs 7-2d and 7-2e** Definitive mandibular prosthesis in occlusion presenting the right (d) and left (e) sides.

## Case 2: Immediate loading in conjunction with bone grafting in the maxilla with fixed distal cantilever restorations

A 60-year-old edentulous woman presented with insufficient retention of her mandibular full denture. About 6 months prior to her visit, the patient had received new dentures. The full dentures were in acceptable functional and esthetic condition, but she was unhappy with the denture retention in her mandible. The radiologic examination showed sufficient bone quality in the vertical dimension, and both the vertical and horizontal dimensions were acceptable. Ultimately, the patient decided to get a fixed implant-supported denture. An impression of the mandibular denture was taken so that a prosthetic guide could be fabricated for the mandible.

*Note: The prosthetic guide represents the position of the planned implants and determines for the surgeon the exact area in the middle of the fossae for the replacement teeth, according to the customized wax-up of the case. Therefore, the author uses the term* prosthetic guide *in lieu of* surgical guide *because it better describes its purpose.*

A midcrestal incision was performed under local anesthesia with 1:200,000 epinephrine. A mucoperiosteal flap was elevated and the alveolar ridge was exposed. The thin alveolar ridge in the anterior mandible was reshaped using a diamond bur under sterile saline cooling. A bilateral preparation of the mental nerve was performed to avoid damaging the nerve during implant placement.

The plateau of the alveolar ridge in the symphysis was sufficient to place six Ankylos implants in the areas of the right and left lateral incisors to first premolars without any bone augmentation. The prosthetic guide was used during drilling, and the implants were placed with high primary stability because of the progressive thread design especially at the apical part of the implant. The implants also had a sand-blasted surface, a machined 2-mm collar, a diameter of 3.5 mm, and a length of 14 mm.

Standard straight abutments were seated on the implants with a torque of 20 Ncm as recommended by the manufacturer (Fig 7-2a). The Periotest values were determined to record implant stability. Provisional caps were fixed in place with TempBond cement, and the mucoperiosteal flap was sutured with 4-0 silk sutures.

Immediately after surgery, the provisional fixed restoration was fabricated chairside with ProTemp acrylic material using the prosthetic guide. A provisional restoration with occlusal contacts only in centric occlusion was cemented on the abutments (Fig 7-2b). Relining of the template was performed in centric occlusion in the correct vertical dimension. A radiograph was taken to evaluate the postoperative peri-implant crestal bone level.

The patient was advised to adhere to a soft or liquid diet for the first 4 to 6 weeks following surgery. Rinsing of the oral cavity with chlorhexidine digluconate (0.12%) for sufficient plaque control was indicated until the sutures were removed 10 days after surgery. Four weeks after implant placement and loading, the peri-implant soft tissues showed a healthy color. Impressions were taken using Impregum and special transfer caps in custom trays (Fig 7-2c). Two weeks later, an implant-supported metal-ceramic fixed restoration was fabricated and provisionally cemented with TempBond (Figs 7-2d and 7-2e). Distal cantilevers were used for the second premolar and first molar in order to establish first molar occlusion.

# 7 Immediate Loading in Edentulous Jaws

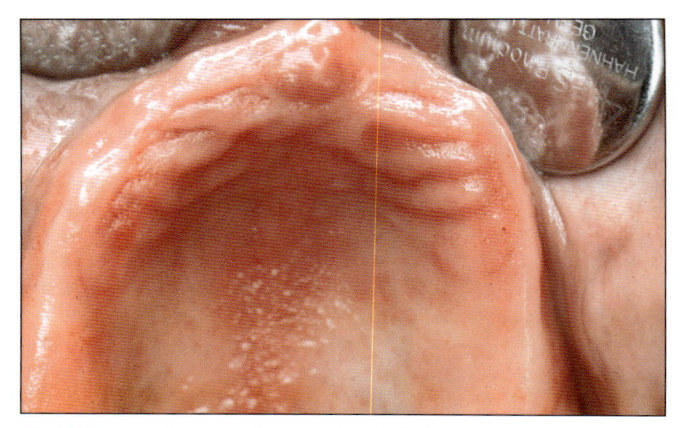

**Fig 7-2f** Edentulous maxilla immediately before surgery.

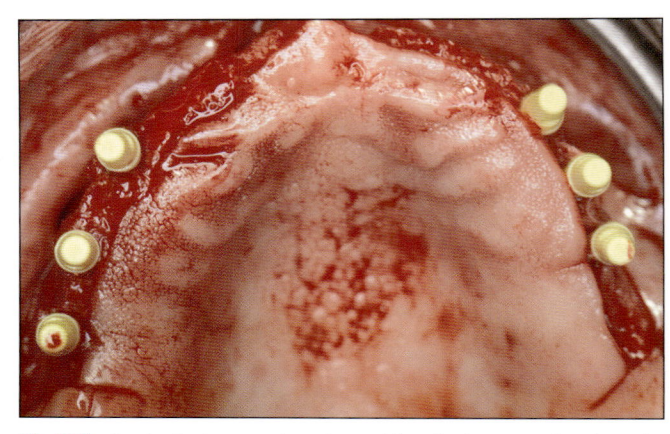

**Fig 7-2g** Implant placement and provisional abutments in place for correct selection of the final abutments before immediate loading.

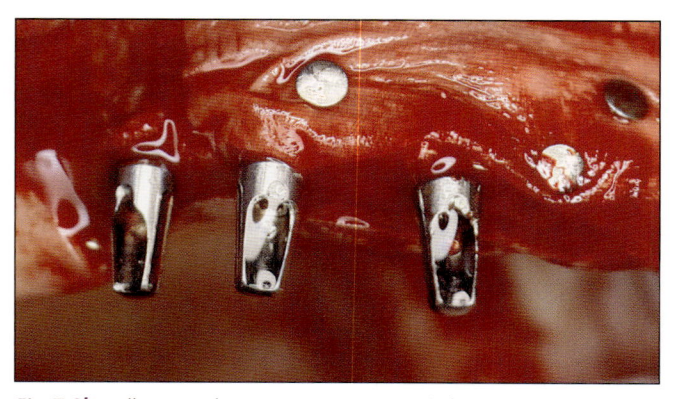

**Fig 7-2h** Following abutment connection with final torque, bone augmentation is performed to cover the exposed implant threads. The autogenous bone was covered with a collagen membrane.

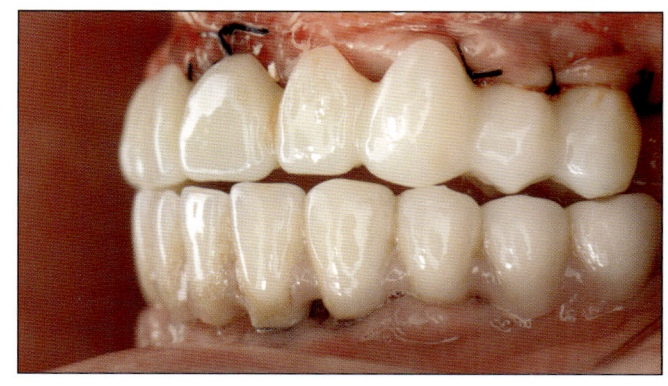

**Fig 7-2i** Provisional maxillary bridge in occlusion. Note the small contacts used to avoid excessive forces on the immediately loaded implants right after surgery.

Four months after loading, the patient asked for a similar treatment in the maxilla (Fig 7-2f). A prosthetic guide similar to the one used for the mandible was employed. A mucoperiosteal flap was elevated following a midcrestal incision under local anesthesia. The alveolar ridge was too narrow (less than 3-mm width) and the bone quality too compromised (very weak) to achieve optimal implant placement.

The implants were placed using the protocol for the Ankylos implant system in the areas of the left and right canines through second premolars. All implants were 3.5 mm in diameter and 14 mm in length. They had excellent primary stability, but some of the threads in the buccal aspect were exposed. Autogenous bone graft was harvested from the two tuberosities using a trephine and milled with a bone mill. Temporary resin abutments were placed (Fig 7-2g) to check the parallelism and then replaced with the definitive angulated abutments using controlled torque. All implants were covered buccally with one Bio-Gide (Geistlich) collagen membrane, which was fixed in place with titanium Frios tacks (Fig 7-2h). The flap was sutured in place, and a provisional cross-arch–shaped fixed prosthesis without any distal cantilevers was fabricated chairside (Fig 7-2i).

*Note: Special attention is given to ensure that the provisional prosthesis is well polished and has open areas for sufficient plaque control and food debris removal during the initial stages of healing. A provisional prosthesis should be good but not perfect to ensure that the patient will return for follow-up visits. Missing follow-up visits could have a deleterious effect on the patient's implant prognosis.*

The Periotest values were determined immediately before placement of the provisional prosthesis, and the same postoperative care instructions were given to the patient as she had received for the mandibular treatment. A symmetric balanced occlusion was used for the provisional fixed restoration in centric occlusion with only group contacts in the lateral movements of the mandible. One week after surgery, the sutures were removed. The impression for the definitive fixed implant-supported restoration was taken 4 weeks after surgery using a similar impression technique (without removing the abutments) as that used for the mandible. Finally, a radiologic examination was used to determine the crestal bone level at the time of the prosthesis delivery.

The patient was re-examined every 3 months. The restorations were removed, and the Periotest values were determined. The follow-up examination 3 years after loading in the mandible (2.5 years after loading in the maxilla) showed excellent soft tissues in all peri-implant areas as well as an esthetic result (Figs 7-2j to 7-2q).

Case Reports

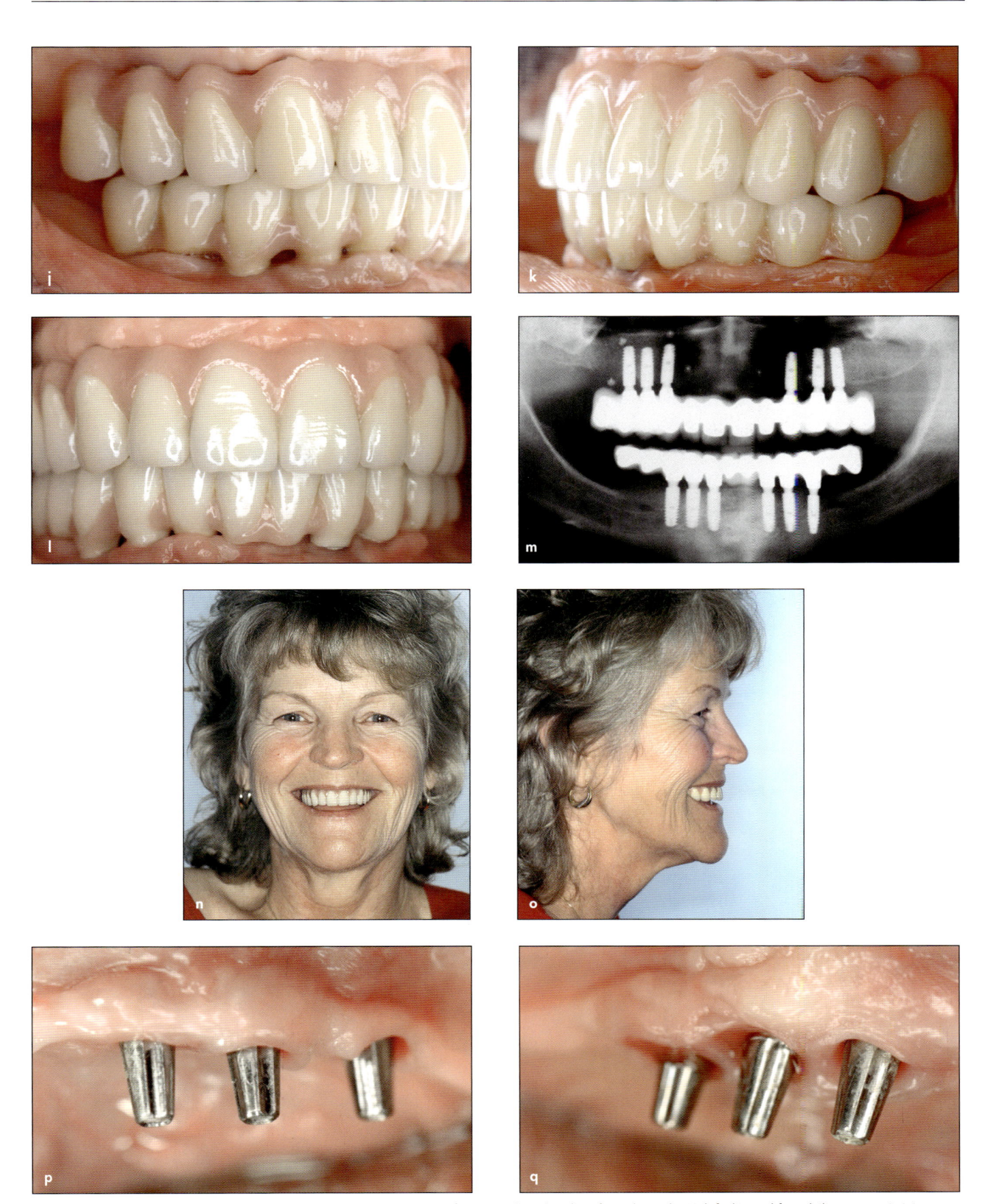

**Figs 7-2j to 7-2q** Definitive implant-supported restorations 3 years after immediate loading from the right *(j)*, left *(k)*, and facial *(l)* aspects. *(m)* A panoramic radiograph showing the bone stability after 3 years. *(n and o)* The esthetic result of the restorations after 3 years of loading presents harmony with the smile line. Patient comfort was much improved. *(p and q)* The peri-implant soft tissues are in excellent condition.

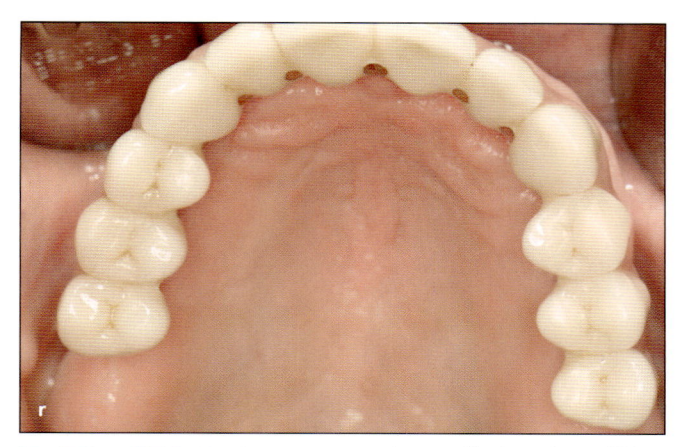

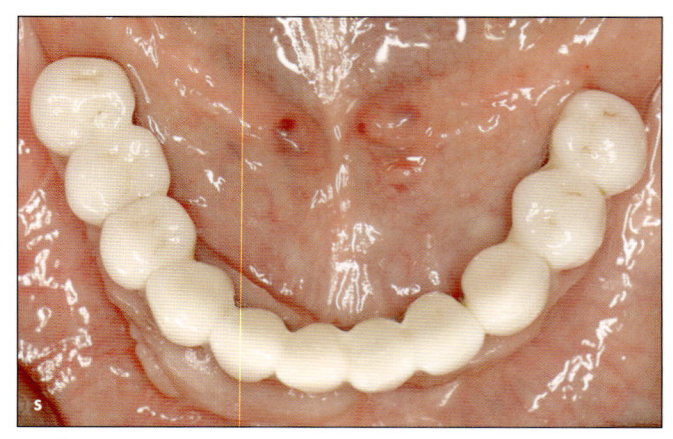

**Figs 7-2r and 7-2s** Final restorations in the maxilla *(r)* and mandible *(s)* 5 years after successful immediate loading.

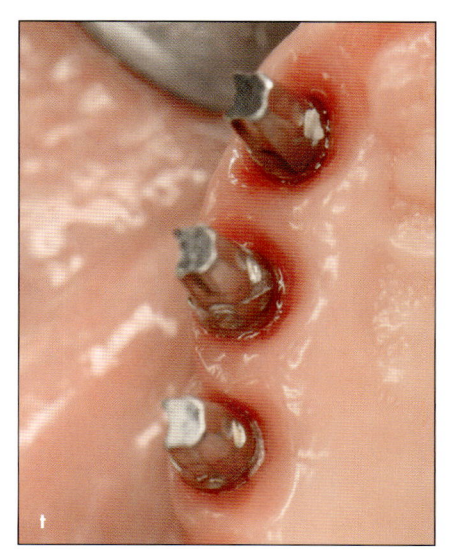

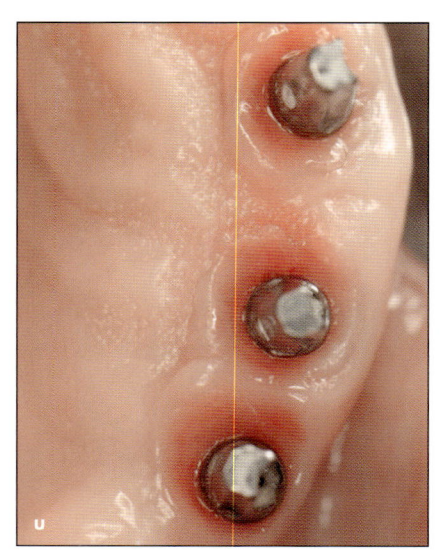

**Figs 7-2t and 7-2u** Excellent soft tissues around implants in the maxilla 5 years after successful immediate loading. (Dental technician: Mike Funk, Reichelsheim, Germany.)

No marginal bone loss was observed at any of the implants. The mean Periotest value was 2.00 ± 3.83 at baseline, −1.33 ± 2.50 at the time of the prosthesis delivery, and −1.41 ± 2.75 at the 3-year follow-up examination after removal of the prosthetic restorations.

The result 5 years after immediate loading was excellent and presented healthy soft tissues around all implants in the maxilla as well as the mandible (Figs 7-2r to 7-2u).

# Case Reports

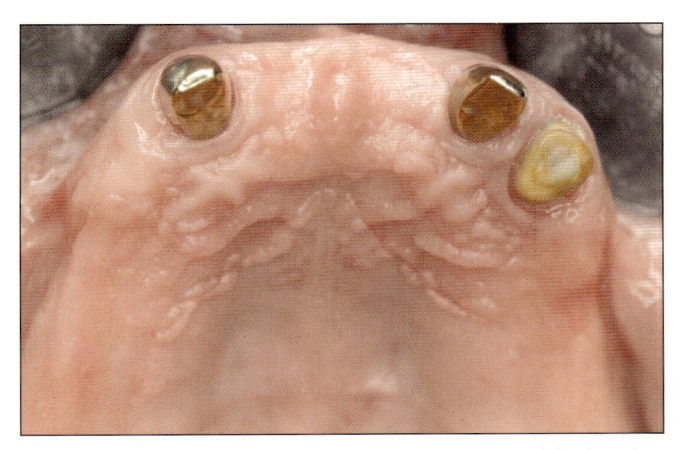

**Fig 7-3a** Partial edentulous maxilla prior to extraction of the hopeless teeth and implant placement.

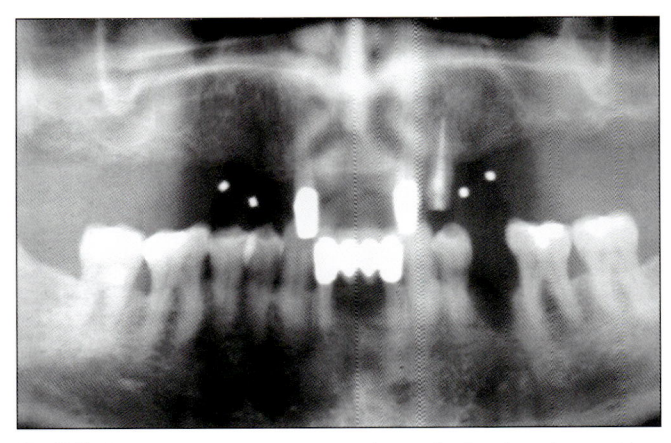

**Fig 7-3b** Preoperative panoramic radiograph showing the positions of the implants.

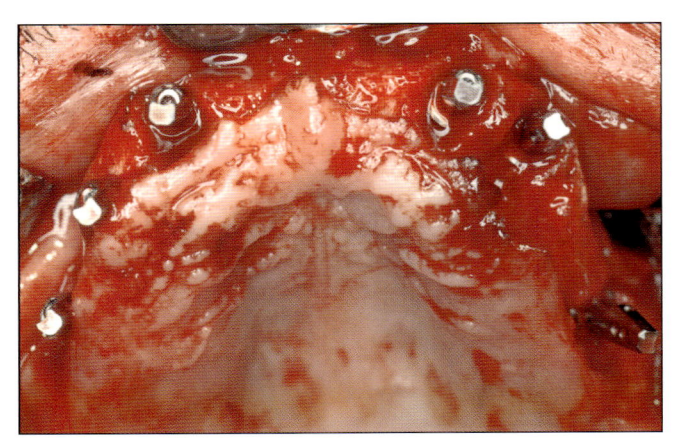

**Fig 7-3c** Implant placement and final abutment connection (Morse taper) with a final torque of 15 Ncm.

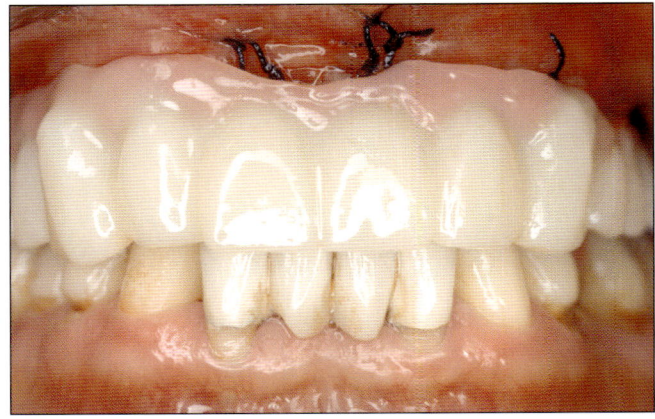

**Fig 7-3d** Provisional prosthesis in place following surgery for immediate functional loading.

## Case 3: Advanced immediate loading in the maxilla with poor bone quality using a fixed restoration

A 60-year-old man presented with insufficient retention of his maxillary partial denture. The maxillary lateral incisors had some mobility because of advanced attachment loss, and his maxillary left canine was compromised because of a root canal treatment and placement of a post and core restoration (Fig 7-3a). The long-term prognosis and predictability of dental implants and the different treatment alternatives were explained to the patient. He accepted the proposed treatment plan to extract the remaining maxillary teeth and place six implants, three to be placed in the alveolar sockets immediately after extraction (immediate implants). After a duplicate of the partial denture was fabricated, radiographs were taken to evaluate the height of the alveolar ridges (Fig 7-3b). The width of the ridge was determined using bone sounding and a final transfer of the soft tissue thickness measurements to the study casts.

A mucoperiosteal flap was elevated, and the maxillary teeth were removed atraumatically and with special care to avoid fracture of the buccal bony plate. After a careful cleaning of the sockets, six Ankylos implants were placed in the maxillary right and left lateral incisor and the left canine sites (immediate implants) and in the maxillary right second premolar and canine and left first molar sites. Angulated abutments were connected immediately after implant placement and fixed with a final torque of 15 Ncm according to the manufacturer guidelines (Fig 7-3c). With the aid of a template, a provisional fixed implant-supported restoration (Fig 7-3d) with excellent occlusal contacts was fabricated chairside, and the vertical dimension was maintained. Finally, a radiographic examination was performed to determine the exact crestal bone level at baseline. The patient was advised to adhere to a soft or liquid diet for the first 2 to 3 months postoperatively.

# 7 Immediate Loading in Edentulous Jaws

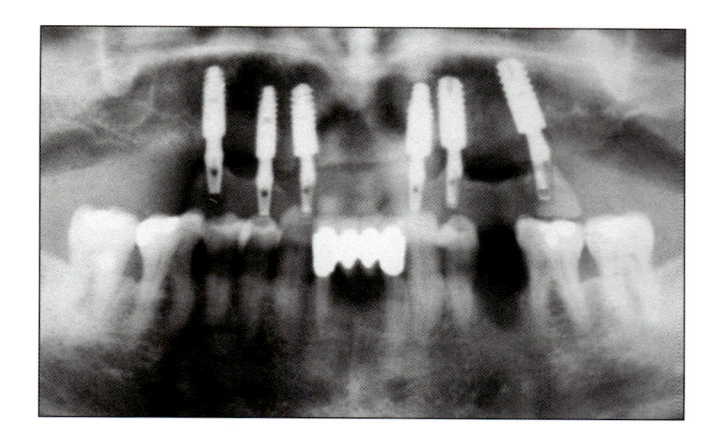

**Fig 7-3e** Crestal bone stability 3 months after immediate loading prior to impression for final restoration.

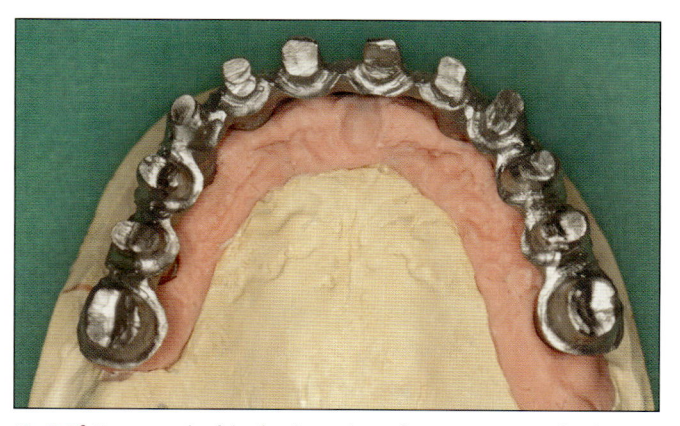

**Fig 7-3f** Framework of the final prosthesis for cementation of individual crowns.

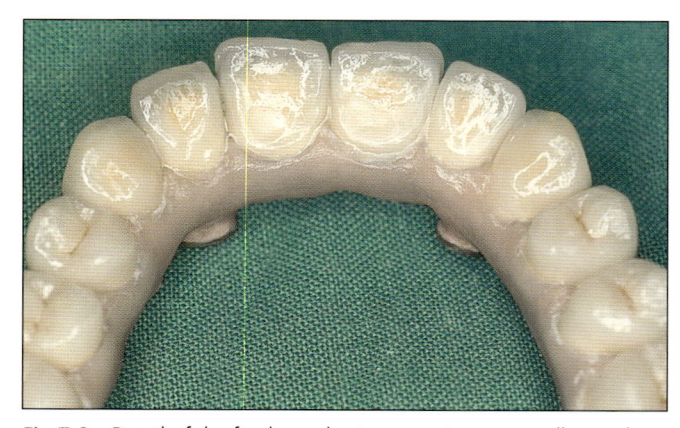

**Fig 7-3g** Detail of the final prosthesis presenting an excellent esthetic result.

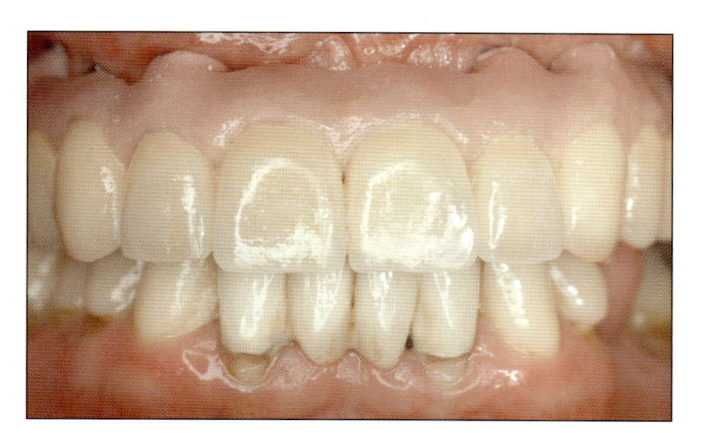

**Fig 7-3h** Final prosthesis in place after cementation.

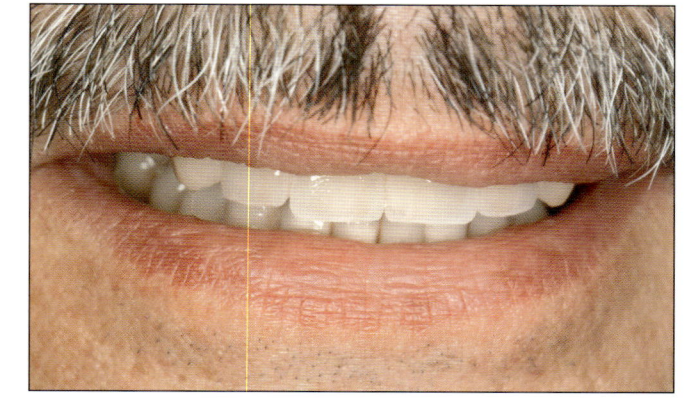

**Fig 7-3i** Excellent esthetic result of the prosthetic rehabilitation 6 months after treatment.

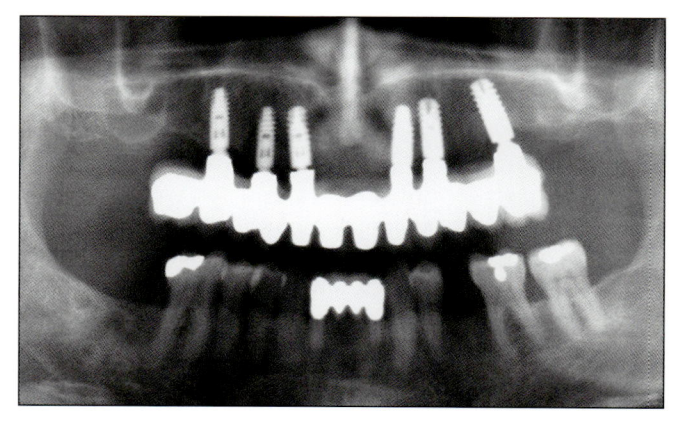

**Fig 7-3j** Panoramic radiograph 8 years after immediate functional loading presenting crestal bone stability around all implants.

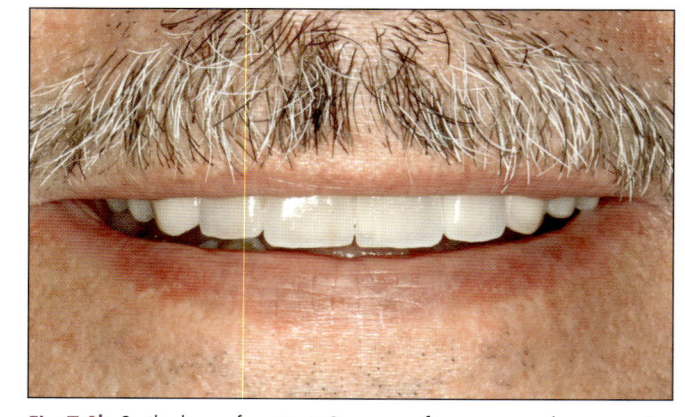

**Fig 7-3k** Smile line of patient 8 years after surgery demonstrating a highly esthetic result. (Dental technician: Susanne Roth, Frankfurt, Germany.)

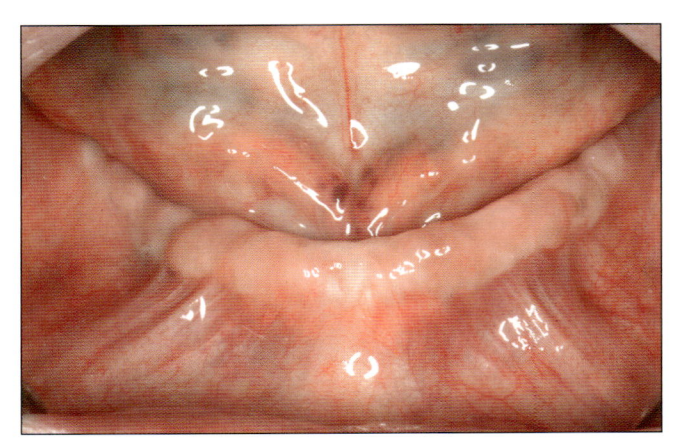

**Fig 7-4a** Edentulous mandible immediately before surgery.

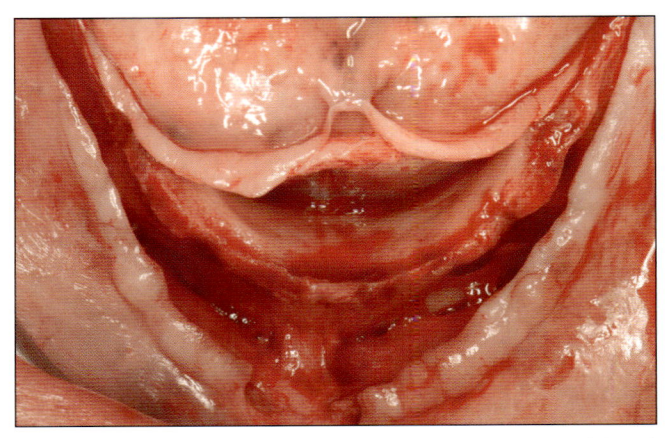

**Fig 7-4b** Flap elevation revealing the advanced resorption of the alveolar ridge and the extreme undercuts in the anterior mandible.

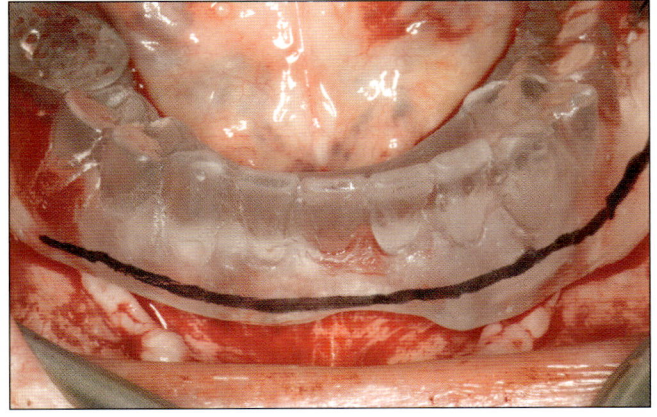

**Fig 7-4c** Prosthetic guide in place and marked to show the exact bone level for planing.

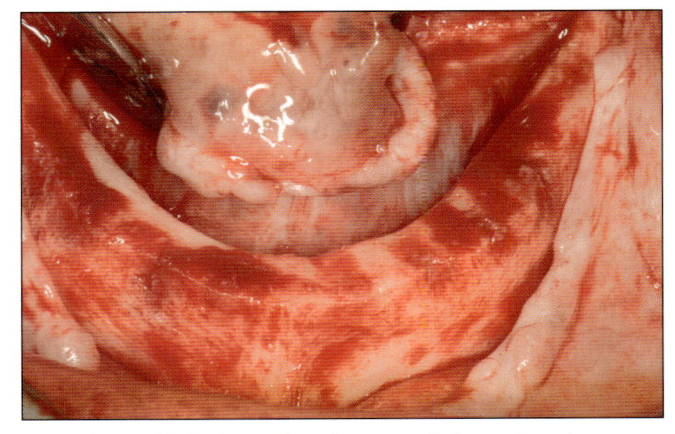

**Fig 7-4d** Mandibular bone after planing ready for implant placement.

After a 3-month healing period, the final steps for delivery of the definitive restoration were performed. The soft tissues around all implants were healthy and the Periotest values were low (Figs 7-3e). A metal-ceramic fixed prosthesis was fabricated with individual crowns for cementation on the framework (Figs 7-3f to 7-3h). The patient was very happy with the final esthetic result and function of the new prosthesis (Fig 7-3i). One year after loading, the prosthesis was removed and the clinical situation of the implants was evaluated. All implants were clinically stable and showed excellent peri-implant soft tissue conditions. The panoramic radiograph showed that the crestal bone level was stable without resorption or inflammatory reactions in the tissues. The same results were observed at every annual follow-up examination, and the bone stability esthetic result were the same 8 years after loading (Figs 7-3j and 7-3k).

The Periotest values at the time of delivery of the definitive prosthesis and at the follow-up examination 8 years after loading (after removal of the prosthetic restorations) were negative, which demonstrates the excellent implant stability.

## Case 4: Advanced immediate loading protocol in the atrophic mandible

The following case demonstrates the use of an advanced treatment protocol for a woman with an edentulous mandible who wanted a fixed implant-supported restoration (Fig 7-4a). The patient, a smoker, tried to quit smoking before implant surgery. Elevation of a mucoperiosteal flap revealed a thin mandibular alveolar ridge with undercuts in submandibular areas (Fig 7-4b). A duplicate of the mandibular denture was fabricated to provide information on the thickness of the anticipated framework and for use as a prosthetic guide. The prosthetic template was placed intraorally to show the necessary level of bone reduction, which was completed with a surgical bur (Figs 7-4c and 7-4d). Straumann Bone Level implants with a 4.1-mm diameter, an SLActive surface, and lengths between 8 and 12 mm were placed and made parallel to each other. The posterior implants were placed with lingual inclinations to avoid sublingual perforations during drilling (Fig 7-4e). After removal of the inserts, multibase abutments were connected parallel

# 7 Immediate Loading in Edentulous Jaws

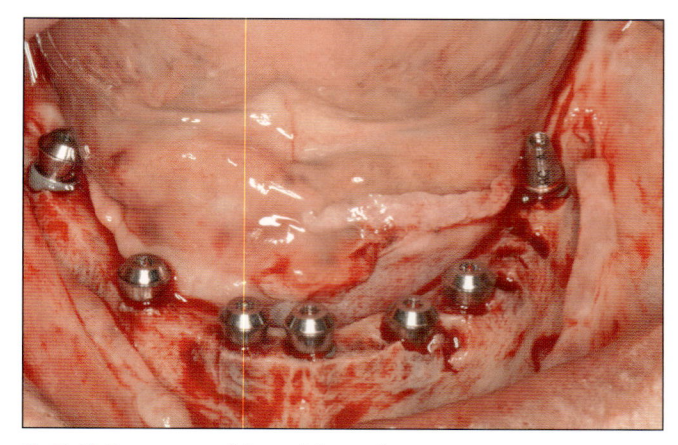

**Fig 7-4e** Implant positions immediately before removal of the inserts.

**Fig 7-4f** Connection of the multibase abutments.

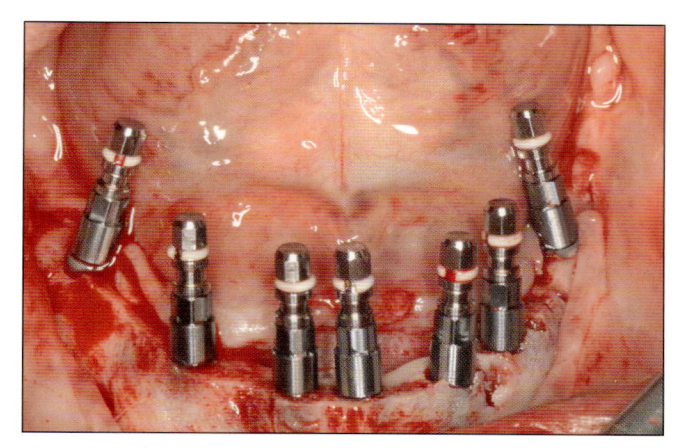

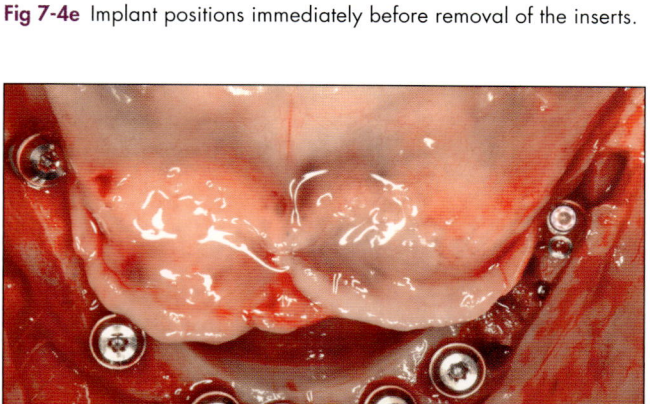

**Fig 7-4g** Occlusal view of the multibase abutments.

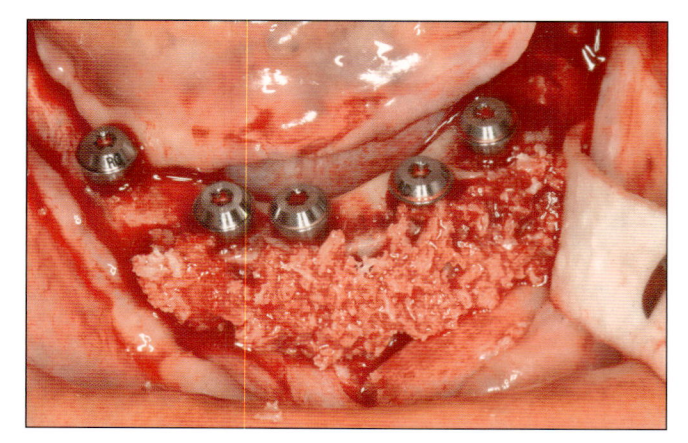

**Fig 7-4h** Lateral bone augmentation with bone allograft.

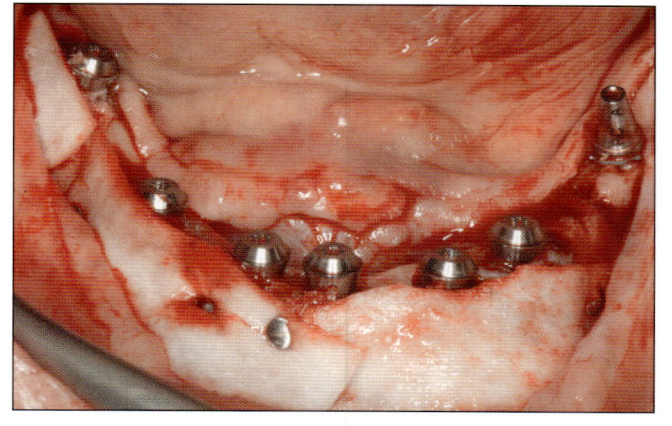

**Fig 7-4i** Collagen membranes in place before flap closure.

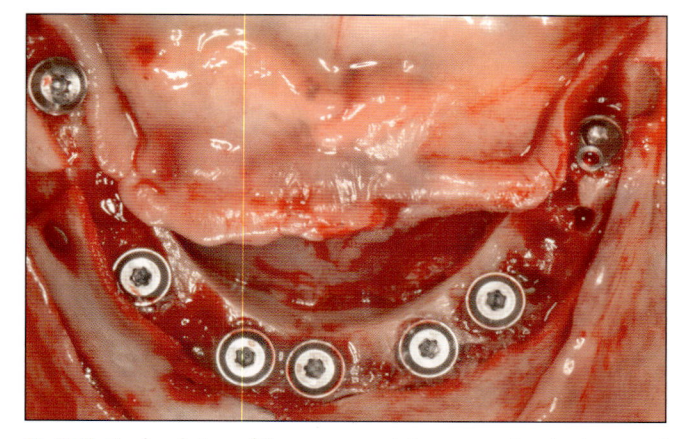

**Fig 7-4j** Occlusal view of the augmented sites presenting the improved shape of the mandibular arch.

to each other (Fig 7-4f and 7-4g). Because of the thin buccal bony plate, bone augmentation was performed using AlloGraft (Straumann) covered with a Mucograft collagen membrane (Osteohealth) secured in place with titanium tacks (Figs 7-4h to 7-4j). Temporary cylinders were connected to the multibase abutments, and the flap was closed with 4-0 silk suture material (Figs 7-4k and 7-4l). The undercuts were closed using rubber dam, and a screw-retained provisional restoration was fabricated with correct vertical dimension and occlusion (Fig 7-4m). The patient was instructed about postoperative antibiotics and analgesics, and a soft/liquid diet was recommended for the first 3 months of healing to avoid complications. The patient was very satisfied with the postoperative clinical outcome (Figs 7-4n and 7-4o).

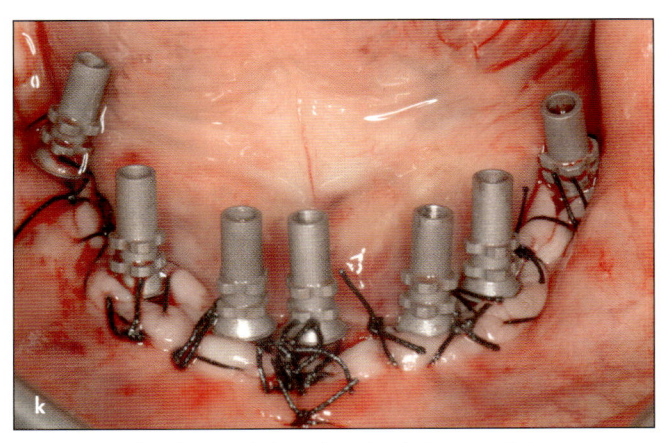

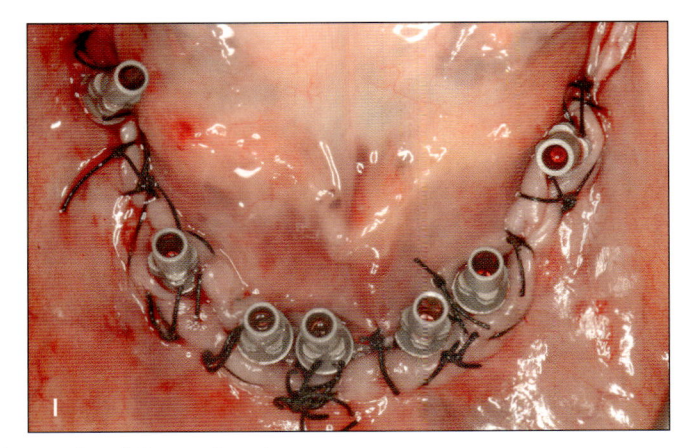

**Figs 7-4k and 7-4l** Frontal *(k)* and occlusal *(l)* views of the temporary cylinders in place following flap closure.

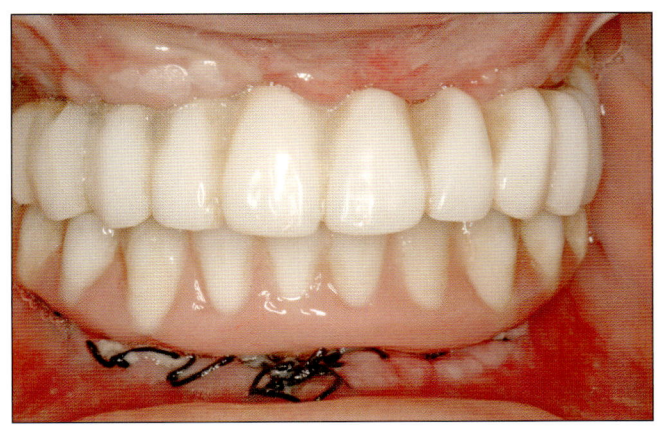

**Fig 7-4m** Provisional restoration in place immediately after surgery.

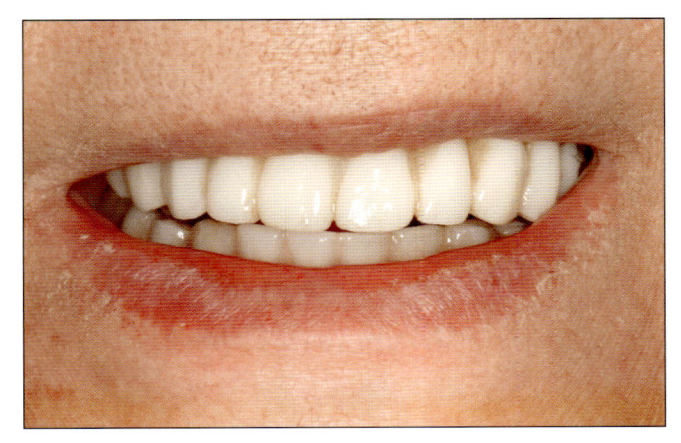

**Fig 7-4n** Smile line of the patient immediately after surgery.

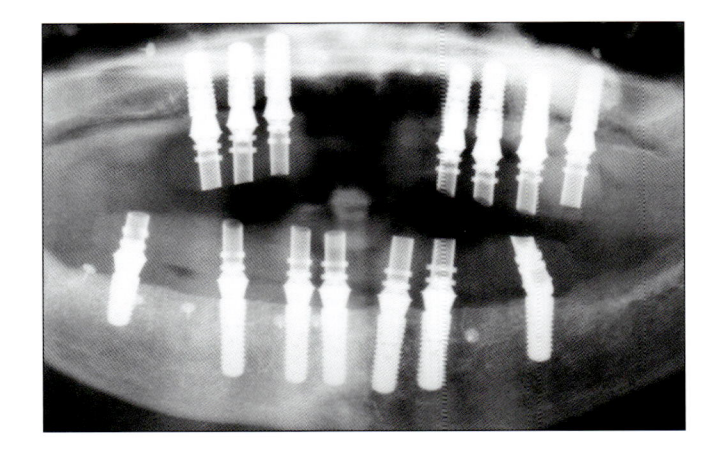

**Fig 7-4o** Panoramic radiograph immediately after surgery demonstrating the baseline crestal bone levels.

## Guidelines for a Successful Immediate Loading Protocol in Edentulous Arches

Based on the protocol illustrated in the above cases, important clinical aspects for surgical treatment using immediately loaded implants include the following:

- A midcrestal incision has to be made and a mucogingival flap must be elevated.
- Based on the surgical and prosthetic guide, the alveolar ridge must be marked precisely at the sites of the osteotomies. A precision wax-up has to be prepared by the dental technician. This represents the prosthetic guide for the implant placement.
- After the implant position is marked (with the use of the prosthetic guide), the osteotomies are carefully prepared. The complete osteotomy should be performed without the use of the surgical guide considering the anatomical landmarks.
- If bone quality is very poor, tapping should be avoided.

- If bone quality is normal or hard (type I or II), tapping should be done in one-third or two-thirds of the osteotomy length, respectively.
- Primary stability is determined using different methods with practicability and efficiency. Periotest or Osstell devices are recommended for this evaluation. The stability of the implant system used is evaluated according to the final torque of the abutment. Implants with high stability (when the abutments are torqued, the implants are stable) can be immediately loaded after their placement. In cases of insufficient stability (the implants become "spinners" when the abutments are connected), a metal-reinforced provisional restoration (for rigid splinting) and a soft or liquid diet must be recommended for at least 3 to 4 months to avoid complications and implant failures.
- Final torque with which the abutments should be connected depends on the bone quality and the type of the implant-abutment connection. If the bone quality is very poor, the final torque cannot be used for the final implant-abutment connection. Implant systems that require a torque greater than 30 Ncm for abutment connection may not be used for immediate loading in cases with compromised (soft) bone quality. If they are used, a gap will be present at the implant-abutment connection that may lead to micromotions, plaque accumulation, and possible implant failure.
- Excessive occlusal contacts of the provisional restoration must be avoided. Group contacts have to be used in the lateral movements of the mandible.
- Distal cantilevers in the provisional prosthesis should be avoided.
- A soft or liquid diet should be used for the first 4 to 6 weeks of healing. In cases with simultaneous bone augmentation, this diet protocol has to be used for the first 3 to 4 months of healing.
- Frequent visits to evaluate the clinical situation are important in the first period of healing before placement of the definitive restoration. Fracture of the provisional prosthesis may be caused by overloading (potential of bruxism); in such cases, the patient should be encouraged to adhere to a soft or liquid diet.
- Provisional restorations must be removed carefully. If the provisional partial prostheses are cemented, a needle holder or a mosquito forceps should be used to take out the cross-arch partial dentures without pressure, using only gentle rotational and tensile forces. Excessive forces due to the use of crown removers may dislodge the implants and lead to failures. As an alternative technique, temporary cylinders and a screw-designed prosthesis would be recommended. However, this requires additional time the day of surgery for fabrication of a more complicated provisionalization.

# Diet Protocol for Patients with Immediately Loaded Implants

Based on the author's clinical experience, the following diet program, in addition to the conventional postoperative surgical recommendations, is suggested for most patients treated with the immediate loading protocol.

- *0 to 5 days:* Soups, salads with soft vegetables, tofu, juices, yogurt, milk, steamed fish, vitamin supplements
- *6 to 14 days:* Soups, salads with soft vegetables, soft pasta, mashed potatoes, soft cheese, tofu, milk, yogurt, juices, tea, vitamin supplements
- *15 to 30 days:* Soups, salads, well-cooked noodles and vegetables, mashed potatoes, steamed fish, soft cheese, tofu, soft breads, juices, tea, coffee
- *2 to 3 months:* Soups, salads, noodles, rice, purees, steamed fish, soft cheese, tofu, well-boiled meat (no barbecue), juices, tea, coffee
- *After 3 months:* Conventional diet

For patients who cannot adhere to this diet program for religious or cultural reasons, the consistency (hardness) of the food should be considered based on the above diet protocol and suggestions. Moreover, the author recommends frequent small meals for enhanced "training" of the surrounding bone at the implant interface. A calcium- and vitamin-enriched supplementary diet may be supportive, especially in older patients.

Oral hygiene has to be performed in the conventional way after suture removal (7 to 10 days after surgery). Normal tooth brushing with toothpaste and toothbrush as well as the use of interdental brushes are necessary for optimal plaque control 3 to 4 weeks after surgery.

# Recommended Reading

1. Romanos GE. Bone quality and the immediate loading of implants—Critical aspects based on literature, research, and clinical experience. Implant Dent 2009;18:203–209.
2. Javed F, Romanos GE. The role of primary stability for successful immediate loading of dental implants. A literature review. J Dent 2010;38:612–620.

# Immediate Loading in Posterior Regions

The immediate loading of dental implants in the posterior part of the jaws is limited by anatomical variations in both the maxilla and the mandible. In the posterior maxilla, the practitioner has to deal with clinical situations in which the remaining bone is insufficient in height because of the proximity of the sinus floor and compromised bone quality. In the posterior mandible, other anatomical limitations hinder the success of immediately loaded implants, such as insufficient height and width, because of advanced bone resorption, close association with the inferior alveolar nerve, high loading forces, and poor bone quality.[1] Moreover, in patients who are partially edentulous in the posterior jaws (ie, a free-end prosthetic situation), the bending moments of loading (masticatory occlusal) forces may overload the implants. For these reasons, placement of a restoration in occlusion immediately after placement of the implants may be an additional risk factor contributing to implant failure that is not warranted by the demands of esthetics in these areas.

Nevertheless, when certain requirements are met, a cross-arch restoration can be immediately loaded with successful, predictable results (see also chapter 7). The main factors affecting the outcome of immediate restorations, especially in the posterior jaws, are the diameter and length of the placed implants, use of the correct implant thread design to increase the primary stability, splinting for better immobilization, and last but not least, the patient's adherence to a soft or liquid diet in the initial stages of healing, which has been recommended in many studies using immediate loading protocols.[2–5]

## Posterior Maxilla

In a study conducted by Testori et al,[6] immediately loaded provisional prostheses without occlusal contacts with the opposing dentition were placed in the posterior area of both the maxilla and the mandible in partially edentulous patients. The implant-supported fixed partial prostheses were delivered within 24 hours after surgery. Two months after loading, the immediate restorations were replaced by definitive prostheses. The implant used most often for this protocol was 4 mm in diameter and 11.5 mm in length; implants wider than 3.2 mm and longer than 8.5 mm were recommended and splinted together using provisional partial dentures. The centric or eccentric contacts were verified with interposition of 200-μm articulating paper.

The survival rate was approximately 96% after 2 years of loading, and failed implants were lost in the first 6 months of loading. Based on these clinical data, the authors concluded that immediately (nonocclusally) loaded implants can be restored with predictable results, similar to those achieved with early loaded implants (loaded after 8 weeks of healing). The results suggest that this protocol may be used in everyday clinical practice when the cases are well selected. Exclusion criteria for the Testori et al[6] study included heavy smoking, an active infection or inflammation in the site intended for implant placement, the need for simultaneous augmentation, and the placement of implants in fresh extraction sockets.

Without doubt, biomechanical characteristics are critical, and several predictors play an important role in achieving a favorable outcome with this treatment protocol. The presence of adjacent teeth for occlusal protection has been recommended in order to distribute and com-

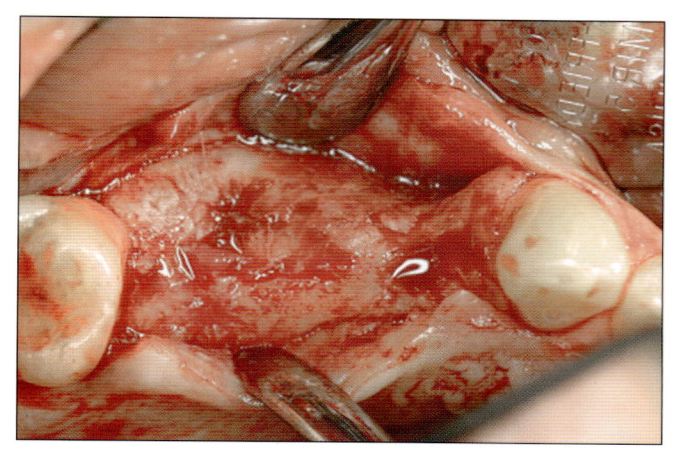

**8** | Immediate Loading in Posterior Regions

**Fig 8-1a** Narrow alveolar ridge in the posterior maxilla immediately after elevation of a mucoperiosteal flap.

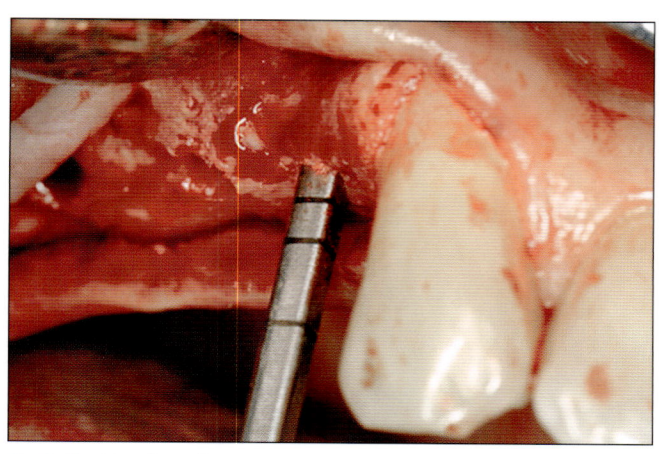

**Fig 8-1b** Alveolar ridge expansion using an osteotome in the area of the implant placement (bone spreading).

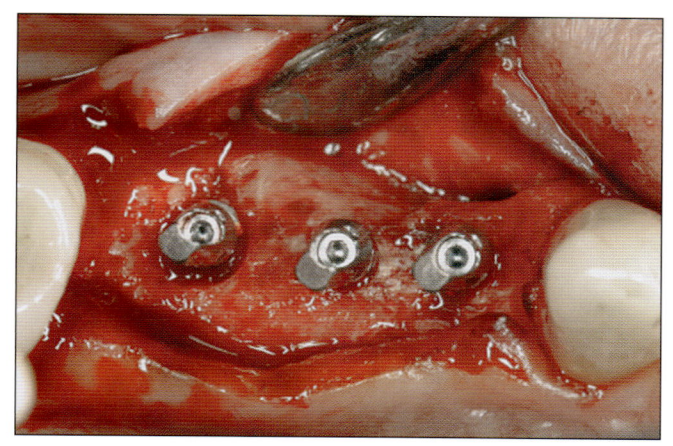

**Fig 8-1c** Implant placement and abutment connection for immediate loading.

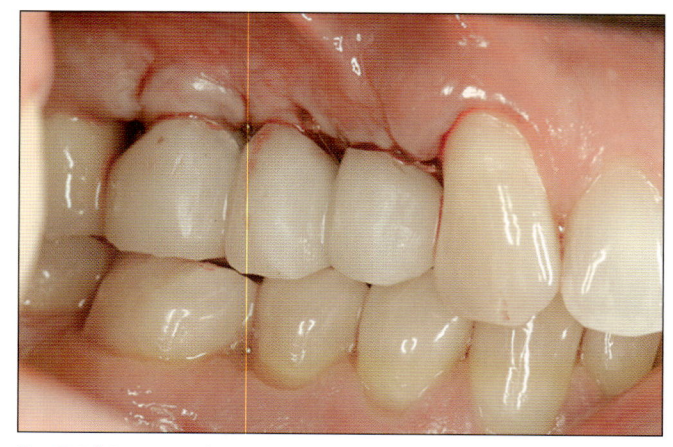

**Fig 8-1d** Provisional restoration in occlusion (immediate functional loading).

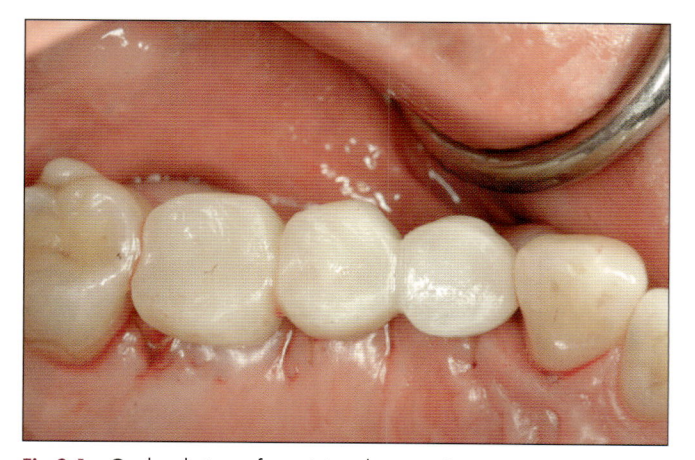

**Fig 8-1e** Occlusal view of provisional restoration.

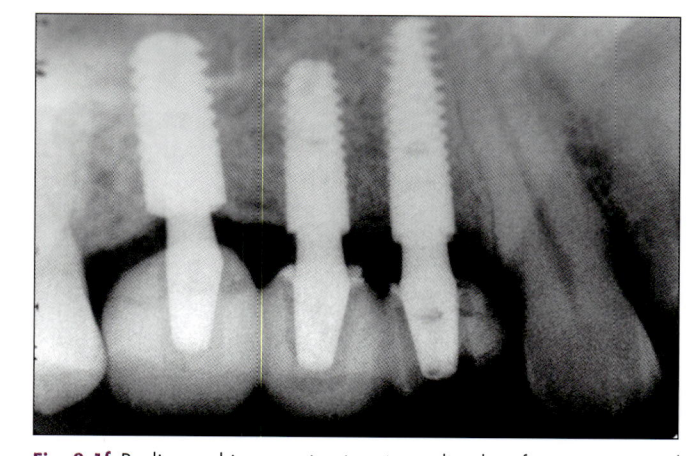

**Fig 8-1f** Radiographic examination immediately after surgery and loading.

pensate for the loading forces. Furthermore, the use of tapered implants is advantageous when immediate loading protocols are applied because their primary stability is 27% higher than that of their cylindric counterparts.[6] The increased primary stability has even been observed in type 4 bone quality.[7] The increased insertion torque of tapered implants compared with that of standard implants has been documented (see also chapter 4).

Figures 8-1 and 8-2 present two cases of immediate loading in the posterior maxilla.

Posterior Maxilla

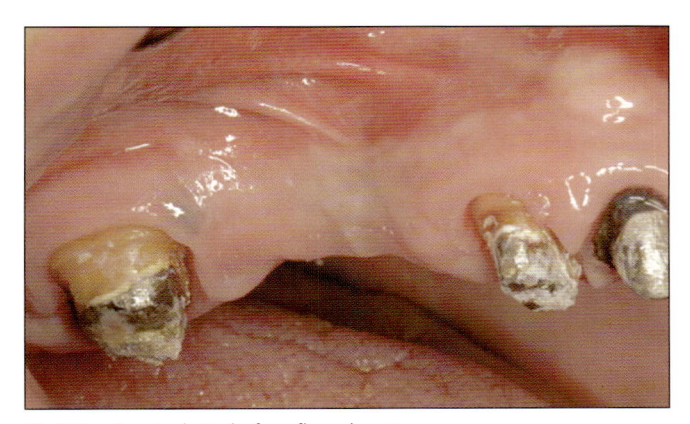

Fig 8-2a Surgical site before flap elevation.

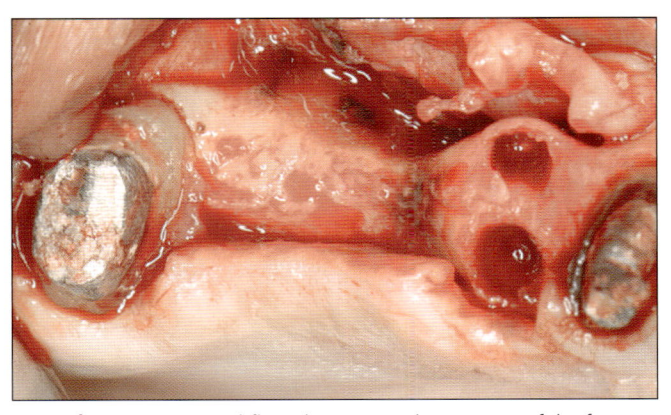

Fig 8-2b Mucoperiosteal flap elevation and extraction of the first premolar.

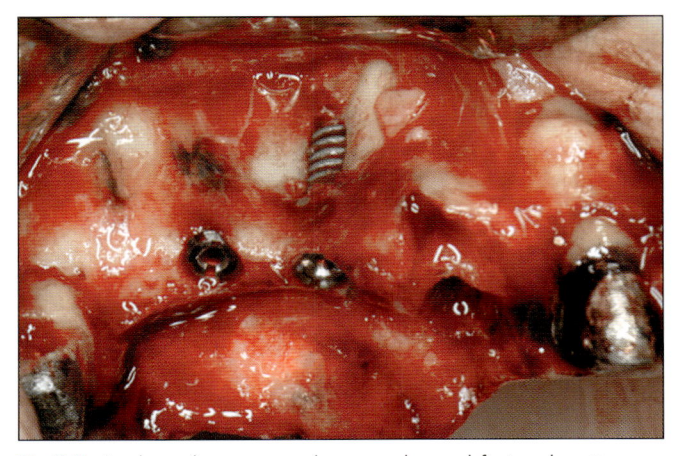

Fig 8-2c Implant placement at the premolar and first molar sites presenting fenestrations in the alveolar bone.

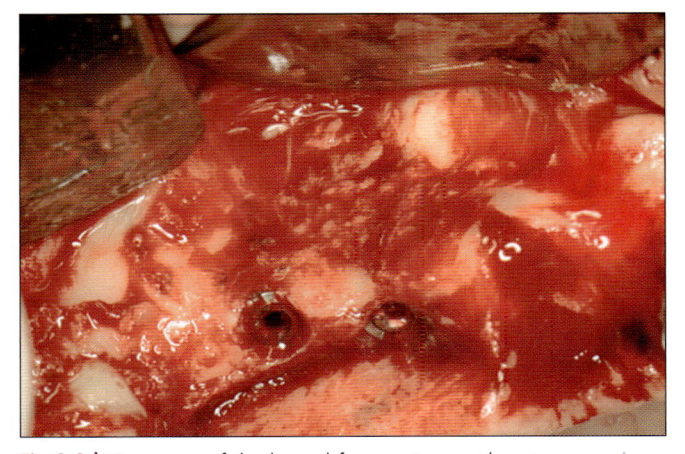

Fig 8-2d Coverage of the buccal fenestrations with autogenous bone harvested from the tuberosity.

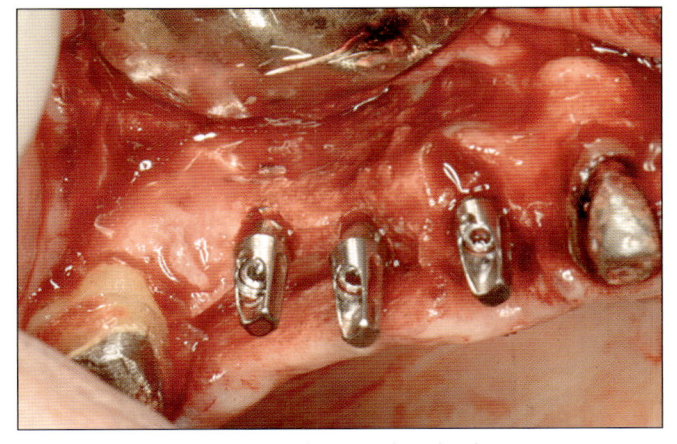

Fig 8-2e Abutment connection for immediate loading.

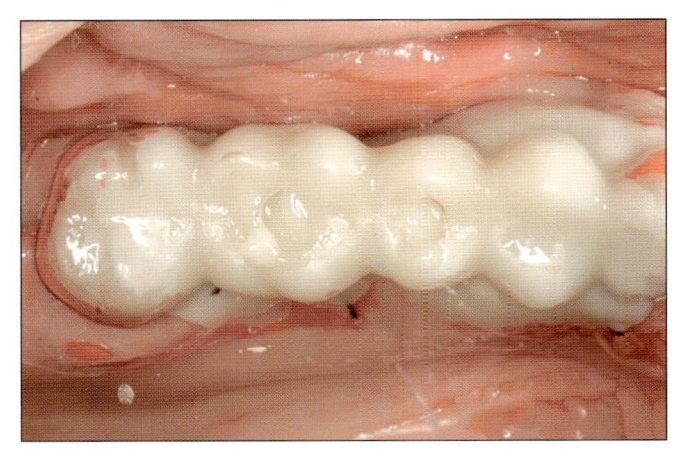

Fig 8-2f Fabrication of the provisional restoration chairside using the shell vacuum technique.

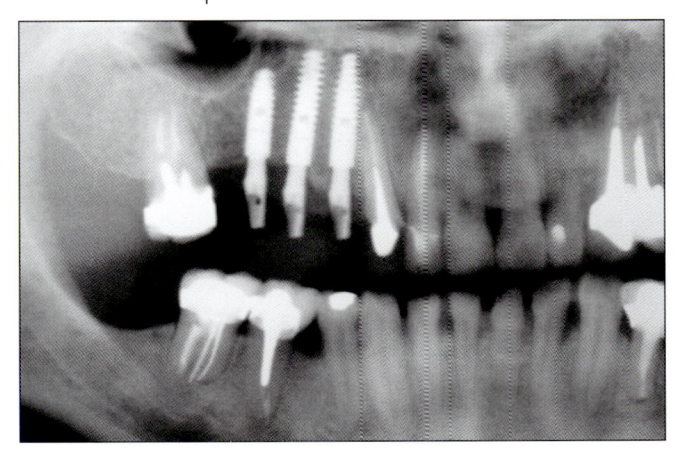

Fig 8-2g Radiographic examination performed just after implant placement for immediate loading to evaluate the implant position and crestal bone levels. (Surgery by G. E. Romanos and G. Bilalis; restoration by G. Bilalis, New York, NY.)

**Table 8-1** Mean clinical values obtained at test (immediately loaded) and control (delayed loaded) implant sites

| Parameter | Test implants | Control implants |
|---|---|---|
| Plaque index | 0.4 ± 0.6 | 0.8 ± 0.7 |
| Sulcus bleeding index | 0.5 ± 0.6 | 0.3 ± 0.5 |
| Probing pocket depth (mm) | 1.9 ± 0.2 | 2.1 ± 0.2 |
| Keratinized mucosa width (mm) | 2.5 ± 1.2 | 3.3 ± 1.4 |
| Periotest value | −3.7 ± 0.9 | −3.2 ± 1.3 |

**Table 8-2** Periotest values for test and control implants at various time points

| Time point | Implant group | Median | Minimum | Maximum |
|---|---|---|---|---|
| T0 | Test | −3 | −7 | 22* |
|  | Control | −3 | −6 | 1 |
| T1 | Test | −3 | −8 | 18* |
|  | Control | −4 | −8 | 3 |
| T2 | Test | −3 | −5 | 7 |
|  | Control | −3.5 | −7 | 0 |
| T3 | Test | −3 | −8 | 2 |
|  | Control | −3 | −5 | 0 |
| T4 | Test | −3.7 | −6 | −1 |
|  | Control | −3.2 | −8 | 0 |

T0, baseline; T1, 6 weeks; T2, 6 months; T3, 12 months; T4, 24 months
*Represents the same implant placed in extremely poor bone quality.

## Posterior Mandible

Implant prognosis in the posterior mandible is associated with many problems because of insufficient bone quality and quantity[8-10] as well as anatomical limitations that necessitate the placement of shorter implants. In addition, biomechanical factors, such as increased loading forces in this location, may be associated with higher rates of failure.[11] Frequent cases of peri-implantitis have also been reported in the posterior mandible.[12]

The immediate loading of implants placed in the posterior mandible may be associated with more failures because of the additional risk of micromotions at the interface, which may lead to fibrous tissue formation[13] and, finally, implant failure. From a biomechanical point of view, increased bending moments can occur when implants are placed and loaded in the posterior part of the jaws.[14] The clinical studies on immediate loading in the mandible report a high number of failures in the posterior section caused by poor bone quality in these areas.[15-18]

Tarnow et al[19] placed a high number of implants in the mandible (including the posterior mandible) and did not remove the provisional restoration during the 4- to 6-month healing period. The authors recommended the use of screw-retained provisional and non-cemented restorations for easy removal and to eliminate macromovements during the healing period.[19]

Immediate loading in the posterior mandible was evaluated in 12 consecutive cases using a split-mouth design to compare the traditional loading protocol with the immediate occlusal loading protocol.[4,5] Twelve patients (7 men, 5 women; mean age: 50.75 ± 7.95 years) participated in this study, which was approved by the ethics committee of the University of Frankfurt in accordance with the Declaration of Helsinki. The patients had bilateral free-end prosthetic situations in the mandible and were treatment planned for three implants distal to the canines to replace their missing teeth. One side was randomly selected as the control for placement of three delayed loaded implants with a progressive thread design (Ankylos, Dentsply Friadent) for submerged healing. After 3 months, the implants were exposed and loaded with splinted resin crowns. These provisional splinted crowns were replaced 6 weeks later by definitive splinted restorations. On the contralateral side, three implants that were exactly the same size as the control implants were placed and served as the test group. Abutments were placed, and the test implants were immediately loaded. Provisional crowns splinted the three implants together in each side and had occlusal contacts only in maximal intercuspation (immediate functional loading). Eccentric contacts during lateral movements of the mandible were eliminated. Canine, anterior guidance, or group function was used in all clinical cases.

Periodontal indices and bone loss were evaluated at frequent follow-up intervals. Healing was uneventful, and all implants were clinically stable. No complications or postoperative infections were observed during the observation period. No visible implant mobility was observed either immediately after surgery or during the loading period in both implant groups. After a mean loading period of 25.3 ± 3.3 months, the findings presented normal clinical values without differences between the test and control implants ($P < .05$), as presented in Table 8-1. The Periotest values (Medizintechnik Gulden) at the different time intervals are presented in Table 8-2. Twenty-nine of the 72 sites examined did not show any bone loss. These results confirm that immediate functional loading of dental implants with a progressive thread design has the same prognosis as delayed loading in the posterior mandible 2 years after loading.

Figures 8-3 and 8-4 present case examples of patients treated in the study described above. Implants placed in fresh extraction sockets (immediate implants) with immediate loading in the posterior mandible are shown in Figs 8-5 (unilateral partial denture) and 8-6 (distal cantilever partial prosthesis). Figure 8-7 presents the response of alveolar bone in a case of controlled overloading.

## Posterior Mandible

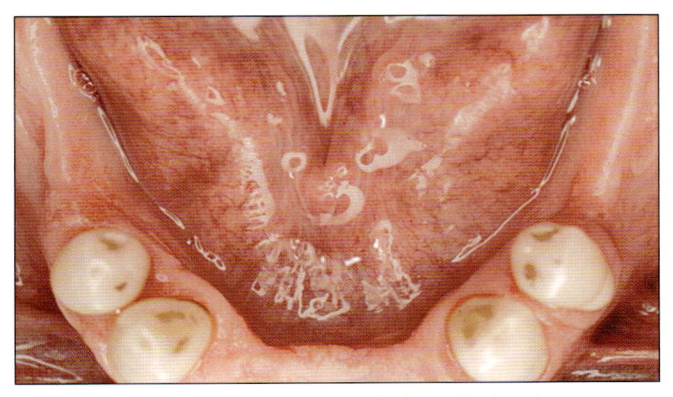

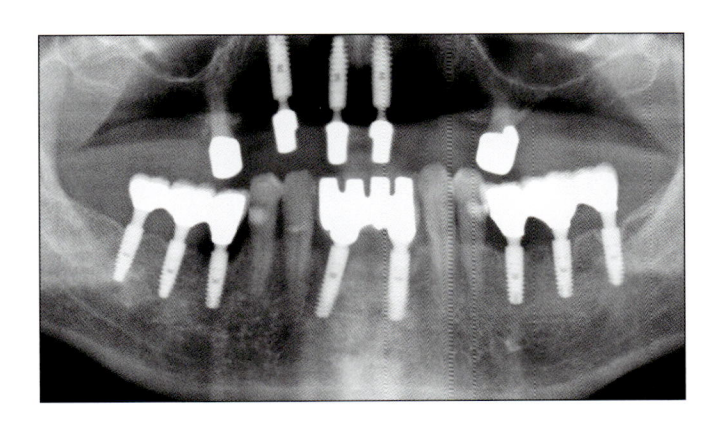

**Fig 8-3a** Preoperative occlusal view of bilateral edentulous posterior mandible of a 59-year-old man.

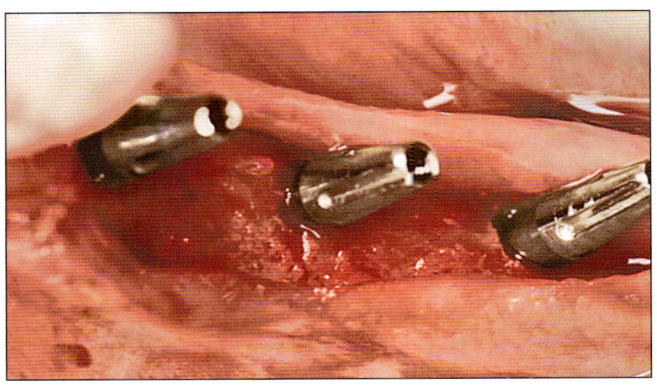

**Fig 8-3b** Three implants placed on the left side and connected with their abutments for immediate loading with provisional splinted crowns.

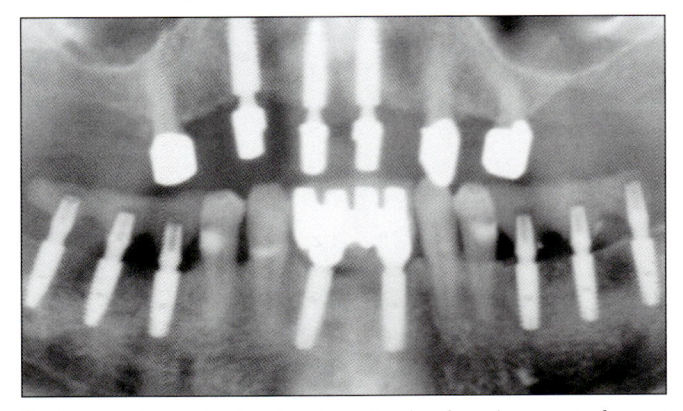

**Fig 8-3c** Radiograph showing bone levels after placement of provisional restorations bilaterally.

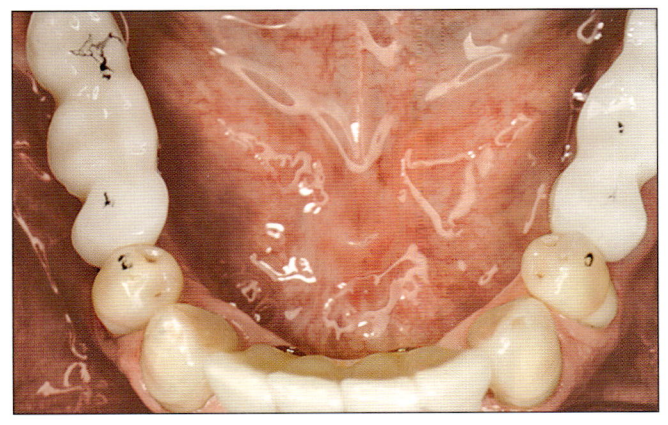

**Fig 8-3d** Occlusal view of provisional splinted restorations.

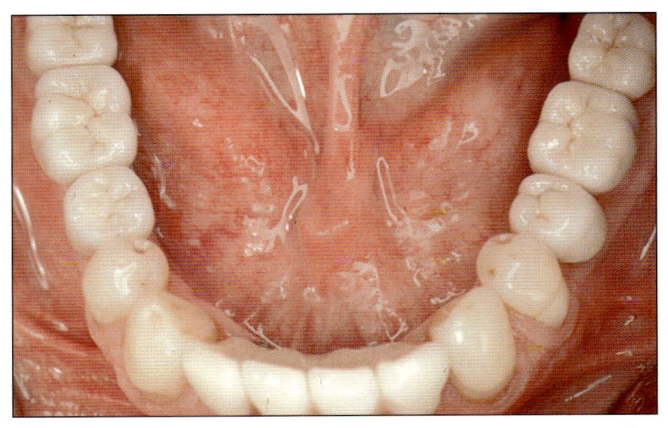

**Fig 8-3e** Occlusal view showing definitive restorations 5 years after placement. The left side was immediately loaded and the right side underwent delayed loading.

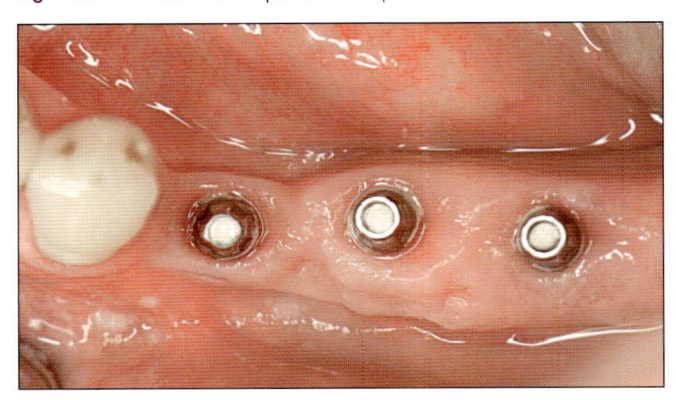

**Fig 8-3f** Follow-up photograph taken 5 years after loading demonstrating the healthy condition of the soft tissues around the immediately loaded implants.

**Fig 8-3g** Panoramic radiograph 12 years after loading. Note the marginal bone loss on the right side around the implants that underwent delayed loading compared to the immediately loaded implants on the left side.

83

**8** | Immediate Loading in Posterior Regions

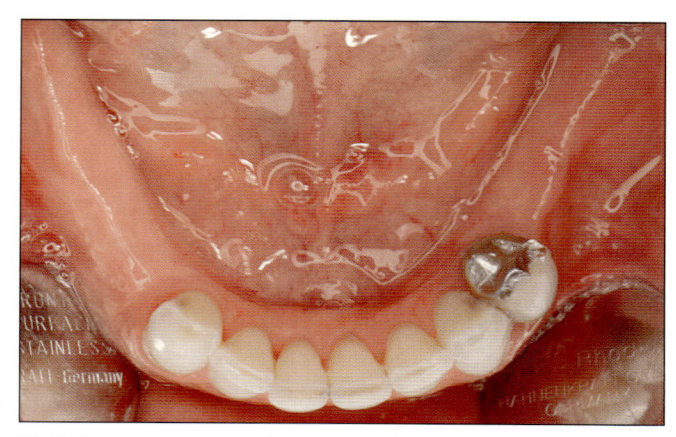

**Fig 8-4a** Preoperative occlusal view of bilateral edentulous posterior mandible.

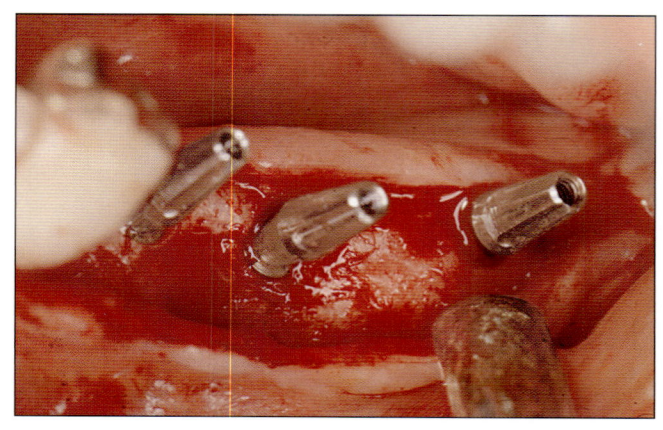

**Fig 8-4b** Three implants on the left side connected with their abutments for immediate loading.

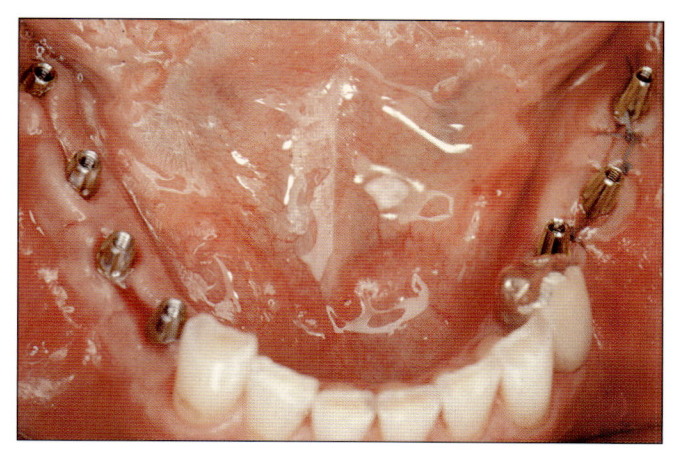

**Fig 8-4c** Occlusal view of implants placed in the posterior mandible. Implants ready for immediate loading are on the left side, while the healed (osseointegrated) implants with planned delayed loading are on the contralateral site.

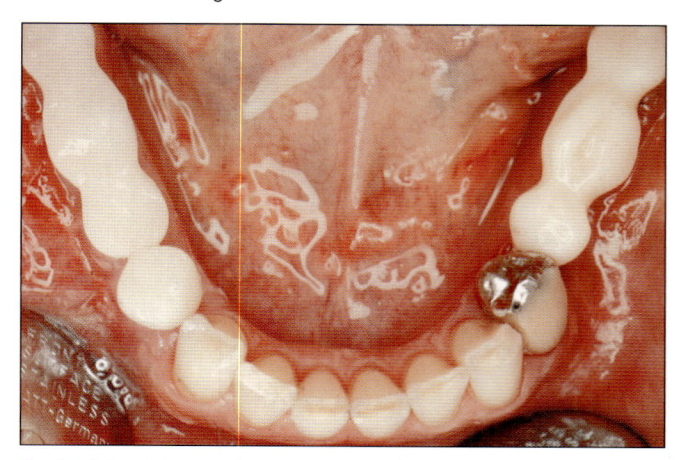

**Fig 8-4d** Provisional splinted crowns in place.

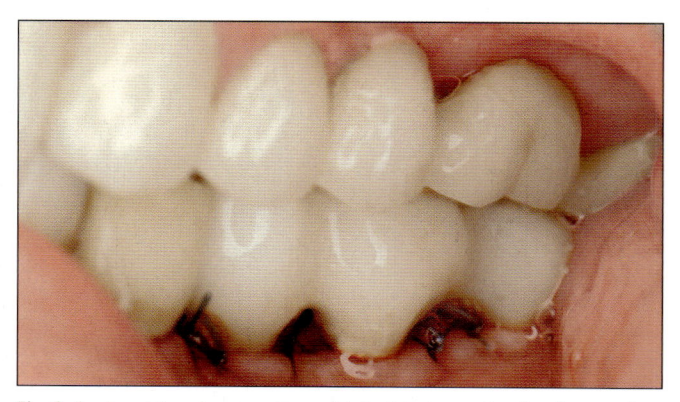

**Fig 8-4e** Provisional restoration of left side immediately after implant placement (immediate loading).

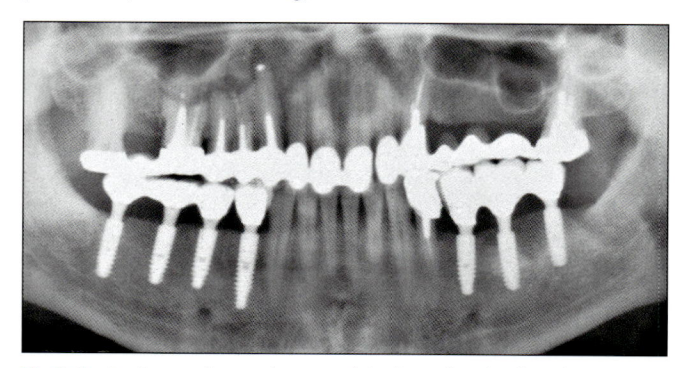

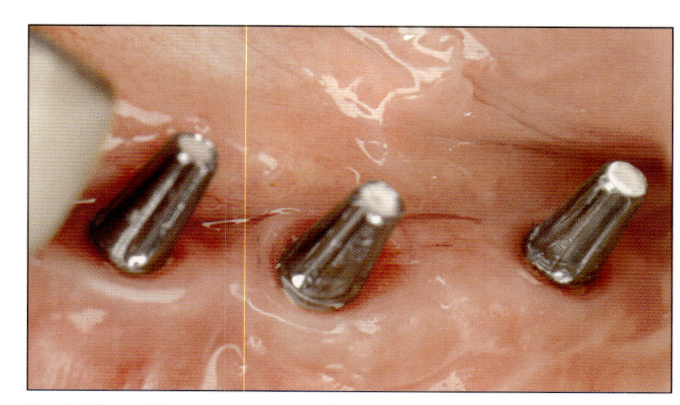

**Fig 8-4f** Healthy peri-implant soft tissues 6 weeks after surgery at the day of the delivery of the definitive restorations.

**Fig 8-4g** Radiographic evaluation of the bone levels after placement of the definitive prosthesis.

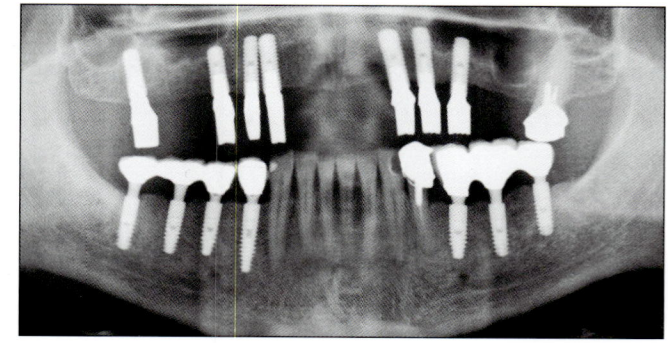

**Fig 8-4h** Follow-up radiographic evaluation performed 12 years after immediate loading on left side and delayed loading on right side. No crestal bone loss was observed around the immediately loaded implants.

Posterior Mandible

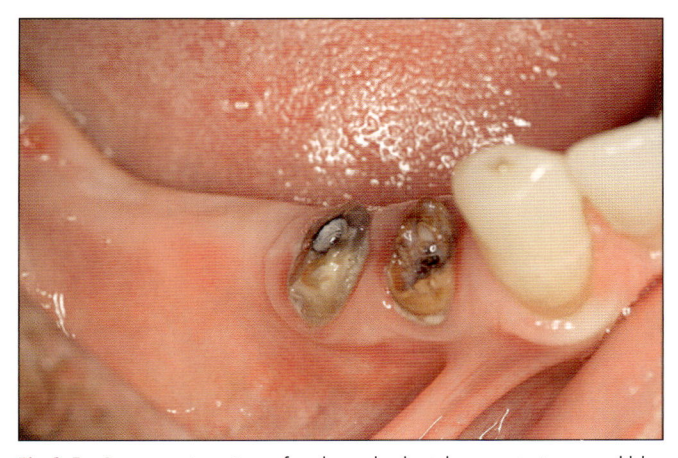

**Fig 8-5a** Preoperative view of unilateral edentulous posterior mandible.

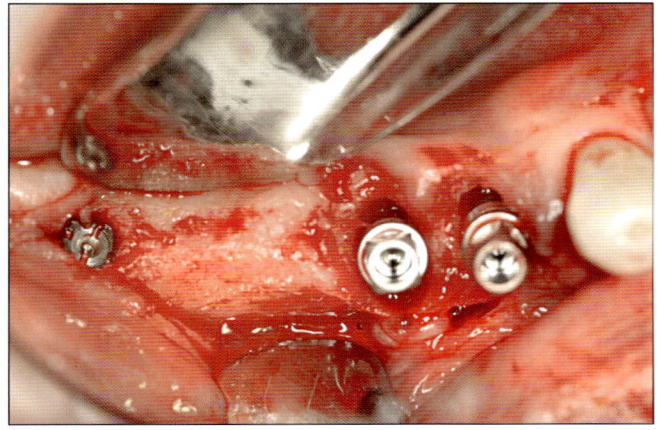

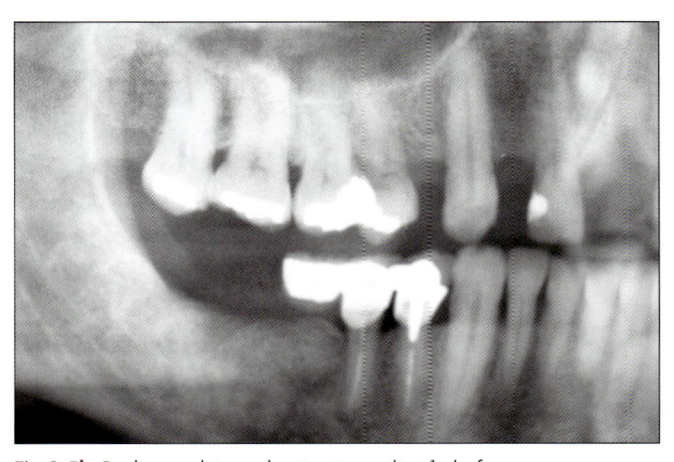

**Fig 8-5b** Radiographic evaluation immediately before surgery.

**Fig 8-5c** Placement of implants at the premolar and first molar sites following extraction of the premolars.

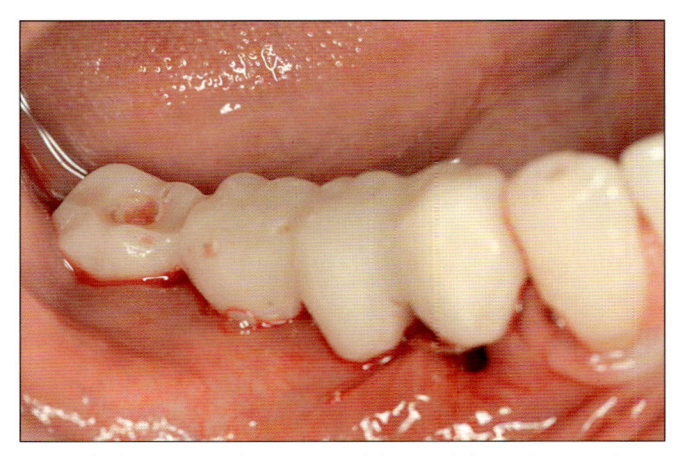

**Fig 8-5d** The provisional restoration, fabricated chairside, in occlusion immediately after implant placement.

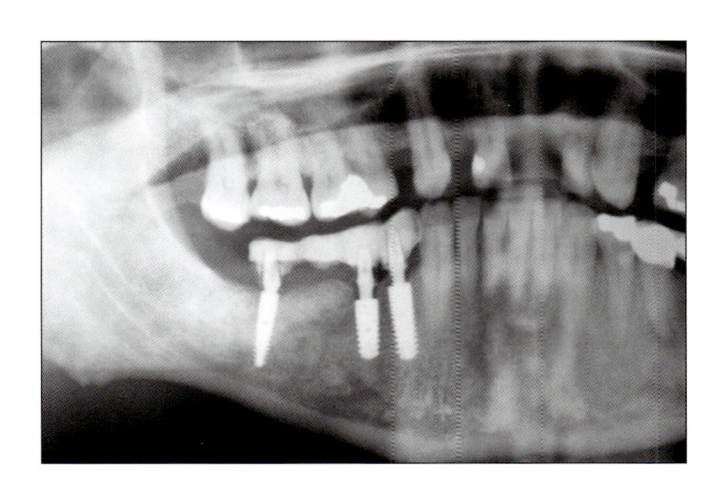

**Fig 8-5e** Radiographic examination performed just after placement of immediately loaded implants. Observe the subcrestal placement of the immediate implants to compensate for crestal bone resorption. (Restoration by S. Shetti, New York, NY.)

# 8 Immediate Loading in Posterior Regions

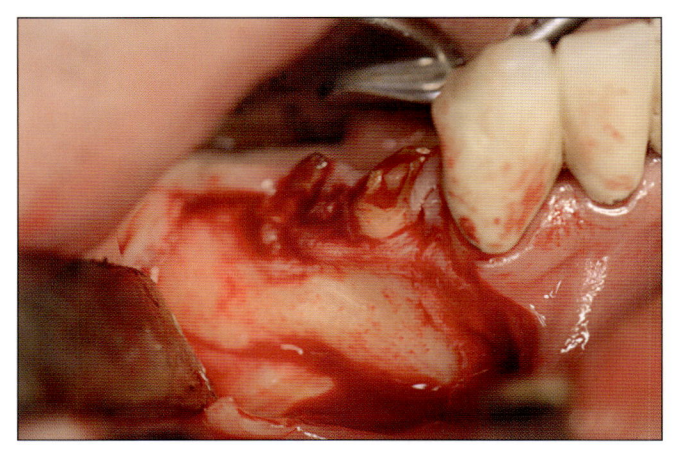

**Fig 8-6a** Remaining roots in the posterior right mandible immediately prior to extraction. Note the preparation of the mental foramen.

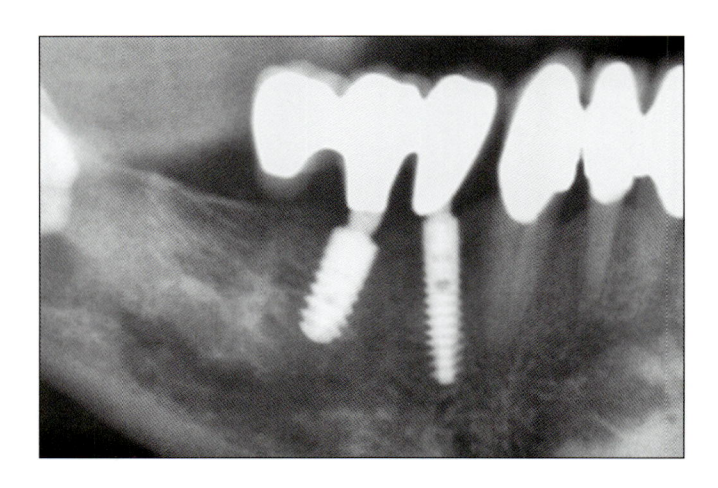

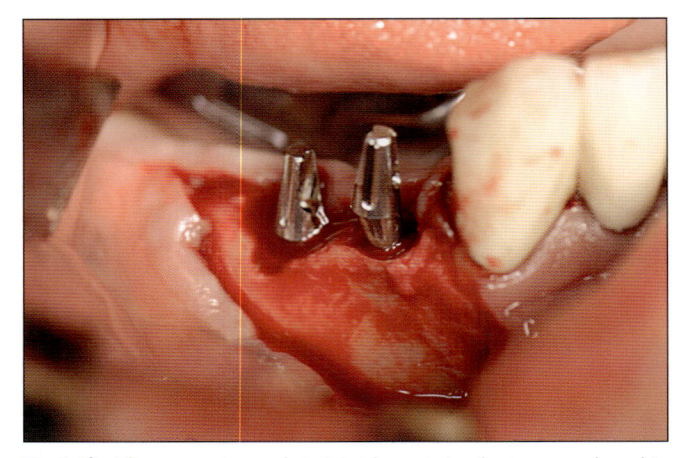

**Fig 8-6b** After extensive socket debridement, implants were placed in the fresh sockets and connected to angulated abutments. To improve primary stability, no tapping was completed.

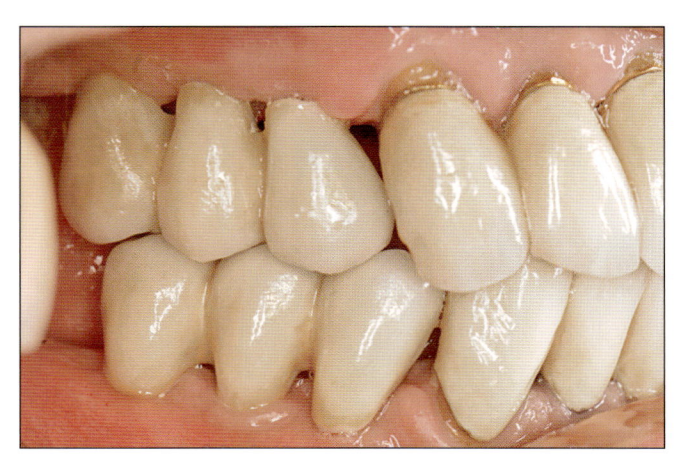

**Fig 8-6c** Follow-up photograph showing right side in occlusion 2 years after immediate loading of the maxillary and mandibular posterior implants.

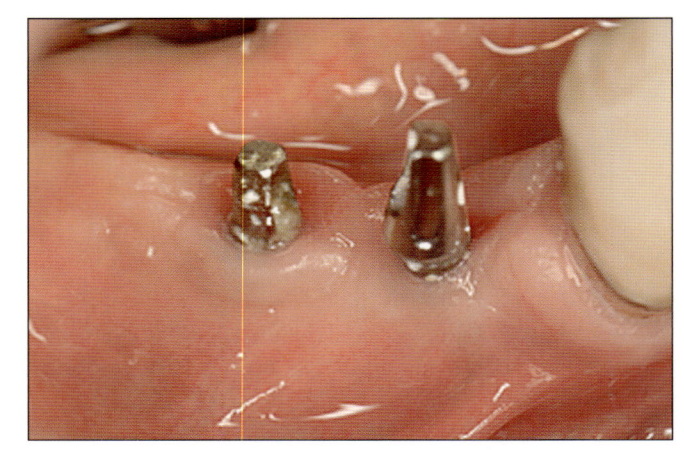

**Fig 8-6d** Peri-implant soft tissues show excellent health (no bleeding on probing or suppuration) immediately after removal of the temporarily cemented definitive prosthesis in the posterior mandible. Implants were stable during the 2-year observation period. The patient was advised to return for frequent professional cleanings to optimize oral hygiene.

**Fig 8-6e** Radiographic evaluation of the peri-implant condition 2 years after immediate loading demonstrating no crestal bone loss and excellent bone growth at the implant interface. Note that the implant connected with the distal cantilever is not associated with crestal bone loss. (Restoration by A. Petre-Veropol, Frankfurt, Germany.)

Posterior Mandible

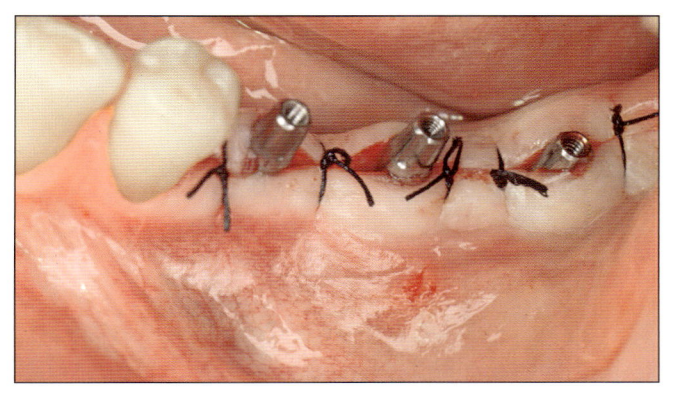

**Fig 8-7a** Implant placement and abutment connection immediately after surgery for immediate loading. (Patient had no history of bruxism at this time.)

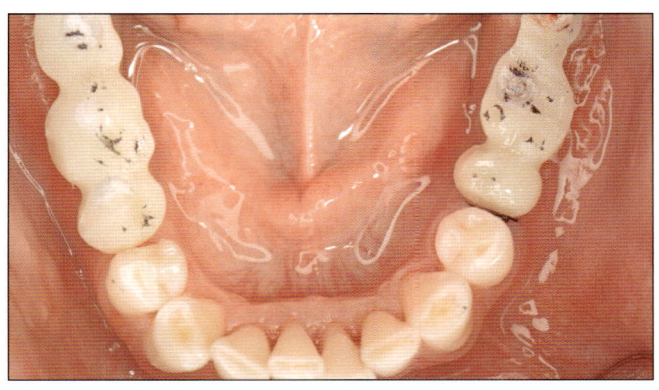

**Fig 8-7b** Occlusal view of the provisional splinted crowns immediately after placement with immediate loading on the left side and delayed loading on the right side.

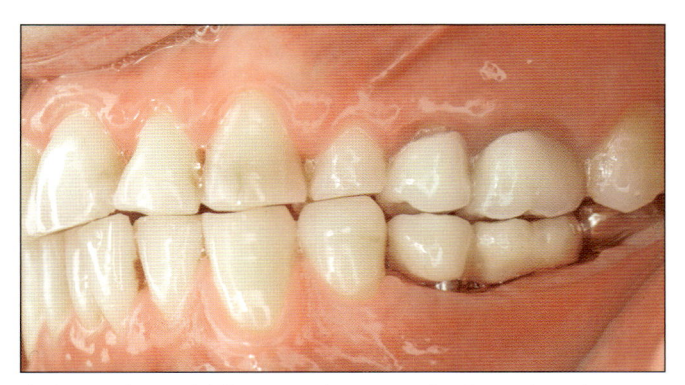

**Fig 8-7c** Delivery of definitive prosthesis 6 weeks after implant placement.

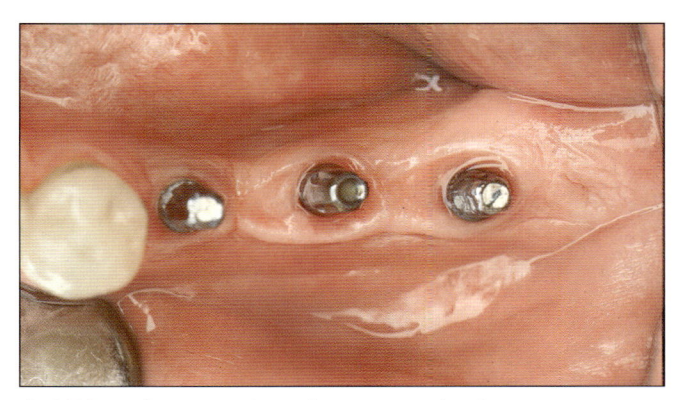

**Fig 8-7d** Excellent peri-implant soft tissues 6 weeks after surgery.

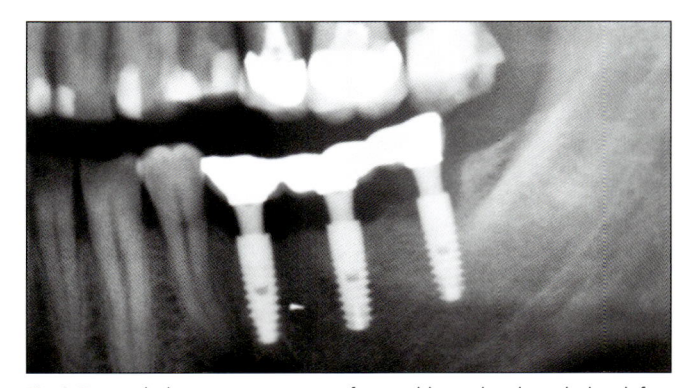

**Fig 8-7e** Radiologic examination of crestal bone levels with the definitive prosthesis in place on immediately loaded implants 6 weeks after surgery.

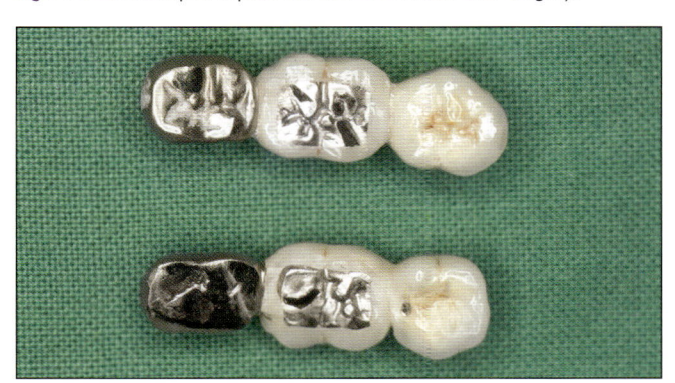

**Fig 8-7f** One year after loading, the final prostheses presented flat occlusal surfaces and holes due to overloading. At that time, the patient was diagnosed as a bruxer. New restorations were fabricated with a stronger metal framework, and a nightguard was applied.

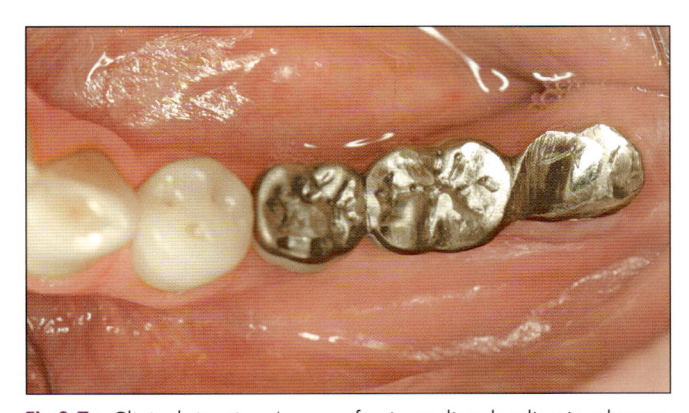

**Fig 8-7g** Clinical situation 4 years after immediate loading in a bruxer. The occlusal surfaces of the teeth and restorations show clear signs of clenching. No mobility was observed in the implants.

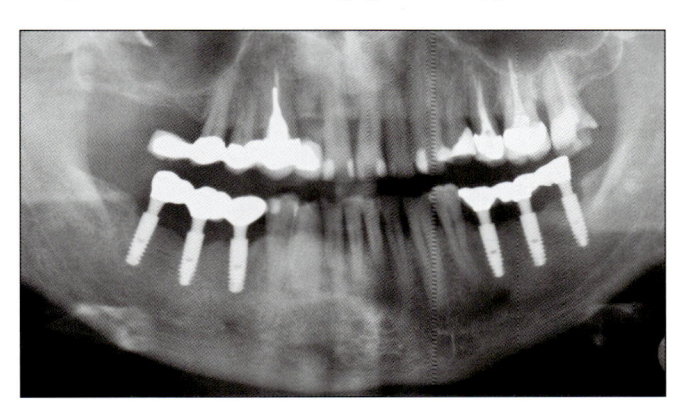

**Fig 8-7h** Radiologic evaluation of the peri-implant bone levels 9 years after loading in a bruxer. The left posterior mandible shows implants that underwent immediate loading and present no crestal bone loss. The right posterior mandible shows implants that underwent delayed loading.

87

## Conclusion

The general requirements for successful immediate functional (occlusal) loading in the posterior part of the jaws are:

- Patients who will comply with recommendations.
- Use of implant systems with high primary stability.
- Use of implants with a tapered design and a rough surface.
- Careful preparation of osteotomy sites without tapping, especially in areas with compromised (poor) bone quality.
- Stabilization of implants by splinting them with a fixed provisional restoration to eliminate possible micromotions, especially in the initial healing stages.
- Replacement of each missing tooth by one implant, if possible.
- Minimization of the loading (masticatory) forces. A soft or liquid diet for the initial stages (first 4 to 6 weeks) of loading is strongly recommended.
- No known history of bruxism or presence of hypertrophic masticatory muscles. They are contraindications for this treatment protocol.
- Avoidance of excessive pull-out forces for removal of the cemented provisional prostheses in the first 6 to 12 weeks of healing; if removal is necessary, screw-type restorations should be used.

## References

1. Bass SL, Triplett RG. The effects of preoperative resorption and jaw anatomy on implant success. A report of 303 cases. Clin Oral Implants Res 1991;2:193–198.
2. Jaffin RA, Kumar A, Berman CL. Immediate loading of implants in partially and fully edentulous jaws: A series of 27 case reports. J Periodontol 2000;71:833–838.
3. Ganeles J, Rosenberg MM, Holt RL, Reichman LH. Immediate loading of implants with fixed restorations in the completely edentulous mandible: Report of 27 patients from a private practice. Int J Oral Maxillofac Implants 2001;16:418–426.
4. Romanos GE. Immediate Loading in the Posterior Area of the Mandible. Animal and Clinical Studies. Berlin: Quintessence, 2005.
5. Romanos GE, Nentwig GH. Immediate versus delayed functional loading of implants in the posterior mandible: A 2-year prospective clinical study of 12 consecutive cases. Int J Periodontics Restorative Dent 2006;26:459–469.
6. Testori T, Bianchi F, Del Fabbro M, Szmukler-Moncler S, Francetti L, Weinstein RL. Immediate non-occlusal loading vs. early loading in partially edentulous patients. Pract Proced Aesthet Dent 2003;15:787–794,796.
7. O'Sullivan D, Sennerby L, Meredith N. Measurements comparing the initial stability of five designs of dental implants: A human cadaver study. Clin Implant Dent Relat Res 2000;2:85–91.
8. Von Wowern N. Variations in bone mass within the cortices of the mandible. Scand J Dent Res 1977;85:444–455.
9. Von Wowern N. Variations in structure within the trabecular bone of the mandible. Scand J Dent Res 1977;85:613–622.
10. Friberg B, Jemt T, Lekholm U. Early failures in 4,641 consecutively placed Brånemark dental implants: A study from stage 1 surgery to the connection of completed prostheses. Int J Oral Maxillofac Implants 1991;6:142–146.
11. Jemt T, Lekholm U. Oral implant treatment in posterior partially edentulous jaws: A 5-year follow-up report. Int J Oral Maxillofac Implants 1993;8:635–640.
12. Esposito M, Hirsch JM, Lekholm U, Thomsen P. Biological factors contributing to failures of osseointegrated oral implants. (II). Etiopathogenesis. Eur J Oral Sci 1988;106:721–764.
13. Hansson HA, Albrektsson T, Brånemark PI. Structural aspects of the interface between tissue and titanium implants. J Prosthet Dent 1983;50:108–113.
14. Rangert B, Krogh B, van Roekel N. Bending overload and implant fracture: A retrospective clinical analysis. Int J Oral Maxillofac Implants 1995;10:326–334.
15. Schnitman PA, Rubenstein JE, Wöhrle PS, DaSilva JD, Koch GG. Implants for partial edentulism. J Dent Educ 1988;52:725–736.
16. DaSilva JD, Wöhrle P, Rubenstein JE, Koch G, Schnitman PA. Four year survival for 137 two-stage implants in partially edentulous patients [abstract 1277]. J Dent Res 1990;69:268.
17. Schnitman PA, Wöhrle PS, Rubenstein JE. Immediate fixed interim prostheses supported by two-stage threaded implants: Methodology and results. J Oral Implantol 1990;16:96–105.
18. Schnitman PA. Brånemark implants loaded with fixed provisional prostheses at fixture placement. Nine-year follow-up. J Oral Implantol 1995;21:235.
19. Tarnow DP, Emtiaz S, Classi A. Immediate loading of threaded implants at stage 1 surgery in edentulous arches: Ten consecutive case reports with 1- to 5-year data. Int J Oral Maxillofac Implants 1997;12:319–324.

# Immediate Loading in Grafted Bone

9

The protocol for immediate loading of dental implants placed in grafted bone is similar to that for immediate loading in natural mature bone. In this chapter, case reports of immediately loaded implants placed after healing in augmented bone are presented, including the long-term results of this protocol. Whether resorption of the augmented bone is reduced under loading conditions is a topic for further research. Histologic and histomorphometric analyses should be done to demonstrate bone remodeling in loading conditions and to measure the bone resorption characteristics. This topic may be of clinical import in trying to control the resorption phenomenon in areas requiring vertical augmentations especially in the posterior mandible. This remains a challenging issue in modern implant dentistry.

## Case Reports

### Case 1: Immediate loading in the maxilla after horizontal augmentation with a corticocancellous block

A 50-year-old man presented for rehabilitation of the maxilla. The maxillary canines were periodontally involved and showed grade III mobility (Fig 9-1a). In addition, a very deep periodontal pocket with vertical bony destruction was found radiographically at the left maxillary canine area, and very deep periodontal infrabony defects were found at the right mandibular first and second molars. The prognosis of these teeth was questionable.

After extraction of the maxillary canines and healing of the sockets (Fig 9-1b), the defect at the maxillary left lateral incisor to first premolar sites was covered with a corticocancellous onlay bone block from the left ramus site and fixed with two osteosynthesis screws (Fig 9-1c). At the same visit, a periodontal flap procedure at the mandibular right first and second molars was performed using an autogenous bone graft from the left side donor site in order to retain these teeth for as long as possible. Four months after healing, the bone condition was evaluated radiographically (Fig 9-1d), and six Ankylos implants (Dentsply Friadent) were placed in the maxilla using a prosthetic guide in the maxillary right first premolar to lateral incisor and left canine to second premolar sites. Finally, the osteosynthesis screws and the implant cover screws were removed, and the final abutments were placed with a 15-degree angulation. The abutments were fixed with a final torque of 15 Ncm, according to the manufacturer protocol (Fig 9-1e). A higher torque is not necessary with this implant system because of its Morse taper (and therefore rigid) implant-abutment connection. This system is preferable to other implant systems necessitating higher torques, which sometimes cannot be used because of weak bone quality. The abutments were covered with temporary resin caps, and the flap was closed using 4-0 silk suture material (Fig 9-1f).

## 9 | Immediate Loading in Grafted Bone

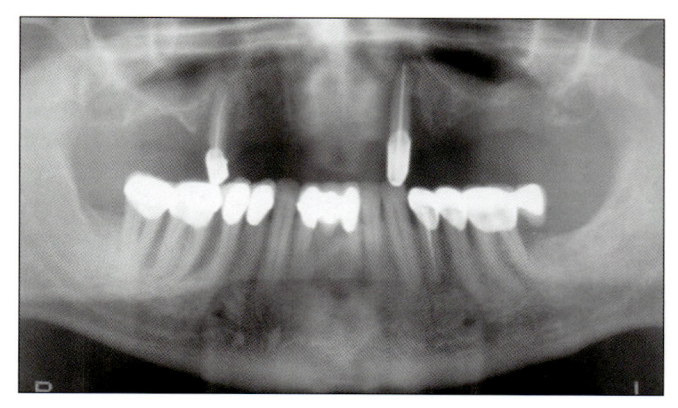

**Fig 9-1a** Radiographic examination presenting advanced periodontal destruction in the maxilla. The remaining maxillary teeth are hopeless.

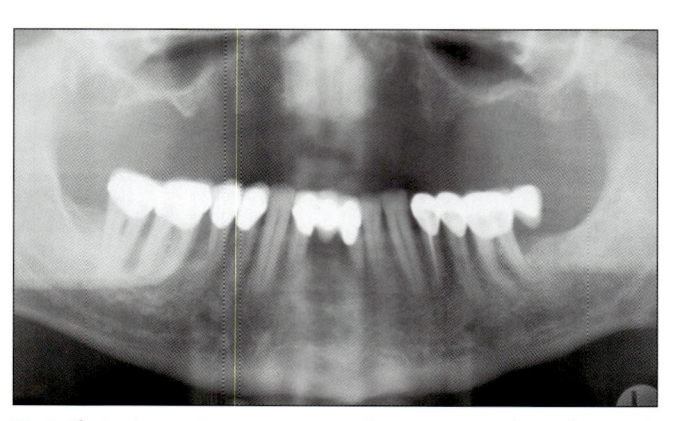

**Fig 9-1b** Radiographic examination after extraction of maxillary teeth and 4 months of healing of the sockets.

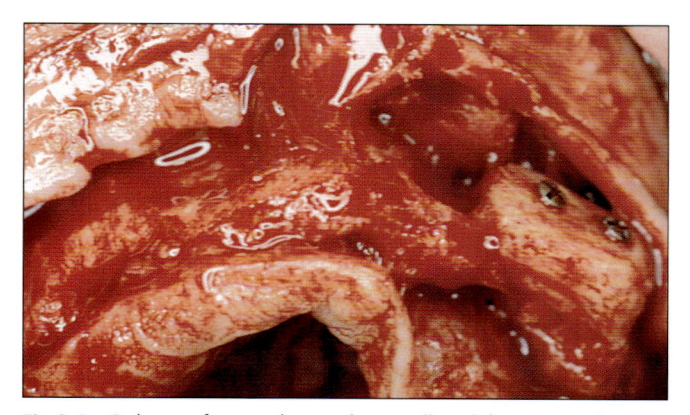

**Fig 9-1c** Onlay graft procedure at the maxillary left canine to first premolar area using a corticocancellous block from the left retromolar site (ramus).

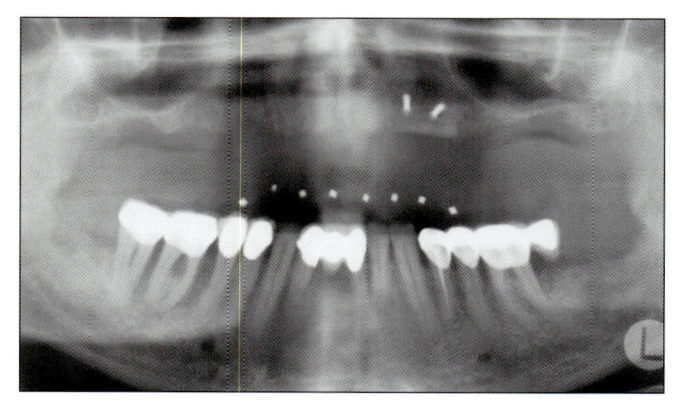

**Fig 9-1d** Radiographic examination 4 months after the grafting procedure presenting excellent integration of the corticocancellous bone graft in the left maxilla.

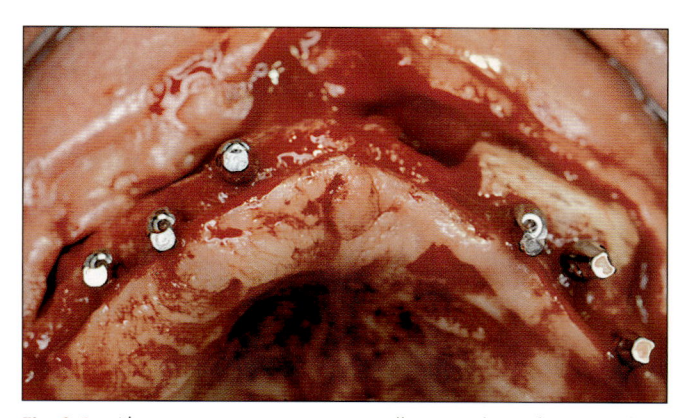

**Fig 9-1e** Abutment connection in maxillary implants for immediate loading using 15 Ncm final torque.

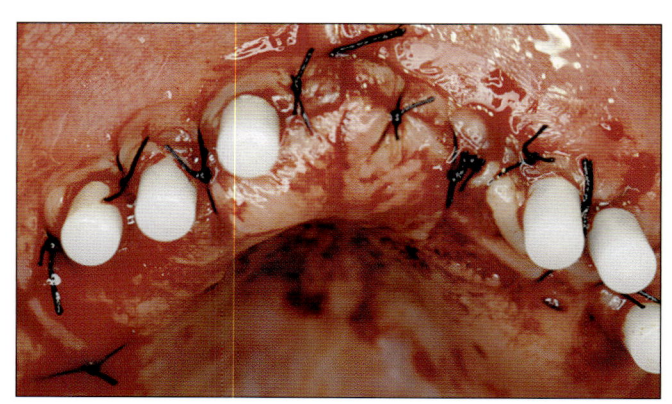

**Fig 9-1f** Flap closure and placement of resin caps for chairside fabrication of provisional restoration.

Case Reports

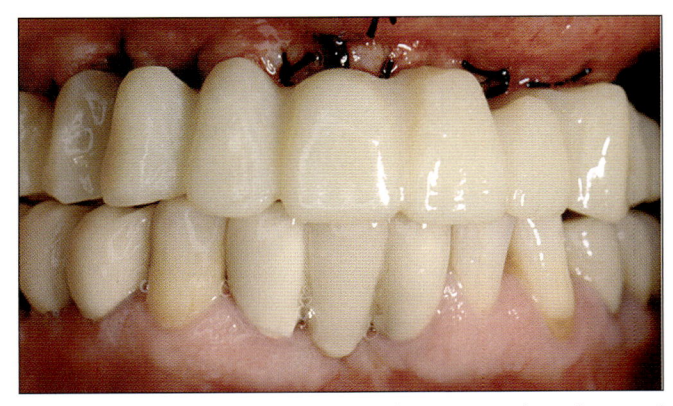

**Fig 9-1g** Provisional restoration in occlusion (immediate functional loading) after surgery using the OST protocol.

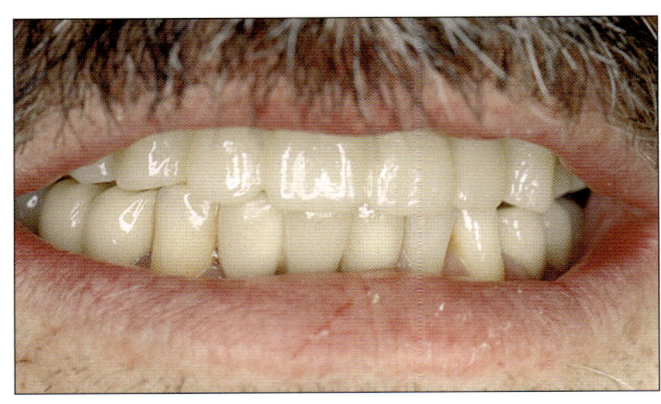

**Fig 9-1h** Moderate smile line after implant placement and immediate functional loading with provisional prosthesis demonstrating a successful esthetic result.

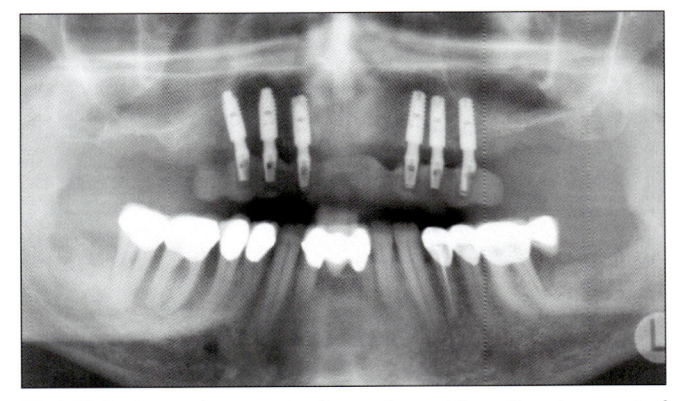

**Fig 9-1i** Radiographic examination performed just after placement of immediately loaded implants in the maxilla with the provisional restoration in place.

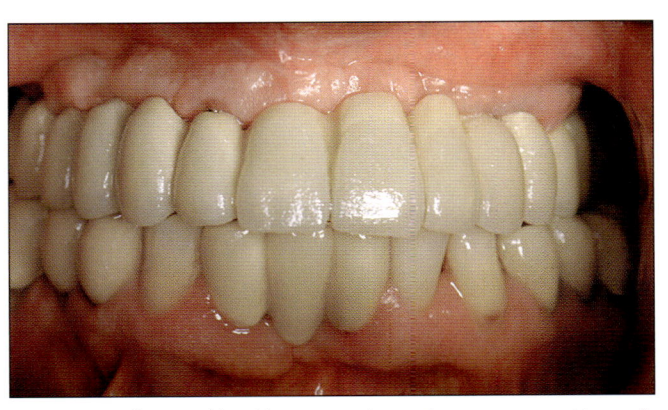

**Fig 9-1j** Excellent and healthy peri-implant soft tissues around immediately loaded implants in the maxilla (at 2-year follow-up).

## Provisional restoration: The Omnivac shell technique

The Omnivac shell technique (OST) was used to fabricate a provisional restoration, which was fixed in place with TempBond (Kerr). The author introduced the OST at the end of the 1990s and published about it in 2003.[1]

With the OST, the implants are splinted together rigidly and the esthetic results are pleasing. The greatest advantage of this technique is that the provisional restoration for cemented partial dentures can be fabricated more quickly than with other techniques. In addition, there is no need for additional materials, and there is a low risk of the restoration locking in the undercuts. When using OST provisionalization, the Omnivac shell with the autopolymerizing resin must be removed before it completely hardens (less than 1 minute) in order to avoid setting the sutures in the resin material. Although there are many different resin materials, the author strongly recommends ProTemp (Espe) because it provides long-term stability and limits micromovements at the implant-abutment interface.

In cases of maxillary provisionalization, the Omnivac shell must cover the entire palatal aspect of the maxilla. The shell is stabilized in the center of the maxilla and maintains the vertical dimension while the resin hardens.

The occlusion was checked for adequate occlusal contacts in intercuspal position as well as group contacts in the lateral mandibular movements (Figs 9-1g and 9-1h). A panoramic radiograph was taken immediately after surgery with the provisional restoration in place to determine the bone level at baseline (Fig 9-1i).

The definitive fixed prosthesis was fabricated from impressions taken 4 to 6 weeks after surgery and fixed with temporary cement material. Three distal cantilevers were fabricated on the right side and two on the left side of the mandible to completely restore the patient's dentition. The patient was advised to replace the anterior mandibular partial denture to improve esthetics, but he rejected the suggestion for financial reasons. Therefore, the shape and color of the maxillary restoration were made to match the mandibular fixed partial denture.

One year after loading, the prosthesis was removed and the implants evaluated for stability. Periodontal clinical indices were performed and showed excellent soft tissue health without bleeding. Radiographs revealed no bone loss around any of the implants. The density of the bone around the implants placed in the augmented area (the maxillary left lateral incisor through first premolar sites) had increased because of the loading forces (dynamic remodeling) applied at the implant-bone interface. Two years after loading (Fig 9-1j) the bone level was

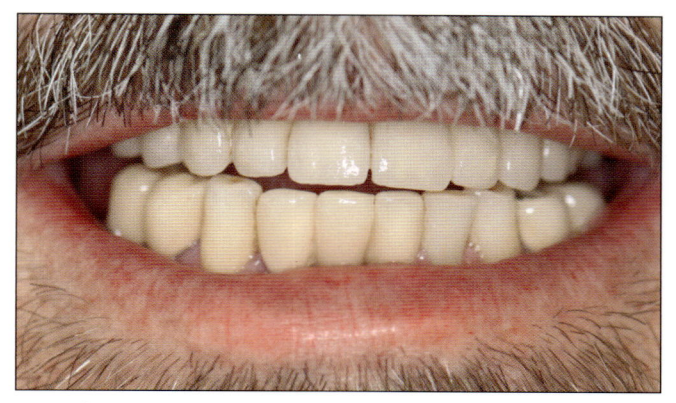

**Fig 9-1k** Excellent clinical result 7 years after immediate loading in the maxilla.

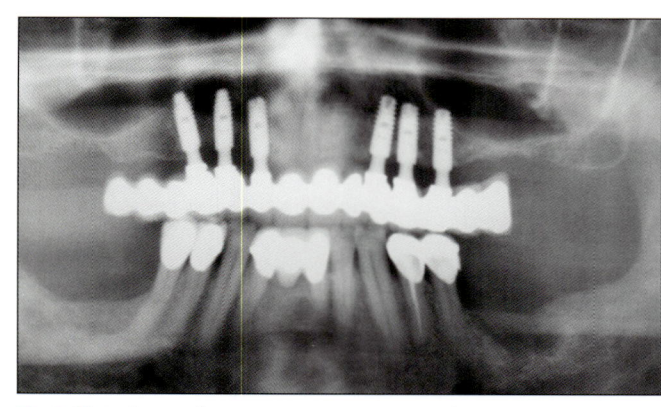

**Fig 9-1l** Radiographic examination 7 years after immediate loading presenting excellent consolidation of the bone at the maxillary site of augmentation.

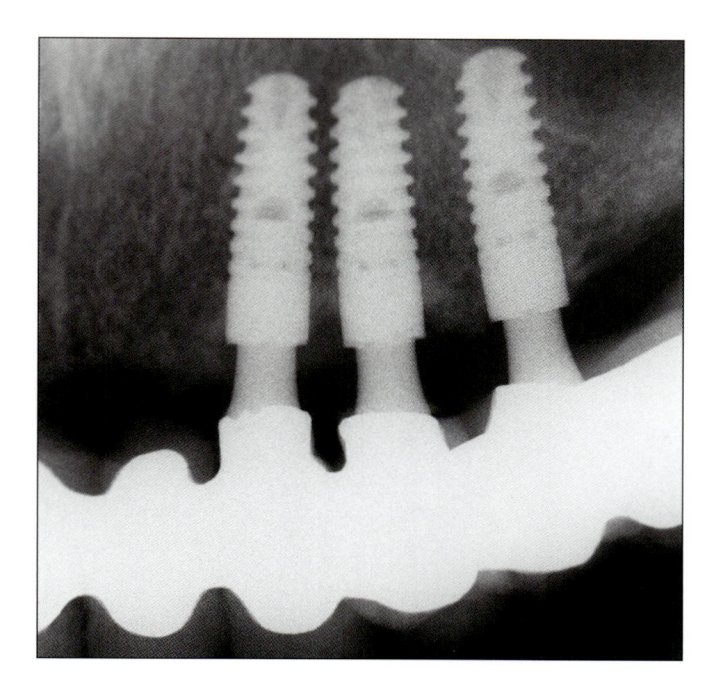

**Fig 9-1m** Periapical radiograph 7 years after loading presenting no differences in the peri-implant crestal bone levels over the entire observation period.

stable and showed no clinical or radiographic signs of resorption. All implants were clinically stable after removal of the restoration, and the soft tissues were healthy.

In addition, newly mineralized bone was evident radiographically at the sites of augmented periodontal tissues at the mandibular right first and second molars when compared with the initial periodontal condition. This is likely because of the loading forces from the distal cantilevers in the maxillary partial denture. These teeth presented some periodontal breakdown 6 years after treatment because the patient was not compliant with periodontal recall appointments. The final clinical and radiographic result after 7 years of loading showed no crestal bone loss around any of the implants (Figs 9-1k to 9-1m).

## Case 2: Immediate loading in the mandible after advanced lateral and vertical augmentation

A woman with advanced bilateral bone resorption in the posterior mandible was interested in fixed mandibular restorations without the removal of her anterior mandibular teeth. Full restoration of the mandible was undertaken, although only the treatment of the mandibular left posterior site is presented here.

The clinical and radiographic examination showed advanced resorption (between 5 and 13 mm) in the posterior mandible (Figs 9-2a to 9-2d). Local anesthesia was administered, and an advanced mucoperiosteal flap

Case Reports

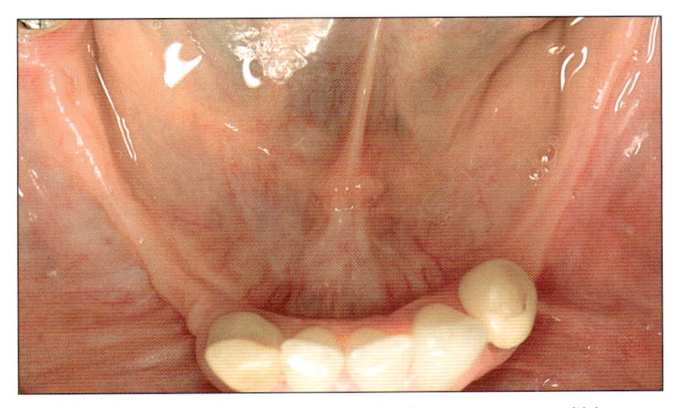

Fig 9-2a Extensive bilateral resorption in the posterior mandible.

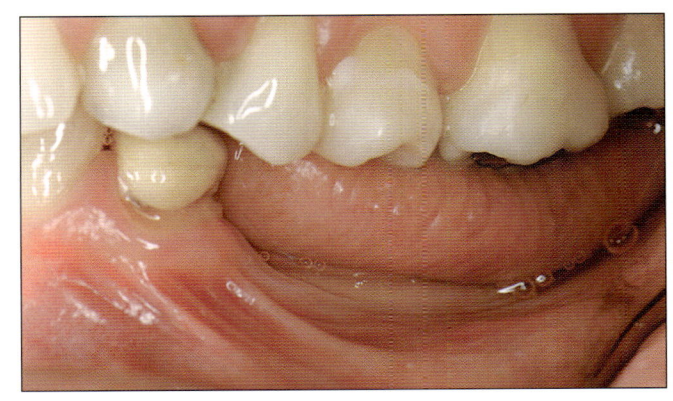

Fig 9-2b Lateral view before augmentation.

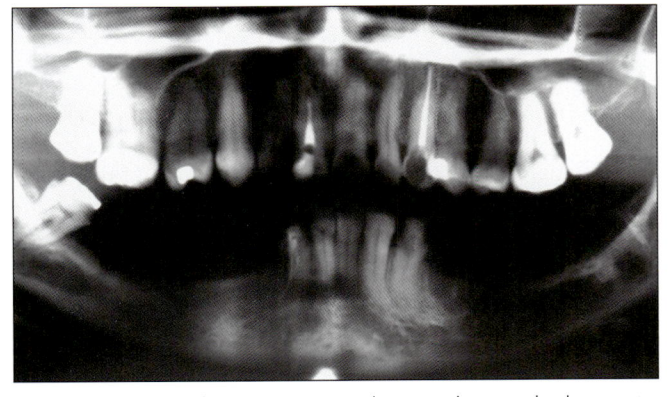

Fig 9-2c Radiographic examination showing the resorbed posterior mandible.

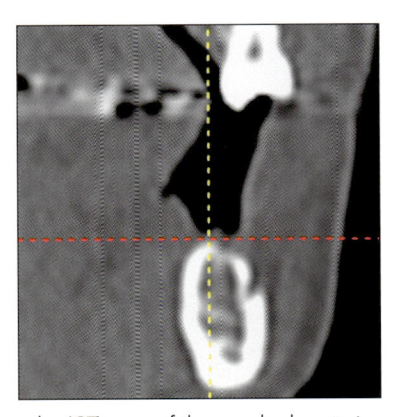

Fig 9-2d Computerized tomography (CT) scan of the resorbed posterior mandible.

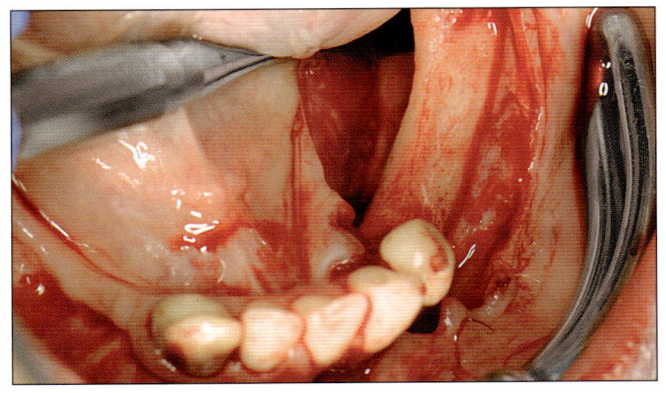

Fig 9-2e Mucoperiosteal flap elevation for augmentation in the posterior mandible. Observe the extensive flap elevation and lingual nerve preservation.

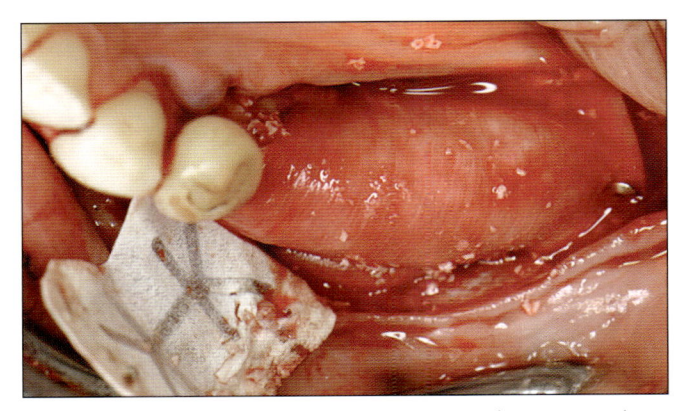

Fig 9-2f Augmentation with cancellous Bio-Oss and autogenous bone graft from the ramus covered with an absorbable collagen membrane.

was elevated (buccally and lingually) (Fig 9-2e). After decortication, vertical and horizontal bone augmentation was undertaken with placement of particulate autogenous bone (from the posterior mandible) in combination with large-particle cancellous Bio-Oss (Geistlich) for guided bone regeneration (GBR). The augmentation material was condensed sufficiently in the areas of decortication. The size of the defect was bigger than the largest size of the titanium-reinforced Gore-Tex regenerative membrane (W. L. Gore). The grafted site was covered with an absorbable Biomend Extend membrane (Zimmer) and fixed in place under tension lingually and buccally with bone tacks (ACE) (Fig 9-2f). A second Gore-Tex membrane was used to support the entire augmented site in the area of the mandibular left second premolar and first molar (Fig 9-2g). The membrane was also immobilized via tacks. Flap advancement with periosteal releasing incisions was performed to close the flap without tension[2] (Figs 9-2h

93

## 9 | Immediate Loading in Grafted Bone

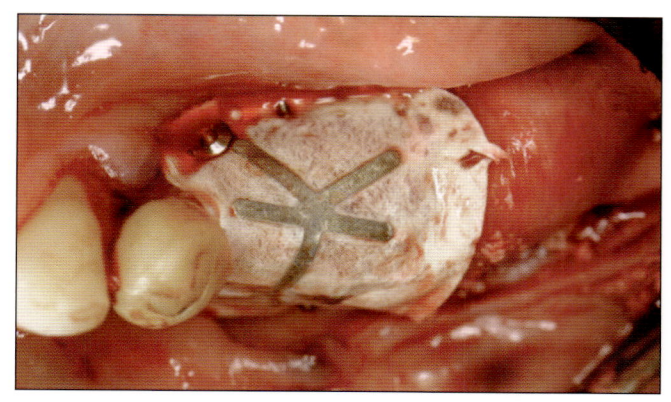

**Fig 9-2g** Augmentation material covered by a collagen membrane and a titanium-reinforced Gore-Tex membrane for better stabilization of the graft. Both membranes were fixed with titanium pins on the buccal and lingual sides of the mandible. Special care was taken with the mental nerve.

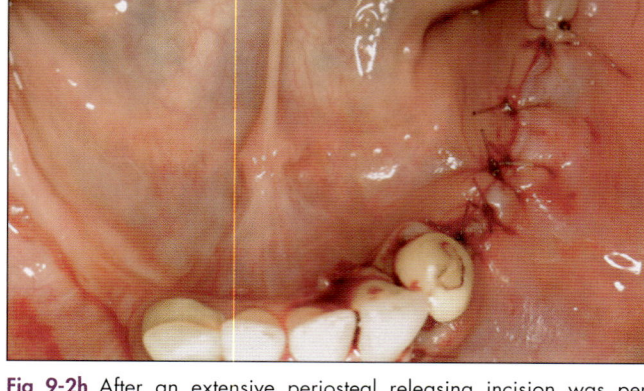

**Fig 9-2h** After an extensive periosteal releasing incision was performed, the augmentation site was completely covered and sutured using chromic gut.

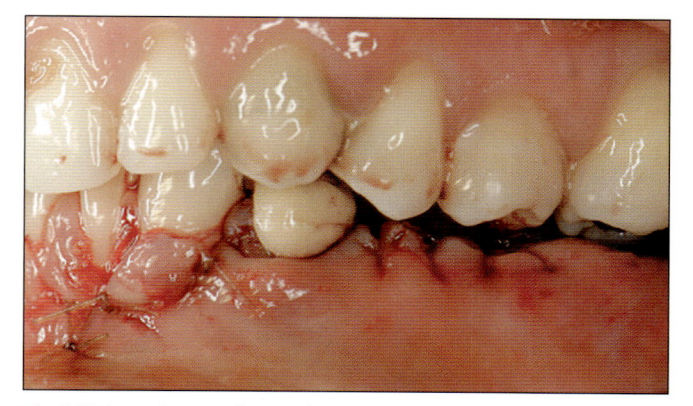

**Fig 9-2i** Lateral view of sutured augmentation site.

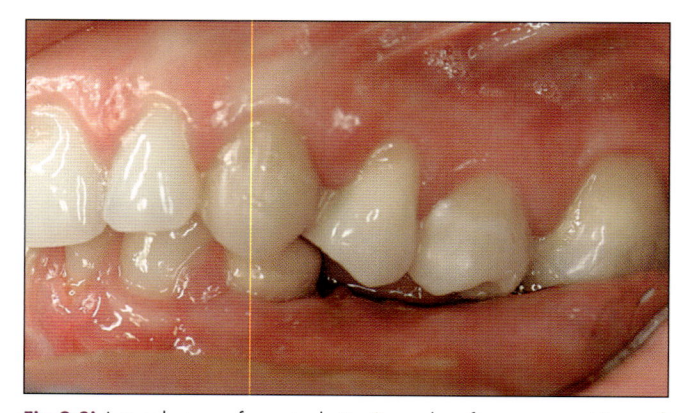

**Fig 9-2j** Lateral view of surgical site 2 weeks after surgery. No graft exposure, flap dehiscence, or other complications were observed.

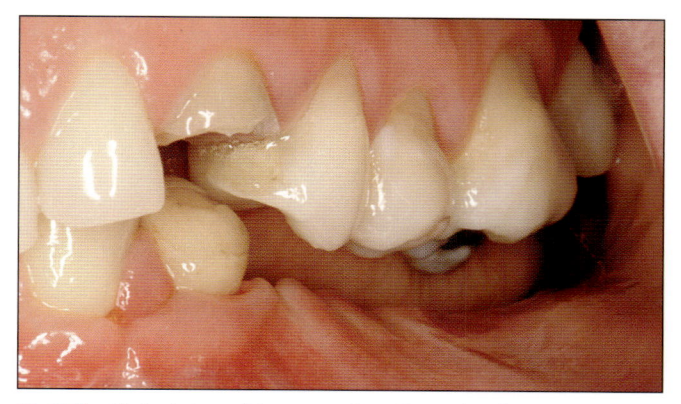

**Fig 9-2k** Clinical view of the surgical site 7 months after surgery. Some vertical resorption of the augmentation is evident. Note the good intraocclusal distance. (The broken maxillary left canine was restored immediately [see Fig 9-2r].)

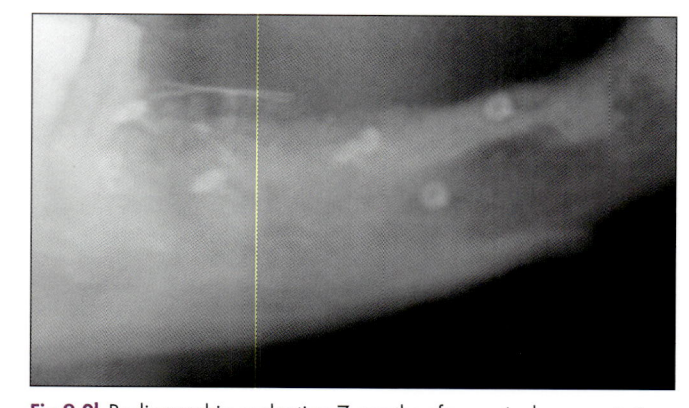

**Fig 9-2l** Radiographic evaluation 7 months after vertical augmentation.

and 9-2i). Postoperative pain medication and sufficient antibiotic coverage was prescribed for the first 10 days after surgery. Chlorhexidine digluconate mouthrinse was used for decontamination of the surgical site, and irrigation with saltwater supported the healing. During the healing period, the patient did not use a partial prosthesis in the posterior mandible.

The healing of the patient was observed weekly for the first month after surgery and then once per month thereafter. Two months after surgery, the soft tissue was healed completely without any type of exposure of the grafting material. The intraocclusal distance was filled with the grafting material and the soft tissues (Fig 9-2j). Seven months after surgery, vertical resorption was observed (Fig 9-2k), and the intraocclusal distance was correct for implant placement. Radiographically, the augmented area did not show any resorption activity (Fig 9-2l).

A flap was elevated very gently (Fig 9-2m), and Ankylos Plus implants (Dentsply Friadent) with lengths of 14 and 11 mm (3.5-mm diameter) were placed in mandibular left second premolar and first molar sites,

# Case Reports

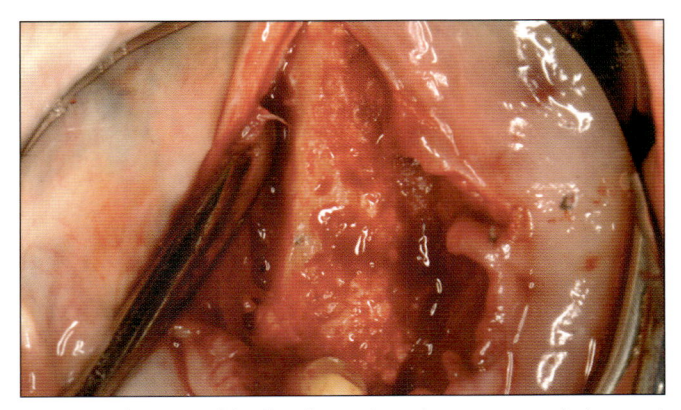

**Fig 9-2m** Elevation of the flap for implant placement reveals the excellent condition of the graft in the horizontal and vertical directions. Note the angiogenesis in the grafted bone indicated by good bleeding.

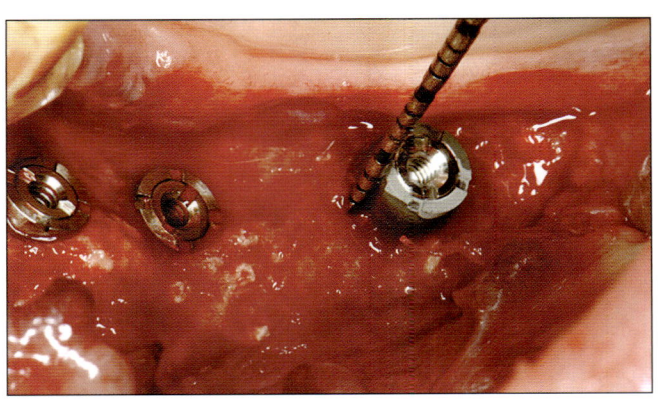

**Fig 9-2n** Implant placement in augmented bone. The distal implant was exposed in the cervical part; therefore, a new augmentation was planned.

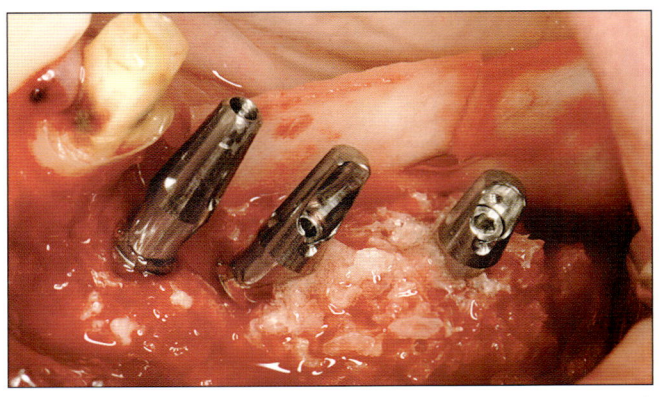

**Fig 9-2o** Augmentation of cervical area of the distal implant with grafting material (Bio-Oss) before coverage with a collagen membrane (Bio-Gide).

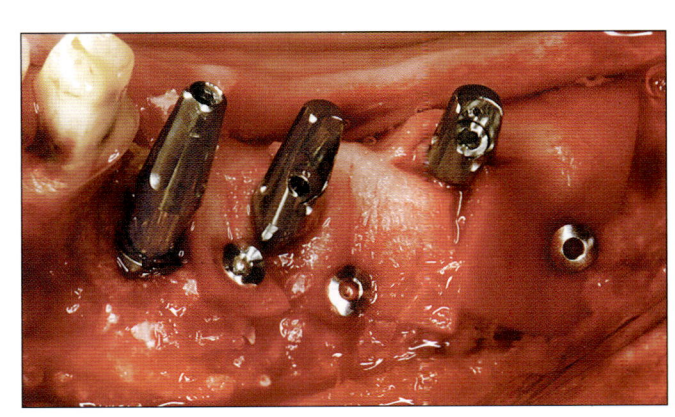

**Fig 9-2p** Fixation of the collagen membrane with titanium pins.

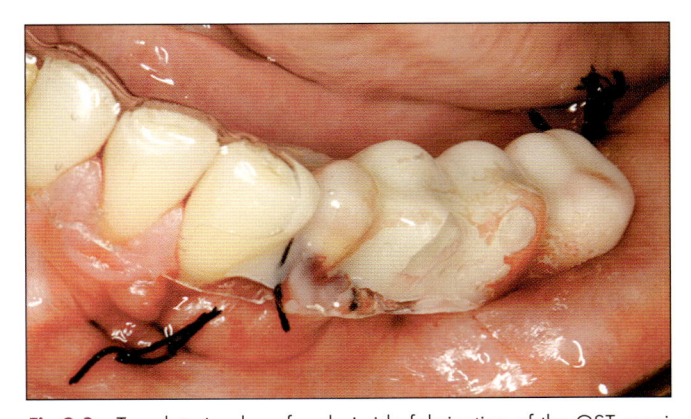

**Fig 9-2q** Template in place for chairside fabrication of the OST provisional restoration.

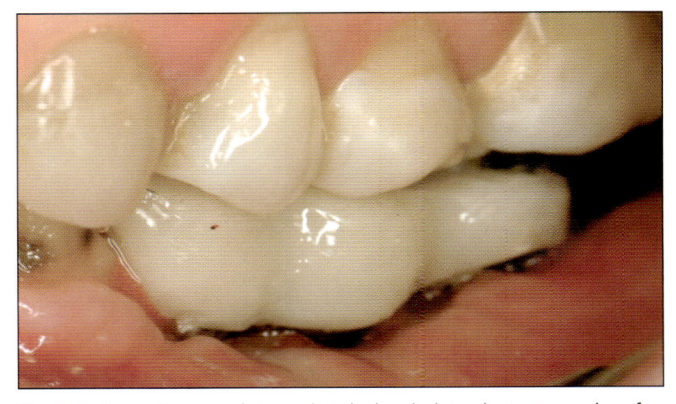

**Fig 9-2r** Lateral view of immediately loaded implants 2 weeks after surgery.

respectively (Fig 9-2n). In the mandibular left second molar site, the implant placed had a length of 9.5 mm with supracrestal placement (3 mm). The supracrestal area was augmented circumferentially with pure cancellous Bio-Oss. The abutments were connected to the implants, and an additional absorbable membrane was fixed around the distal implant to support the new grafting material (Figs 9-2o and 9-2p). The flap was closed with silk sutures, and a provisional restoration was performed using the OST protocol and cemented in place to maintain occlusal contacts for immediate functional loading (Figs 9-2q and 9-2r). The implant position and crestal bone levels were evaluated radiographically after surgery (Fig 9-2s). A soft/liquid diet was recommended for 3 to 4 months. Healing was uneventful.

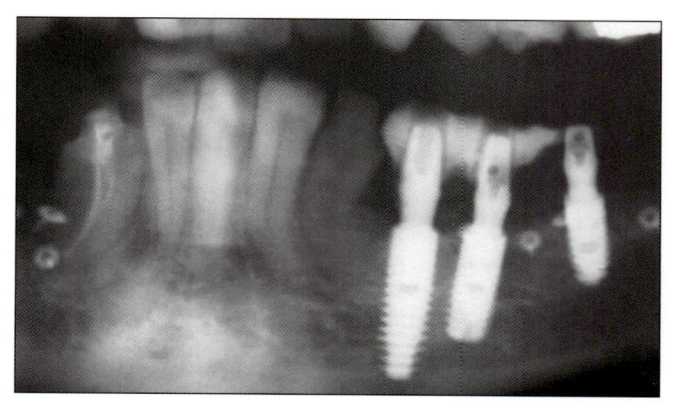

**Fig 9-2s** Radiographic examination immediately after implant placement and loading with the provisional restoration in place.

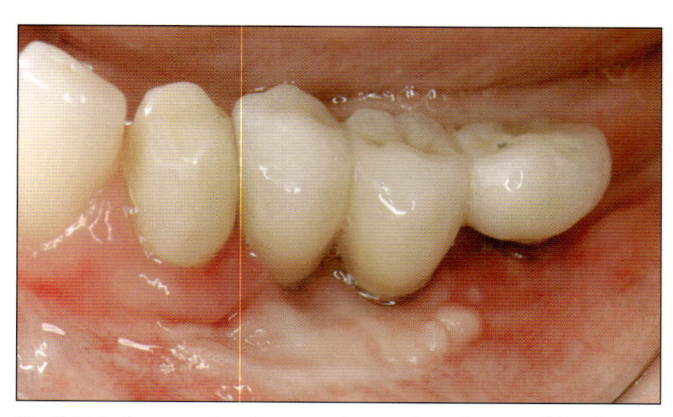

**Fig 9-2t** Follow-up after 2 years of immediate functional loading. A free gingival graft completed after 1 year of loading increased the width of keratinized mucosa.

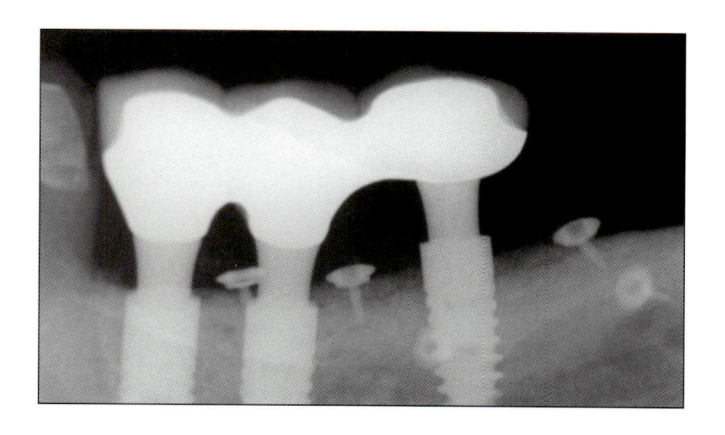

**Fig 9-2u** Radiographic examination 2 years after immediate functional loading presenting increased bone density in the crestal bone (dynamic remodeling). Note the bone loss around the distal implant from insufficient remodeling of the Bio-Oss grafting material. An autogenous bone graft should be used at the second augmentation around the mandibular second molar area.

After 1 year of functional loading, a free gingival graft was completed to increase the keratinized mucosa (Fig 9-2t). At the 2-year follow-up, dynamic remodeling was visible in the radiographic examination with increased bone density in the crestal bone (Fig 9-2u). Bone loss around the distal implant indicated insufficient remodeling of the grafting material used. A composite bone graft with autogenous bone should have been used in this case.

## Case 3: Immediate loading in the maxilla after advanced lateral and vertical augmentation

The following case presents a treatment for a 60-year-old woman who presented with an edentulous maxilla. Advanced augmentative procedures in the maxilla with lateral alveolar ridge augmentation on both sides and a sinus elevation on the left side were performed using particulate autogenous bone from the ramus mixed with Puros human allograft (Zimmer) (Figs 9-3a to 9-3h).

Six months after augmentation, significant gain in alveolar ridge height and width was evident (Figs 9-3i and 9-3j). Bone Level implants (Straumann) with high primary stability were placed and loaded immediately after surgery with a screw-retained, implant-supported hybrid restoration. The implants were connected initially with their multibase abutments, and temporary cylinders were connected for the fabrication of the provisional prosthesis (Figs 9-3k to 9-3n). The patient was advised to follow a soft/liquid diet for the initial 3-month healing period to avoid problems with the osseointegration. The final restoration was delivered 1.5 years after loading because of patient rescheduling (Figs 9-3o to 9-3r).

Case Reports

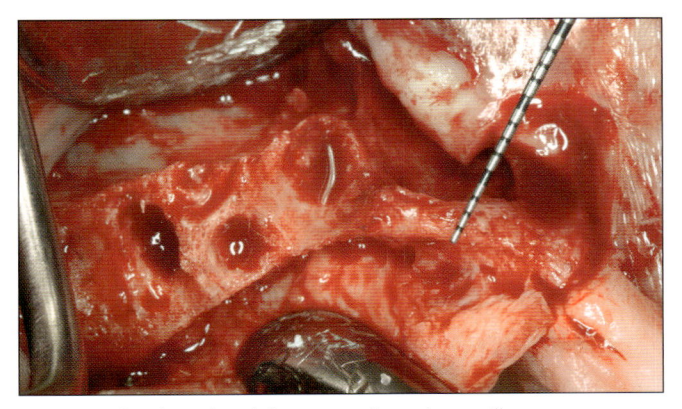

**Fig 9-3a** Alveolar ridge deficiency in the right maxilla.

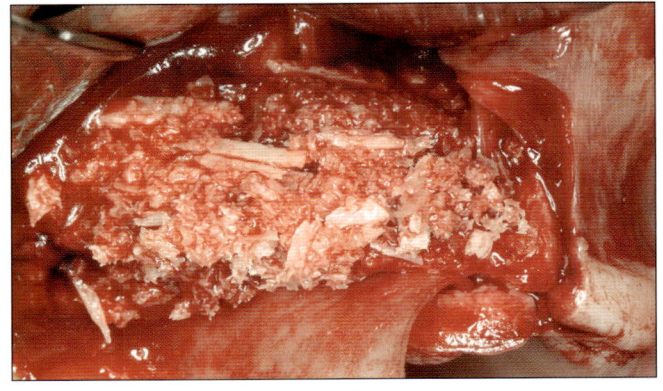

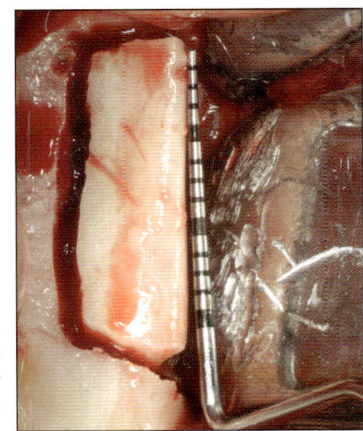

**Fig 9-3b** Corticocancellous bone block from the left ramus harvested for the augmentation in the maxilla.

**Fig 9-3c** Augmentation using particulate autogenous bone and Puros human allograft.

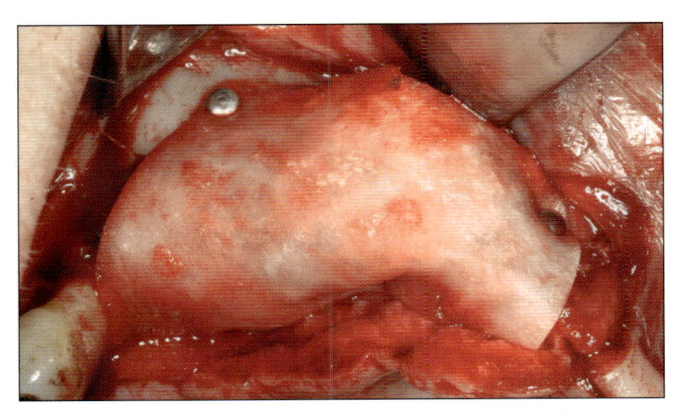

**Fig 9-3d** Coverage of the right maxilla with an absorbable Biomend Extend membrane.

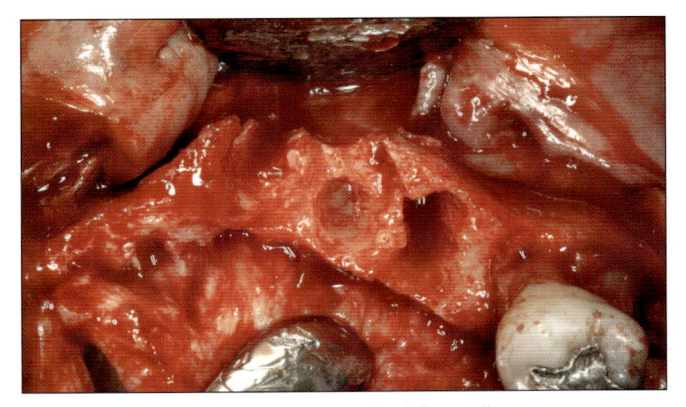

**Fig 9-3e** Alveolar ridge deficiency in the left maxilla.

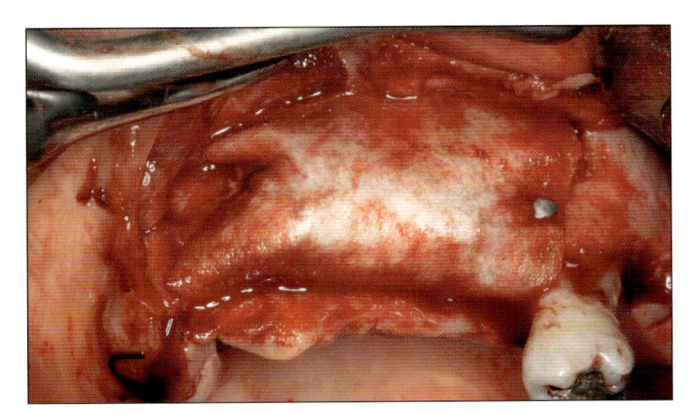

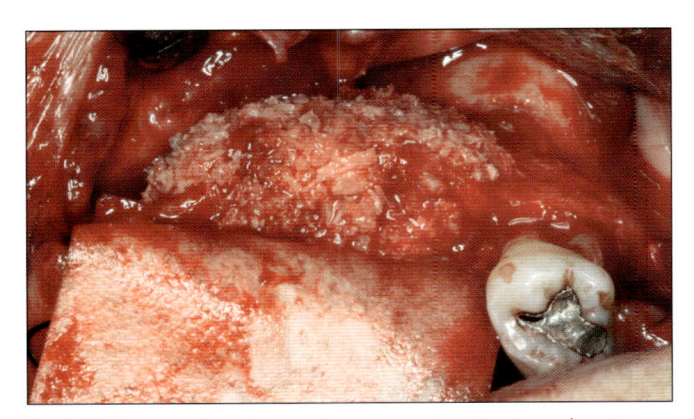

**Fig 9-3f** Horizontal and vertical augmentation via sinus elevation using particulate autogenous bone and Puros human allograft.

**Fig 9-3g** Coverage of the left maxilla with an absorbable Biomend Extend membrane.

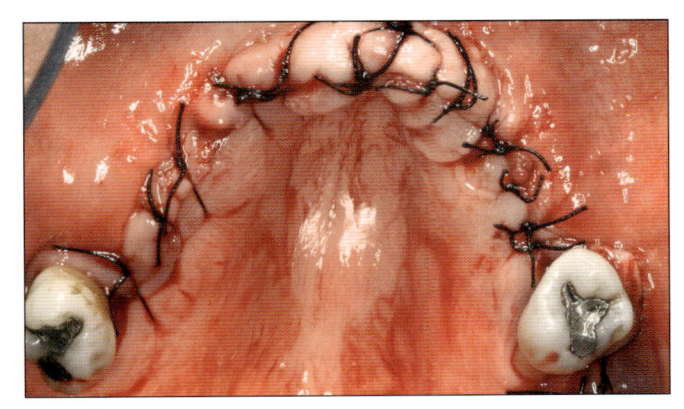

**Fig 9-3h** Flap advancement and primary closure.

97

## 9 | Immediate Loading in Grafted Bone

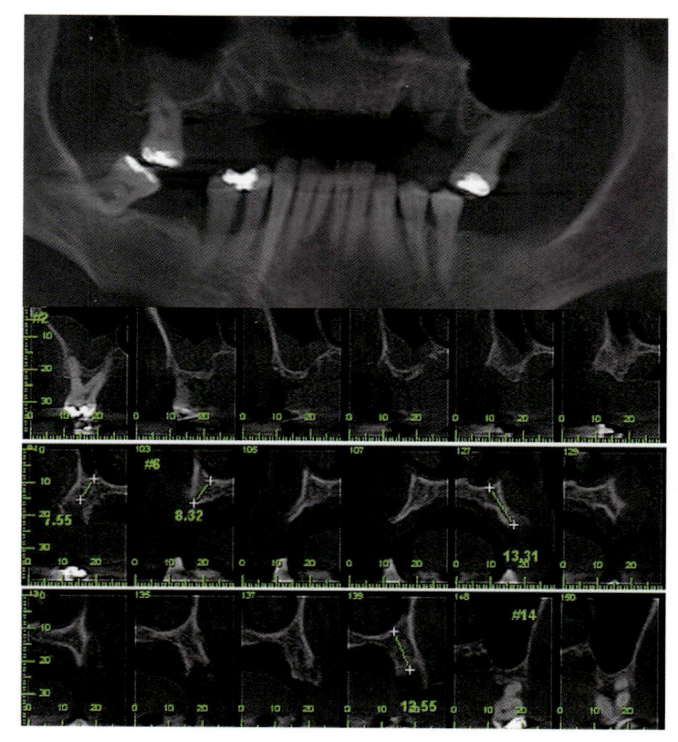

**Fig 9-3i** Cone beam computed tomography (CBCT) scan before augmentation.

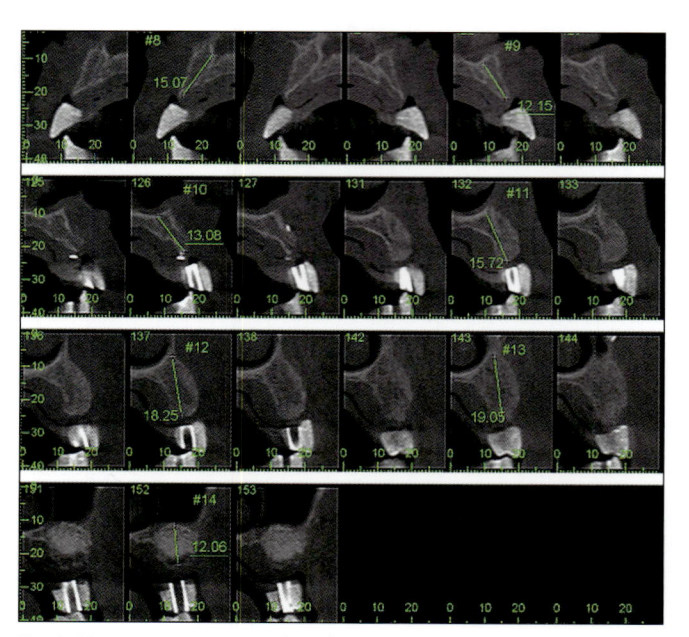

**Fig 9-3j** CBCT scan 6 months after grafting showing the significant gain in alveolar ridge height and width.

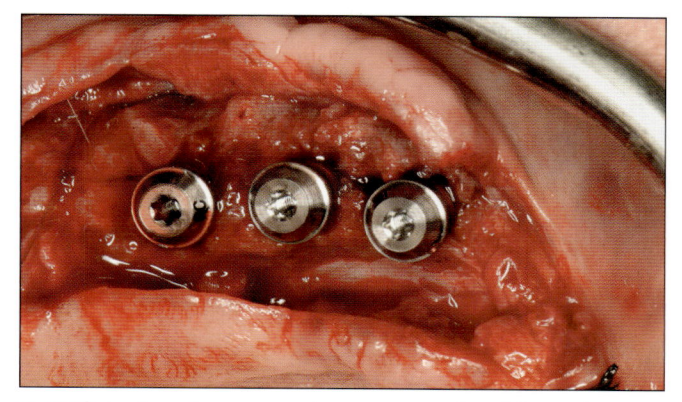

**Fig 9-3k** Implant placement and connection with multibase abutments for immediate loading. Note the excellent bone quality.

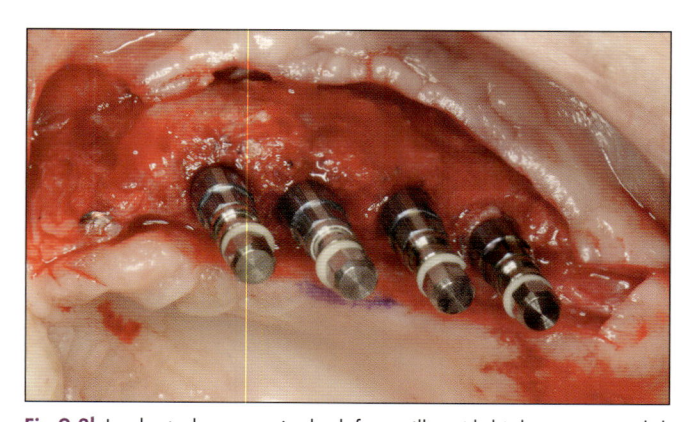

**Fig 9-3l** Implant placement in the left maxilla with high primary stability. Note the excellent bone quality.

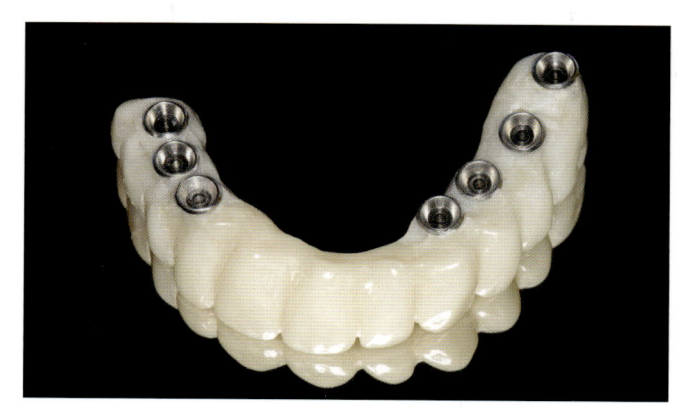

**Fig 9-3m** Provisional restoration for immediate loading.

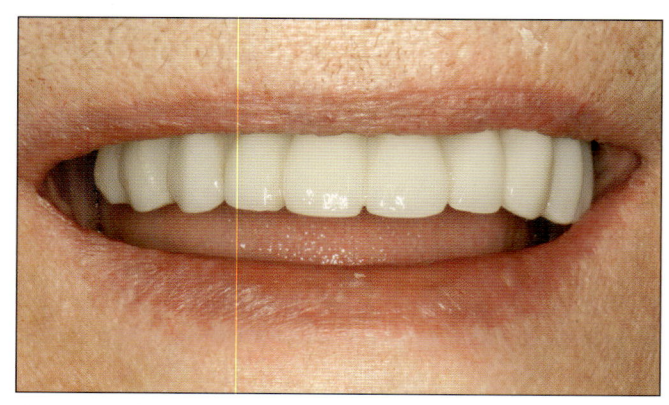

**Fig 9-3n** Smile line of the patient immediately after surgery with a screw-retained provisional prosthesis.

Case Reports

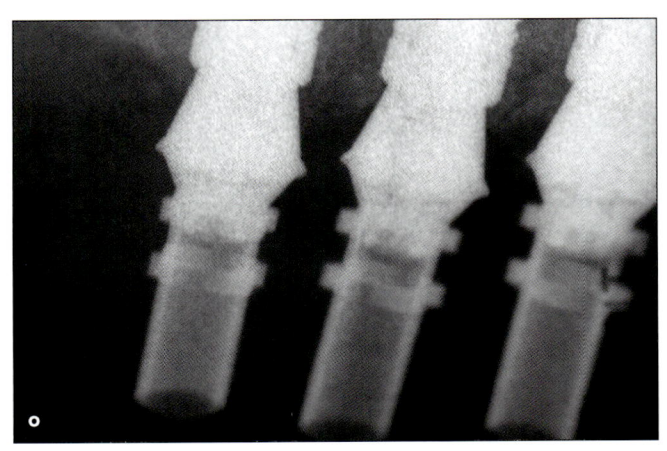

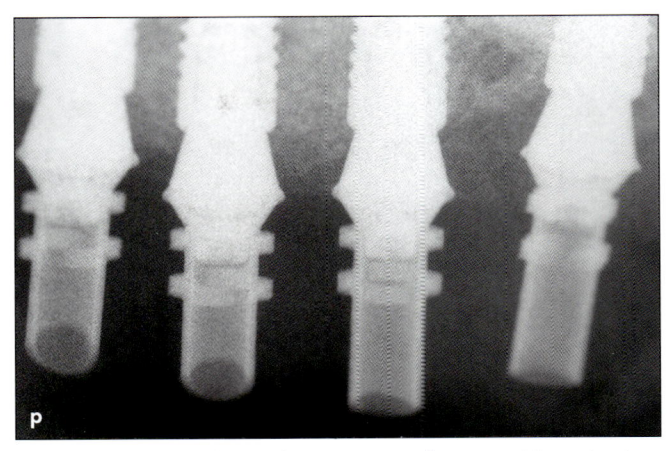

**Figs 9-3o and 9-3p** One year after immediate loading, right-side (o) and left-side (p) periapical radiographs present excellent crestal bone levels.

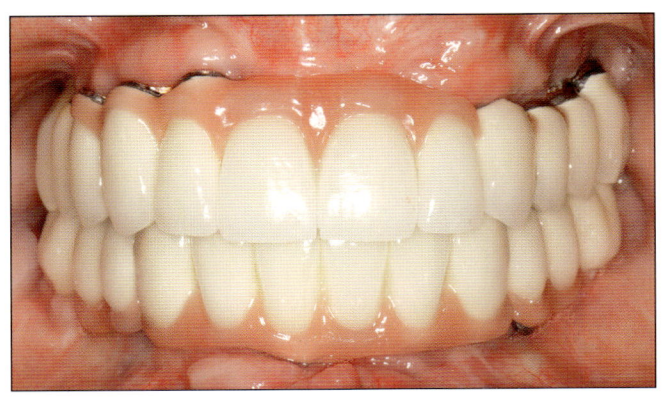

**Fig 9-3q** Final result 2 years after immediate loading.

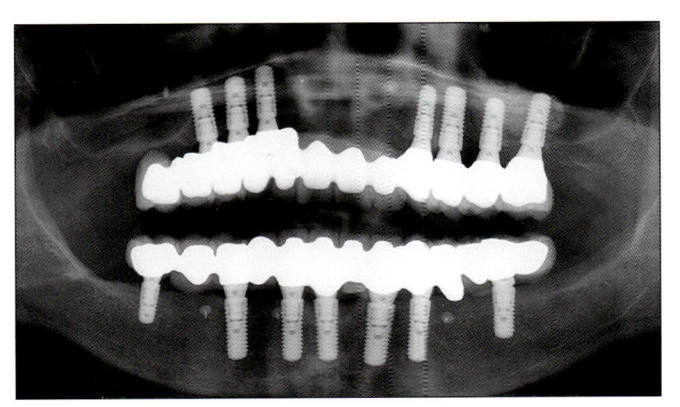

**Fig 9-3r** Radiographic evaluation 2 years after immediate loading presenting excellent crestal bone levels. (Surgery by G. E. Romanos and G. Ciornei, Rochester, NY; restoration by M. Baig, Rochester, NY.)

## Case 4: Immediate loading in the posterior mandible after advanced augmentation

A 60-year-old man presented with advanced resorption in the posterior mandible. Advanced augmentation procedures were performed in the mandible using particulate autogenous bone from the ramus in combination with Puros human cancellous allograft in a 1:3 ratio (Figs 9-4a to 9-4c). The augmented site was covered with absorbable membranes prior to flap advancement, and a postsurgical radiographic examination was completed (Figs 9-4d and 9-4e).

The healing took place with some postoperative complications, including membrane exposure and insufficient follow-up visits by the patient, both of which contributed to some resorption of the grafting material and incomplete bone regeneration at the augmentation site. To avoid further resorption, two Tapered Screw-Vent implants (Zimmer) of 4.7-mm diameter and 10.0-mm length with high primary stability were placed 6 months after augmentation and loaded immediately after surgery with cemented implant-supported (splinted) restorations (Fig 9-4f). Lateral alveolar bone augmentation was accomplished at the same time (Fig 9-4g). The patient was advised to follow a soft/liquid diet for the first 3 months of healing (Figs 9-4h and 9-4i).

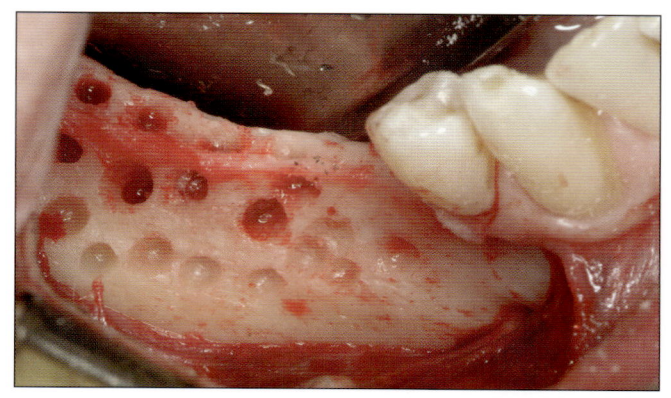

**Fig 9-4a** Decortication of the posterior mandible immediately before augmentation.

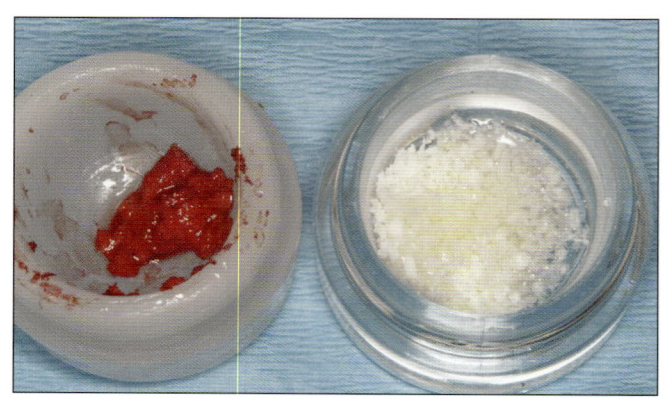

**Fig 9-4b** Composition of the grafting material with autogenous bone from the ramus and human allograft in cancellous form.

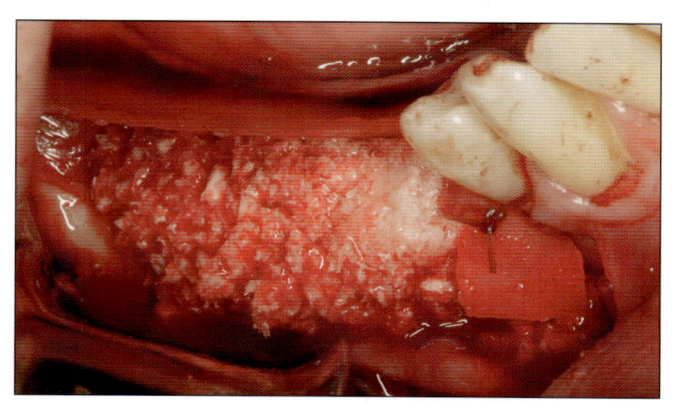

**Fig 9-4c** Augmentation with the composite graft.

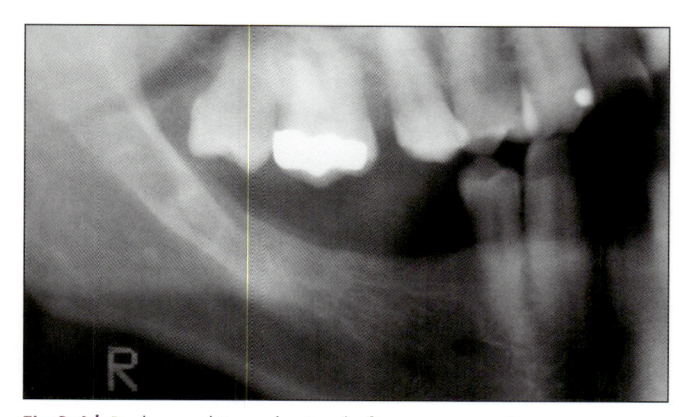

**Fig 9-4d** Radiographic evaluation before augmentation.

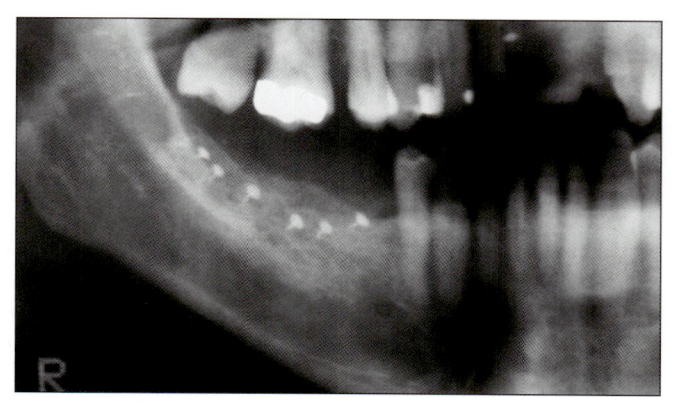

**Fig 9-4e** Radiographic evaluation immediately after bone augmentation.

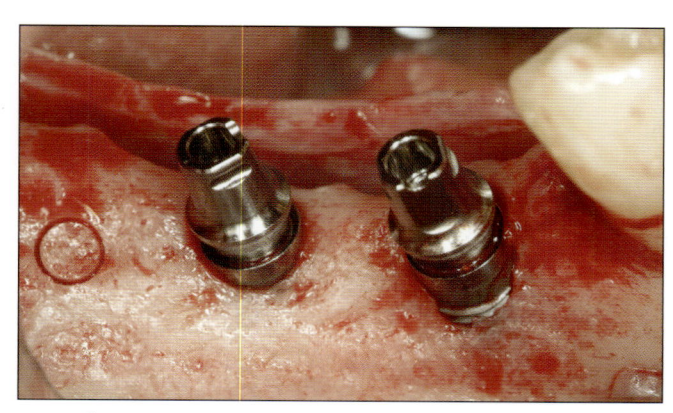

**Fig 9-4f** Implant placement 6 months after augmentation with high primary stability and platform-switching abutment connection for immediate loading.

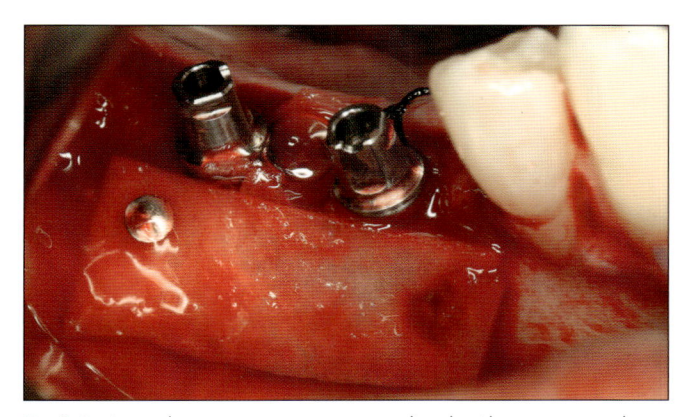

**Fig 9-4g** Lateral augmentation was completed with autogenous bone harvested from the posterior mandible and covered with a collagen membrane. Note the subcrestal implant placement.

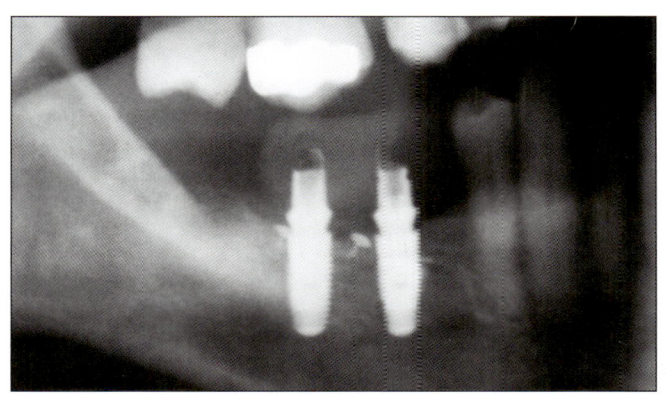

**Fig 9-4h** Radiographic evaluation after implant placement and immediate function. The platform-switching abutments were fixed with a final torque.

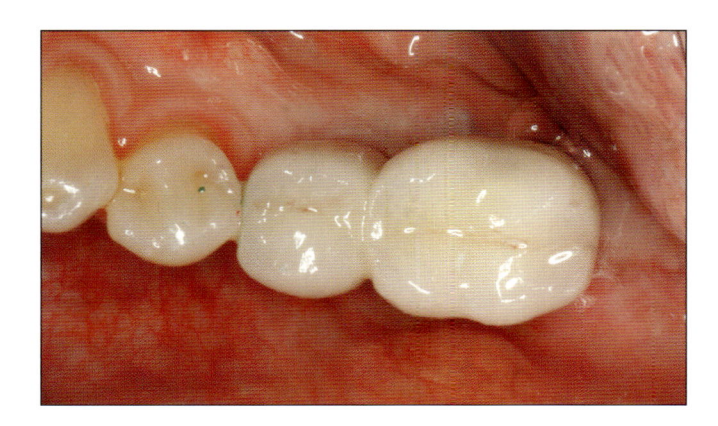

**Fig 9-4i** Final restoration in place. (Restoration by S. Bakeer, Rochester, NY.)

## Case 5: Removal of implants, advanced ridge augmentations, and immediate loading

The following case presents the treatment of a 27-year-old American man who had had implants placed previously in a South Asian country because of tooth agenesis in both jaws. Once the patient was back in the United States, the implants could not been restored because of a lack of Food and Drug Administration clearance for the implant system that had been placed and a lack of compatible prosthetic components in the US. In addition, the implants had not been placed in prosthetically correct positions (Figs 9-5a to 9-5c). Radiographic examination of the implants revealed that they were integrated in the bone. The soft tissue presented a thin tissue biotype. After a comprehensive analysis, a surgical and prosthetic treatment plan was agreed upon in which all implants in the maxilla and anterior mandible would be removed, keeping only the integrated implant in the left posterior mandible. The treatment proceeded in several stages.

All implants in the right maxilla were removed using piezoelectric surgery (Fig 9-5d), and the alveolar ridge was augmented with autogenous bone and Bio-Oss cancellous grafting material (Fig 9-5e). After initial healing of the bone graft in the right maxilla, a similar treatment was completed in the left maxilla, which included a sinus elevation procedure. After healing, Ankylos Plus implants with a progressive thread design were placed with their final abutments and prepared for immediate loading (Figs 9-5f to 9-5h). Fixed provisional prostheses (Fig 9-5i) were made using the OST protocol.

Reconstructive treatment was performed in the mandible with particulate Bio-Oss and Bio-Oss block (Figs 9-5j to 9-5o). After healing, implant placement and OST provisionalization followed a protocol similar to that used in the maxilla (Figs 9-5p to 9-5u). A soft/liquid diet protocol was advised for the first 3 to 4 months of the healing after implant placement.

A couple of months later, the fixed provisional restorations were replaced with the final prostheses (Figs 9-5v and 9-5w). The patient was very satisfied with the final result, and the implants were evaluated every 3 months for the first year of healing. The patient came back 3 years after treatment to evaluate the implant condition, and he presented excellent soft and hard tissues (Figs 9-5x and 9-5y). The final clinical outcome was very successful and the patient was very satisfied.

# 9 Immediate Loading in Grafted Bone

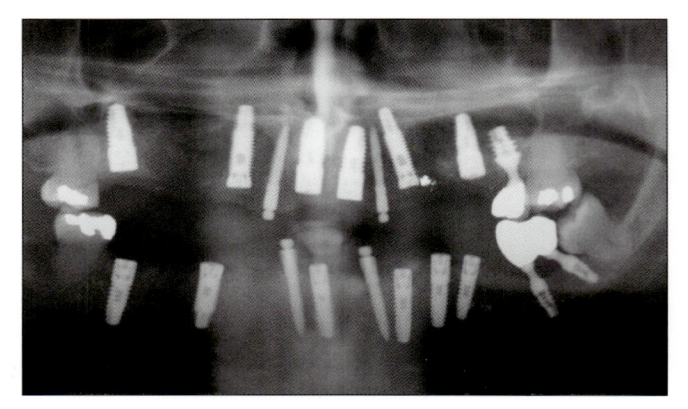

**Fig 9-5a** Radiographic evaluation of the implants previously positioned in the maxilla and mandible.

**Fig 9-5b** Anterior view of the maxilla and mandible before treatment.

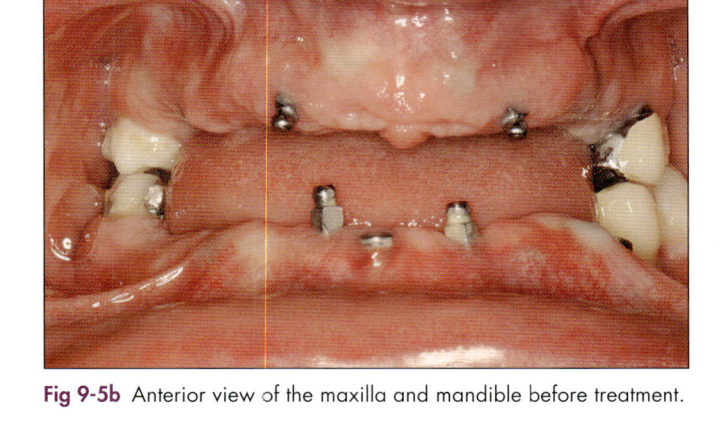

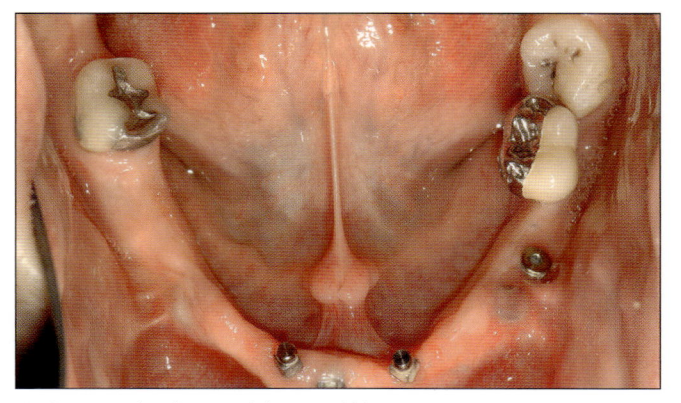

**Fig 9-5c** Occlusal view of the mandible.

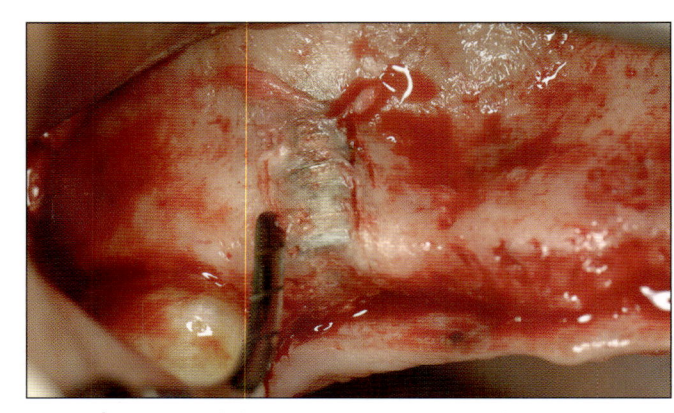

**Fig 9-5d** Removal of the implants using a piezoelectric ENAC OE-W10 ultrasonic unit (Osada).

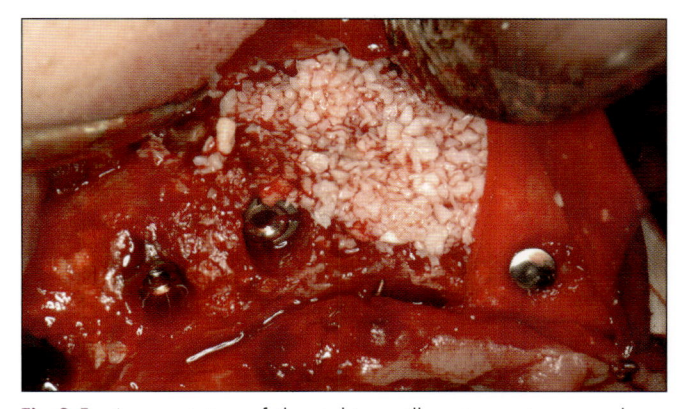

**Fig 9-5e** Augmentation of the right maxilla using autogenous bone and cancellous mineralized bone grafting material (Bio-Oss). It was covered with a Biomend Extend collagen membrane.

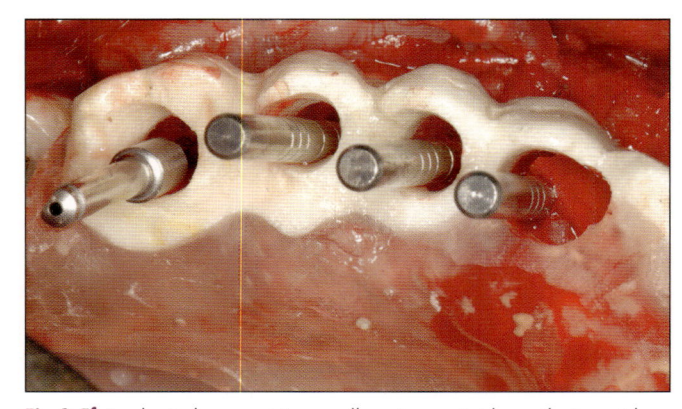

**Fig 9-5f** Implant placement in maxilla using a rigid prosthetic guide.

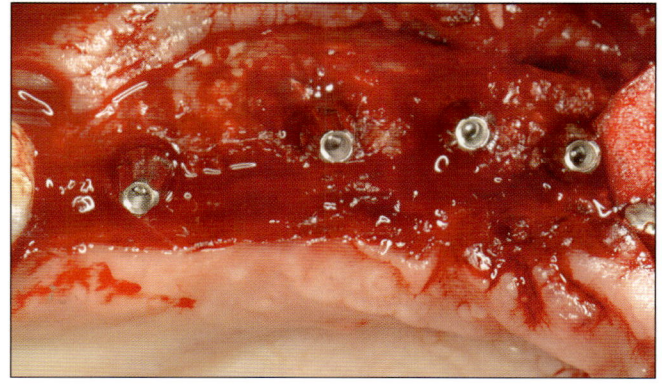

**Fig 9-5g** Abutment connection with final torque immediately after surgery for immediate loading in the maxilla.

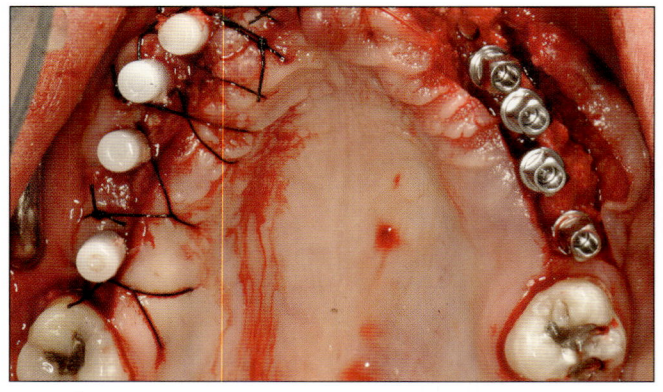

**Fig 9-5h** Plastic caps in place in the right maxilla and implant placement in the left maxilla.

# Case Reports

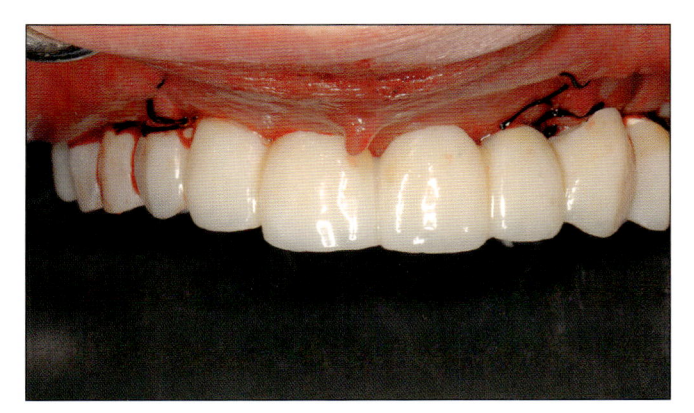

**Fig 9-5i** Provisional restoration in place after flap closure.

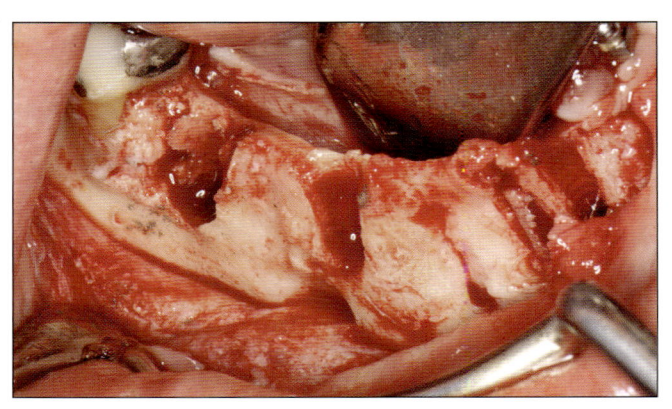

**Fig 9-5j** Intraoperative view of the right mandible before augmentation.

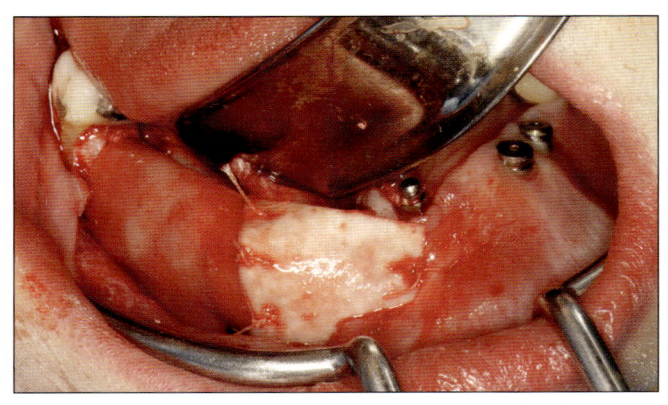

**Fig 9-5k** Vertical and lateral augmentation was completed using autogenous bone and cancellous mineralized bone grafting material (Bio-Oss). The augmented site was covered with two large Biomend Extend collagen membranes fixed buccally and lingually with Salvin titanium tacks.

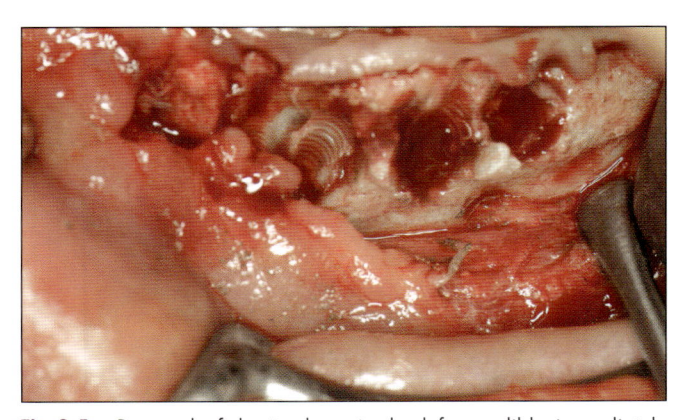

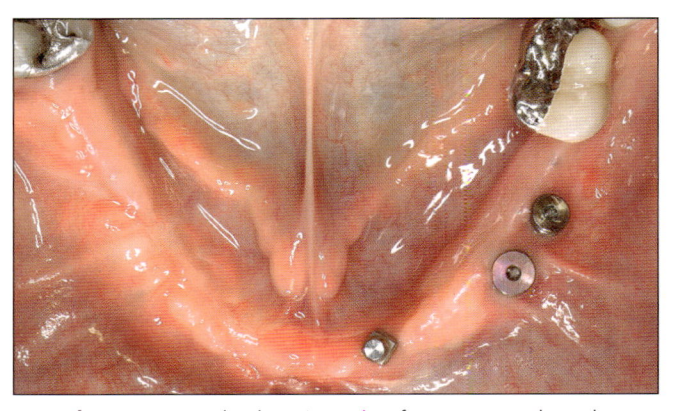

**Fig 9-5l** Postoperative healing 4 months after surgery in the right mandible. Note the incorrect positioning of the implants in the left mandible.

**Fig 9-5m** Removal of the implants in the left mandible immediately before ridge augmentation.

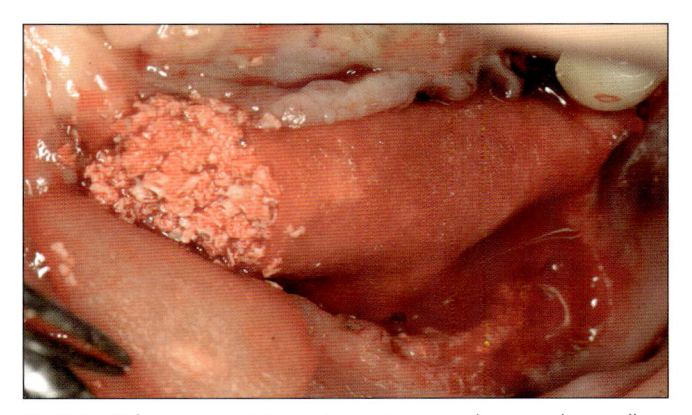

**Fig 9-5n** Ridge augmentation using autogenous bone and cancellous mineralized bone grafting material in a block form (Bio-Oss) covered with two Biomend Extend collagen membranes.

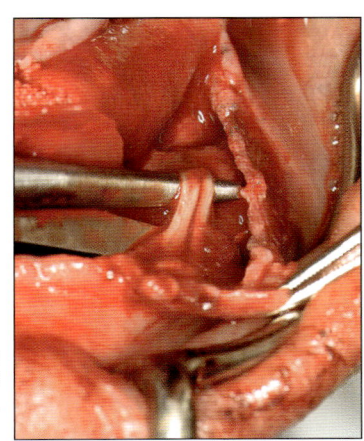

**Fig 9-5o** Flap advancement with required preparation of the mental nerve to avoid permanent nerve damage.

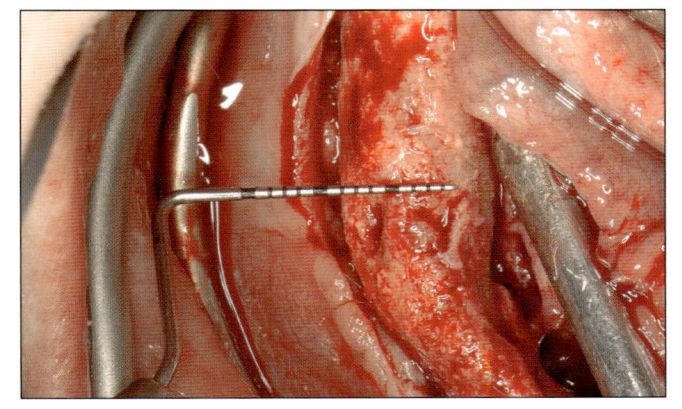

**Fig 9-5p** Gain of bone in the right mandible 6 months after healing.

103

# 9 | Immediate Loading in Grafted Bone

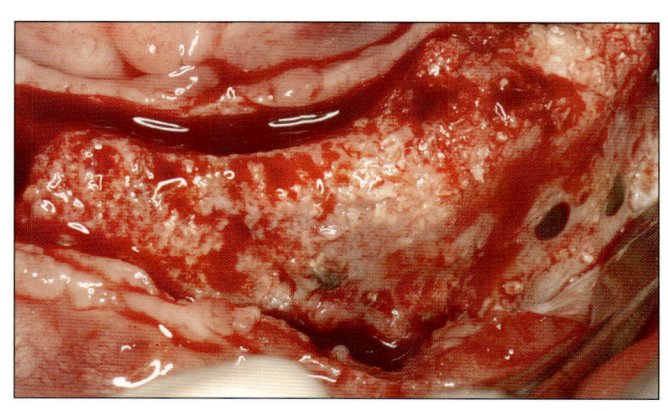

**Fig 9-5q** Sufficient gain of bone in the left mandible 5 months after healing. Note that the new bone also covered part of the fixation tacks.

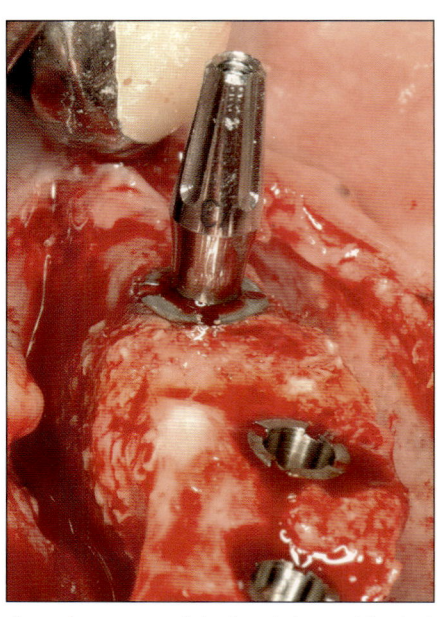

**Fig 9-5r** Implant placement with high stability and final abutment connection in the mandible.

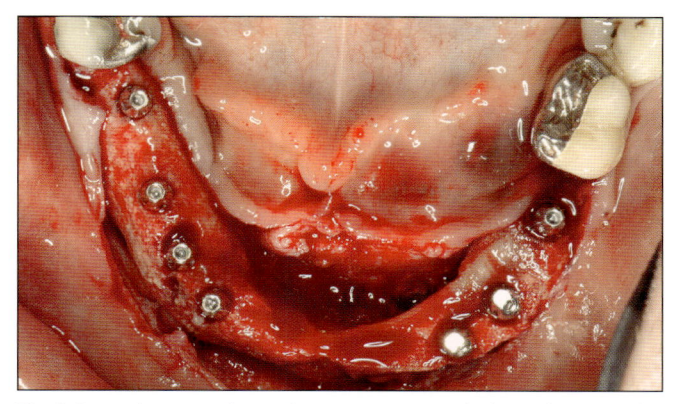

**Fig 9-5s** Implants in place after connection with their abutments for immediate loading.

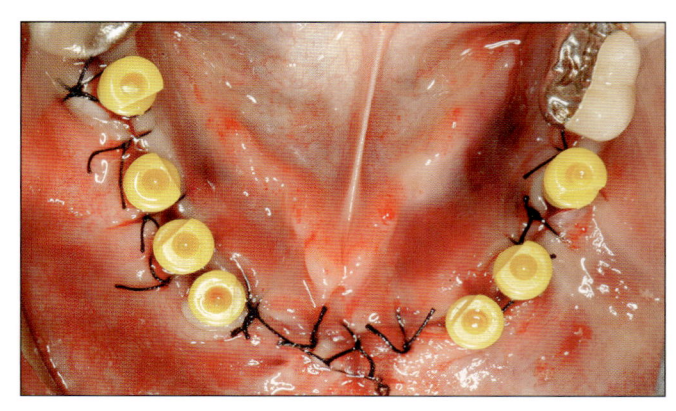

**Fig 9-5t** Flap closure and final impression using impression copings.

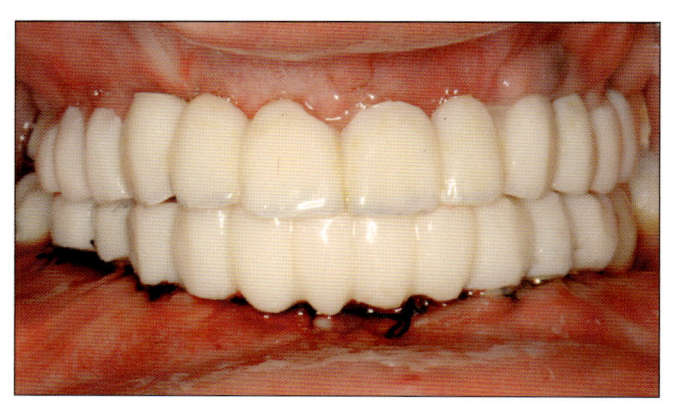

**Fig 9-5u** Provisional restorations in place after cementation with Temp-Bond.

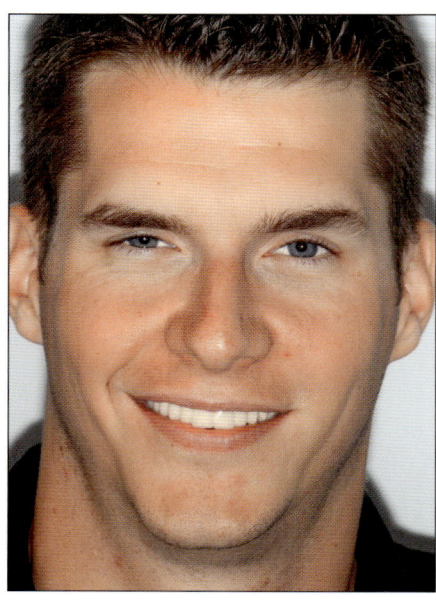

**Fig 9-5v** Facial view of the patient 1 year after complete treatment.

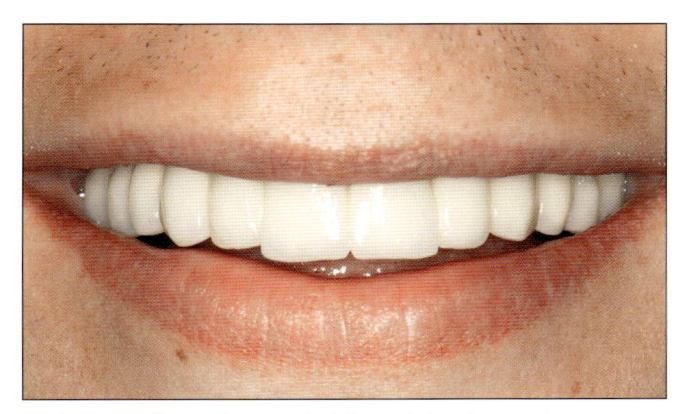

**Fig 9-5w** Excellent esthetic result of the smile line 1 year after treatment.

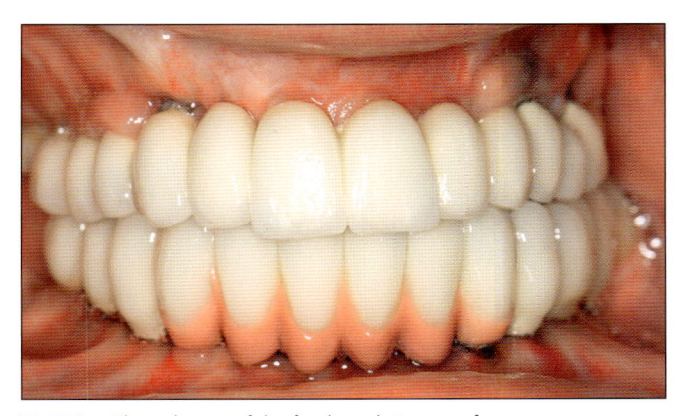

**Fig 9-5x** Clinical view of the final result 1 year after treatment.

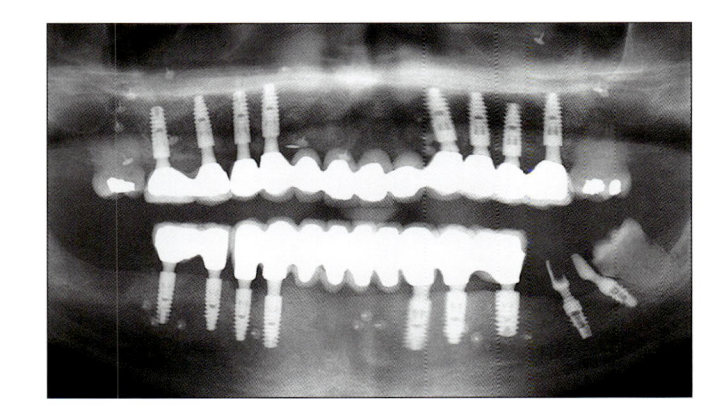

**Fig 9-5y** Radiographic evaluation of the final result 3 years after treatment presenting excellent bone levels and implant integration. (Restoration by M. Palermo, Rochester, NY.)

# References

1. Romanos GE. Treatment of advanced periodontal destruction with immediately loaded implants and simultaneous bone augmentation. A case report. J Periodontol 2003;74:255–261.
2. Romanos GE. Periosteal releasing incision for coverage of augmented sites. A technical note. J Oral Implantol 2010;36:25–30.

# Immediate Loading in Immunocompromised Patients

## Heavy Smokers

### General considerations regarding smoking risk

Heavy smoking has been reported as a risk factor affecting the prevalence and progression of periodontal diseases.[1] Rehabilitation with dental implants in smokers is associated with a higher rate of failure compared with the rate among nonsmokers.[2] Smoking also has been associated with high rates of implant failure and multiple failures in the same patient.[3-7] Data from a 10-year study conducted by Lindquist et al[8] revealed that smokers had greater bone loss around implants placed in their mandibles than did nonsmokers and demonstrated a relationship between the amount of cigarette consumption and the amount of peri-implant marginal bone loss. Similarly, Haas et al[9] showed that, compared with nonsmokers, smokers have a greater gingival bleeding index, increased probing depth, and inflammation with greater marginal bone loss around implants placed in the maxilla. Additional studies have found that patients who smoke have bone loss around implants,[10] reduced bone mineral density,[11] and a 2.5 times greater chance for implant failure. In contrast, interleukin-1 periodontal genotype status was found not to be a significant factor for implant loss.[12]

According to a study of patients with a high number of tooth extractions,[13] wound-healing complications, such as pain and dry sockets, occur more frequently in heavy smokers. Therefore, special care during surgery and more frequent postoperative care visits should be considered for these patients.

One study found cigarette smoking to adversely affect osseointegration of implants placed in grafted maxillary sinuses regardless of the amount of daily nicotine consumption, with the cumulative success rate of implants being lower in smokers (65.3%) compared with nonsmokers (82.7%).[14] Furthermore, the implant success rate in maxillary antral-nasal inlay bone grafts in combination with implant placement is lower in smokers as well.[15]

### Immediate loading in heavy smokers: A prospective clinical study

Although immediate loading with dental implants has been extensively documented in different clinical protocols, heavy smokers have been excluded from most studies.[16-20] However, Romanos and Nentwig[21] applied this protocol in the treatment of nine consecutive patients (five men, four women; mean age: 52.44 ± 8.39 years) who were heavy smokers (ie, smoked more than 20 cigarettes per day for at least 10 years). Patients were included in this study if they (1) were completely edentulous in the maxilla and/or the mandible, (2) signed an informed consent document, (3) were physically and mentally able to tolerate conventional surgical and restorative procedures, and (4) if rehabilitation with dental implants was considered the ideal treatment of choice. Patients were excluded if they (1) had active infection in the sites selected for implant placement, (2) had uncontrolled systemic diseases such as uncontrolled diabetes, (3) were pregnant, or (4) displayed severe bruxism. In the opposing dentitions, the patients had different types of natural tooth and restorative arrangements: implant-supported restorations (three patients), tooth- and implant-supported fixed partial dentures (one patient), healthy teeth (four patients), and a full denture (one patient).

The patients received six implants in the maxilla or mandible (or both), which were loaded using cross-arch provisional partial dentures immediately after surgery. A clinical and radiographic presurgical diagnosis was made by a surgeon who then placed a total of 72 implants with a sand-blasted surface and progressive thread design (Ankylos, Dentsply Friadent) using a prosthetic guide according to the manufacturer guidelines. The implants had a 2.0-mm machined collar. In diameter, they ranged from 3.5 mm (46 implants) to 4.5 mm (25 implants) to 5.5 mm (1 implant), and their lengths varied from 9.5 mm (6 implants) to 11 mm (33 implants) to 14 mm (33 implants). The only 5.5-mm-wide implant was placed in an area of poor bone quality (soft bone and after condensation).

All implants were stable at insertion. In sites with inadequate bone (16 implants at each of the mesial, buccal, and distal sites), exposed threads were covered with autogenous bone harvested from residual donor sites. The augmented areas were covered by a Bio-Gide (Geistlich) collagen membrane, which was fixed in place with Frios titanium pins (Dentsply Friadent). One implant was placed simultaneously with an internal sinus elevation procedure (osteotome technique).

The implants were connected with their abutments and splinted immediately after surgery using cross-arch fixed provisional prostheses having occlusal contacts in centric occlusion and group function in the lateral movements of the mandible (ie, immediate occlusal loading). The provisional prostheses were made chairside with ProTemp (Espe) resin material and a template. Distal cantilevers were avoided. The patients were advised to maintain a soft or liquid diet for the first 6 to 8 weeks of healing to reduce excessive loading of the implants.

The impressions for the fabrication of the definitive prostheses were taken without abutment removal using impression copings. The definitive prostheses were delivered 4 to 8 weeks after surgery (or 3 to 4 months after surgery in cases of augmentation) and cemented with temporary cement (TempBond, Kerr) to make possible peri-implant soft tissue elevation at different intervals after removal of the restoration. Clinical and radiographic indices were evaluated at the start of loading and every 3 months after loading.

After a mean loading period of 33.77 ± 19.08 months (range: 6 to 66 months), only one implant was mobile. All clinical indices had values within normal levels (Table 10-1). The Periotest (Medizintechnik Gulden) values demonstrated a continuous reduction. The crestal bone level was stable, and only the maxillary right second molar and canine sites presented minimal vertical and horizontal bone loss, respectively. In all other sites, no bone loss was observed. Given the high success rate (98.61%) and demonstrated stability of the

**Table 10-1** Peri-implant clinical values around immediately loaded implants in heavy smokers

| Parameter | T0 | T1 | T2 |
|---|---|---|---|
| Plaque index | 1.0 ± 1.2* | 1.2 ± 1.1 | 1.3 ± 1.1 |
| Sulcus bleeding index | 0.3 ± 0.6* | 0.5 ± 0.7 | 0.7 ± 0.1 |
| Probing pocket depth (mm) | NA | 1.7 ± 0.7 | 2.7 ± 0.9 |
| Keratinized mucosa width (mm) | 4.6 ± 1.1* | 4.3 ± 1.4 | 3.3 ± 1.7 |
| Periotest value | 0.9 ± 2.6 | −0.4 ± 3.2 | −1.3 ± 2.5 |

T0, baseline; T1, placement of the definitive prosthesis; T2, final follow-up; NA, not available.
*Measured 2 weeks after surgery.

peri-implant hard and soft tissues around immediately loaded implants restored with fixed, cross-arch implant-supported prostheses in this study, immediate functional loading appears to be as effective in heavy smokers as in nonsmokers.

The following case reports describe the treatment and its results for selected patients in the study.

## Case 1: Immediate loading in the maxilla and mandible of a heavy smoker

This case presents a male heavy smoker with an edentulous maxilla and mandible who wanted better stability for his mandibular full denture. Using the standard immediate loading protocol presented in chapter 7, the patient's edentulous mandible (Fig 10-1a) was treated with the placement of six Ankylos implants using a prosthetic guide. Parallel guides were used to determine correct implant angulation. Immediately after implant placement, the abutments were selected based on the soft tissue height, the angulation of the implant, the distance between the implants, and the interocclusal height (Fig 10-1b). When primary stability of the implants was confirmed, a final torque of 20 to 25 Ncm (for straight, standard abutments) and 15 Ncm (for angulated abutments) was used according to the manufacturer protocol. The temporary resin caps were fixed in place, and the flap was sutured with care. The provisional restoration was fabricated and fixed temporarily with TempBond, and care was taken to allow open spaces for the patient to clean underneath the cross-arch, implant-retained fixed provisional restoration (Fig 10-1c). A radiograph was taken to record the baseline bone levels. The definitive prosthesis was fabricated and placed several weeks later (Fig 10-1d).

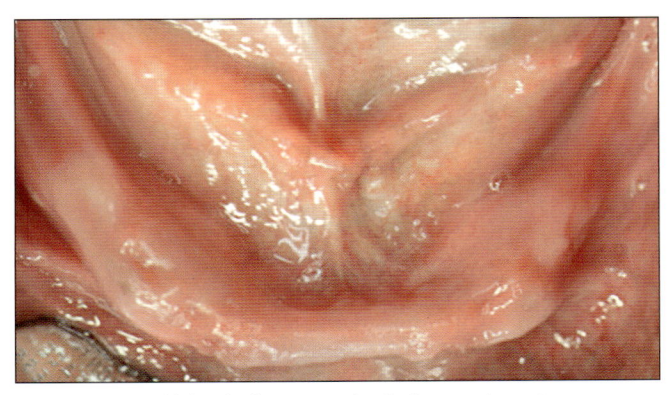

**Fig 10-1a** Mandible of a heavy smoker before implant placement.

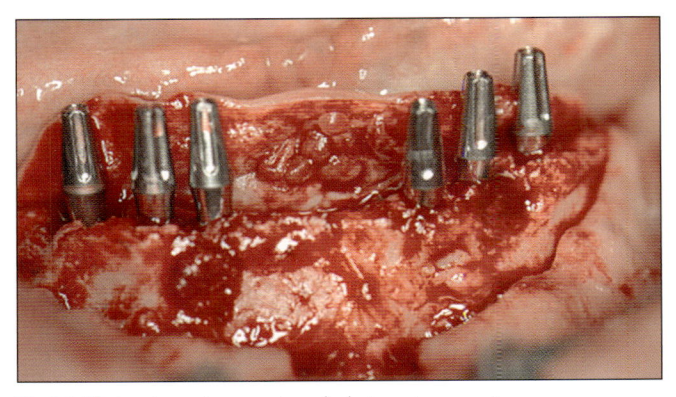

**Fig 10-1b** Implant placement and abutment connection.

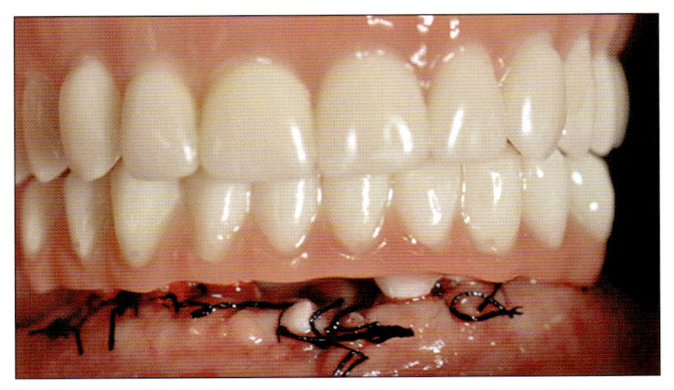

**Fig 10-1c** Provisional restoration in occlusion immediately after surgery.

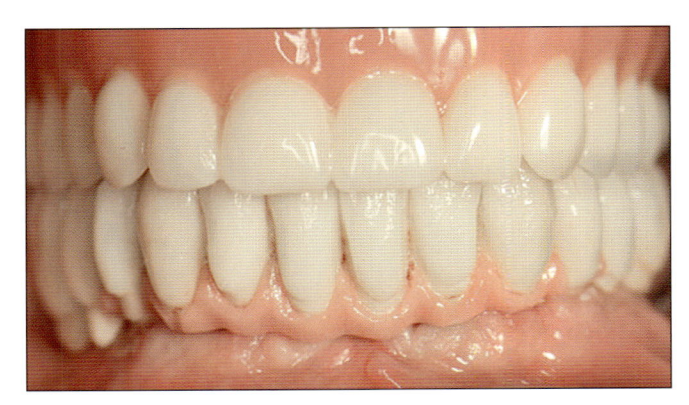

**Fig 10-1d** Definitive restoration on immediately loaded implants in occlusion.

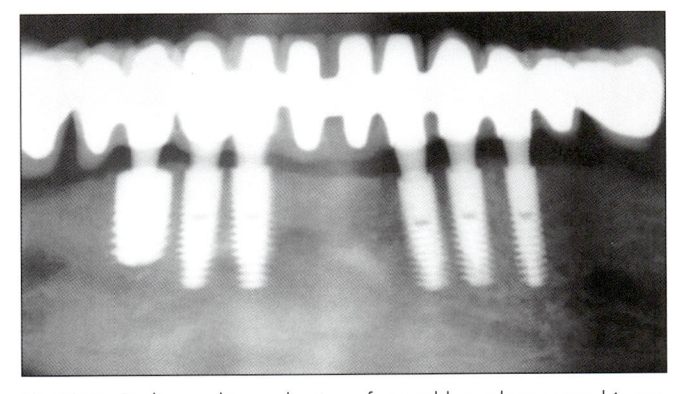

**Fig 10-1e** Radiographic evaluation of crestal bone loss around immediately loaded implants 2 years after loading in a heavy smoker. No changes in peri-implant bone levels were observed.

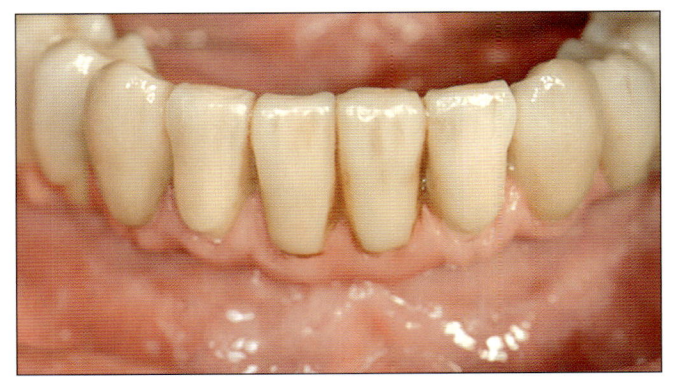

**Fig 10-1f** Clinical evaluation of the definitive implant-supported restoration 2 years after loading presents extensive nicotine staining.

One year after surgery, the definitive restorations presented some staining due to smoking. Therefore, an oral hygiene visit was recommended every 3 to 4 months. Some redness of the peri-implant soft tissues without bleeding was characteristic. The radiographic examination showed no bone loss around any of the implants. All implants were checked for stability using the Periotest device and showed excellent soft tissue health. The patient was very happy with the final functional and esthetic result. The stable radiographic and clinical results achieved at 2 years after loading are presented in Figs 10-1e and 10-1f.

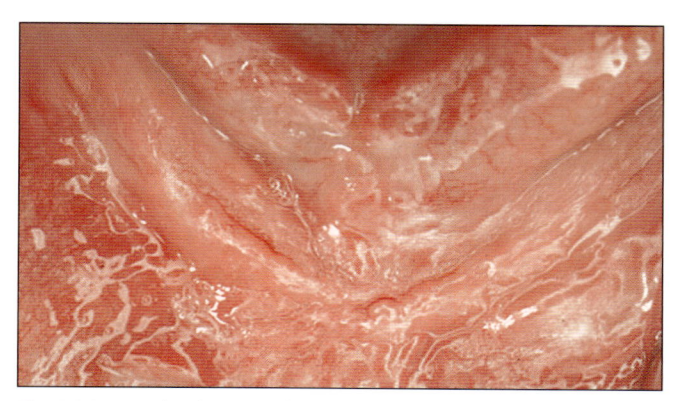

**Fig 10-2a** Occlusal view of the atrophic mandible before implant placement.

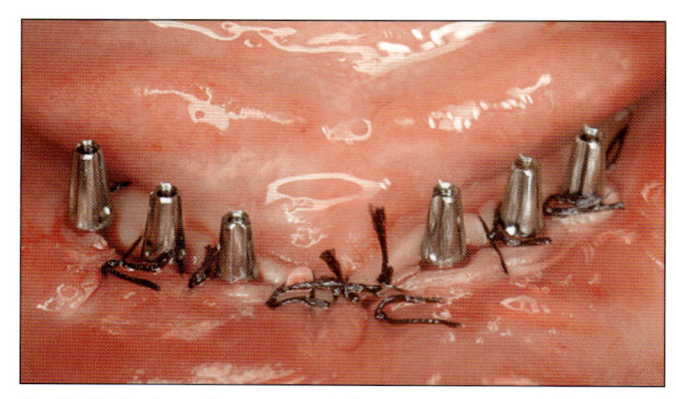

**Fig 10-2b** Implant placement and abutment connection for immediate functional loading.

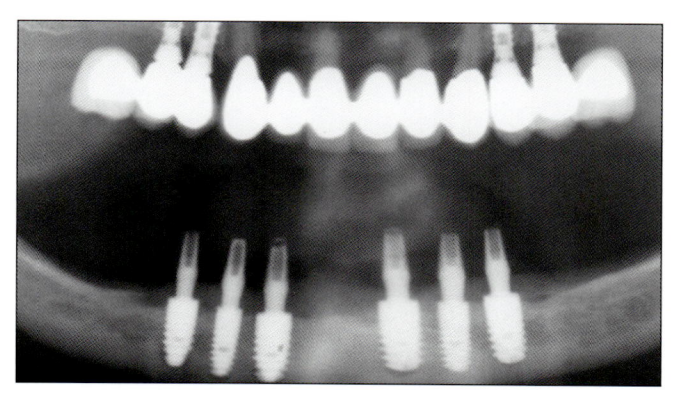

**Fig 10-2c** Radiographic examination after implant placement and abutment connection for immediate loading. Note that implants were placed supracrestally to avoid risk of jaw fracture.

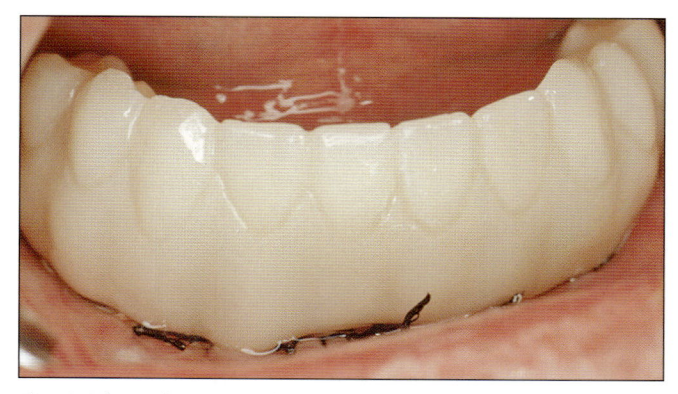

**Fig 10-2d** Fixed provisional restoration in place following surgery.

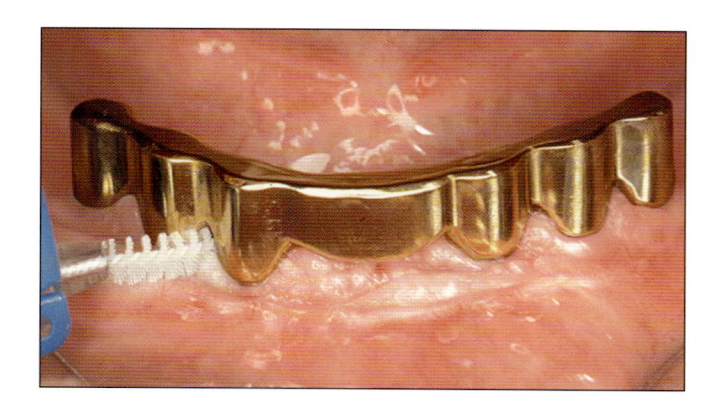

**Fig 10-2e** Delivery of the bar to support the definitive hybrid restoration. The design of the framework should allow for adequate plaque control.

## Case 2: Immediate loading in the advanced resorbed mandible of a heavy smoker

A 51-year-old woman presented for implant-supported mandibular rehabilitation. Extreme atrophy of the mandible was present in the height but not the width of the alveolar ridge (Fig 10-2a). The implants were placed and connected with their abutments for immediate loading (Fig 10-2b), and the bone level at baseline was recorded in a panoramic radiograph (Fig 10-2c). A provisional restoration was fabricated chairside and immediately loaded (Fig 10-2d). The definitive restoration was fabricated several weeks later. The soft tissues presented excellent healing without bleeding. The definitive implant-supported prosthesis was a removable hybrid-type restoration with a customized bar, splinting the implants together (Fig 10-2e).

One year after loading, the bar was removed, the implants were checked for stability using a Periotest device, and clinical soft tissue measurements were taken. The condition of the soft tissues was excellent. The patient was again instructed to use interdental brushes for cleaning the implants underneath the bar reconstruction. Radiographically, the bone level was stable, and no bone resorption was observed compared with baseline. Six years after surgery, the soft tissue continued to show excellent condition, the oral hygiene was acceptable, and no bone loss was present (Figs 10-2f to 10-2h).

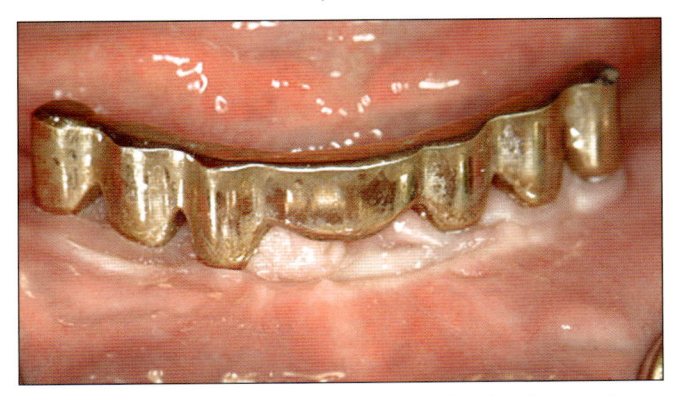

**Fig 10-2f** Clinical situation 6 years after immediate loading in a heavy smoker.

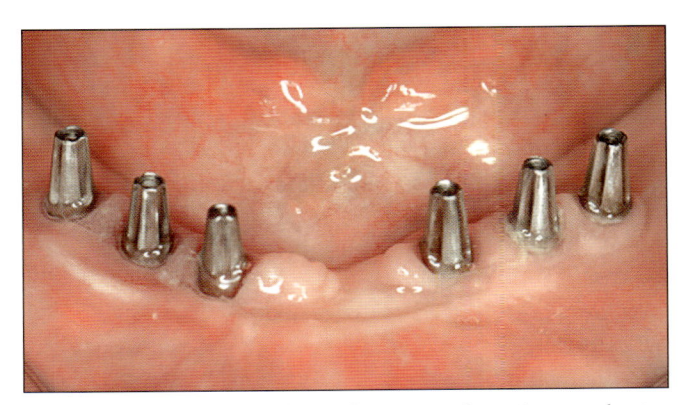

**Fig 10-2g** Excellent peri-implant soft tissue condition 6 years after immediate loading in a heavy smoker. The scar tissue at the buccal aspect of the mandible is associated with earlier implant placement and failure as well as surgical treatment for osteomyelitis.

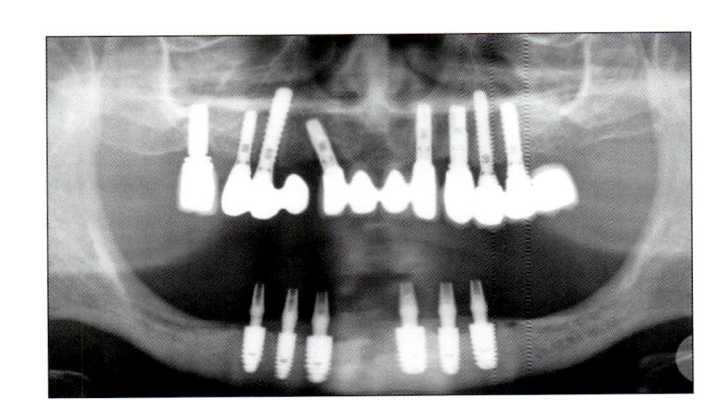

**Fig 10-2h** Radiographic examination of immediately loaded implants in a heavy smoker 6 years after loading. No crestal bone loss occurred during the loading period; the bone level is the same as at baseline. Note the supracrestal implant placement.

## Case 3: Histologic proof of immediate loading in a heavy smoker

A 50-year-old woman presented for prosthetic reconstruction after extraction of her maxillary and mandibular teeth because of advanced periodontal disease (Figs 10-3a and 10-3b). She was working as a flight attendant for an airline and traveled frequently, and she was interested in receiving fixed implant-supported prostheses. She was a heavy smoker (more than 20 cigarettes per day for longer than 10 years) but was considered to be in good general health. The patient was examined clinically and radiographically and was advised to reduce her smoking or quit smoking in order to receive implant therapy. Because of her frequent travel, immediate loading was the recommended treatment protocol.

Alginate impressions of the maxilla and mandible were taken and registered for vertical dimension to fabricate two full dentures. Surgical guides were made with acrylic resin after duplication of the full dentures. In addition, a special splint was made from elastic foil for fabrication of the provisional fixed restoration for postsurgical insertion. A midcrestal incision was made under local anesthesia, followed by elevation of mucoperiosteal flaps in the maxilla and mandible. Twelve Ankylos implants, 3.5 mm in diameter and 11 mm in length, were inserted in the lateral incisor, canine, and first premolar sites in each quadrant (Figs 10-3c and 10-3d). The bone quality was very weak (type 3 or 4). The parallelism of the inserted abutments was examined, and temporary resin abutments were placed on the implants. These abutments were replaced with the final abutments and fixed in place with controlled torque. Periotest values were evaluated to record implant stability immediately after implant placement. The flaps were sutured in place, and temporary fixed restorations were fabricated chairside using the special splint and ProTemp resin material. The provisional restorations had symmetric contacts in centric occlusion, and the vertical dimension was main-

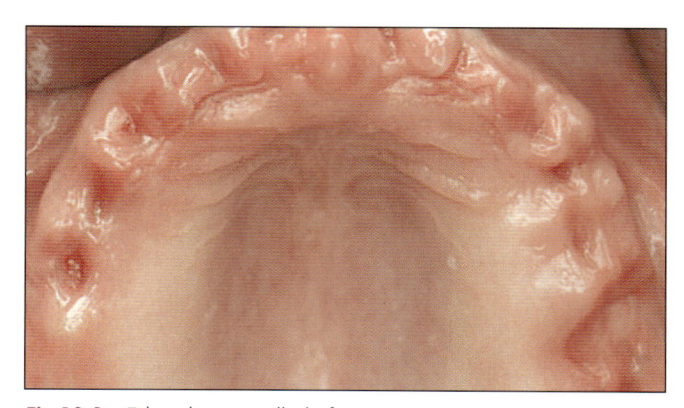

**Fig 10-3a** Edentulous maxilla before surgery.

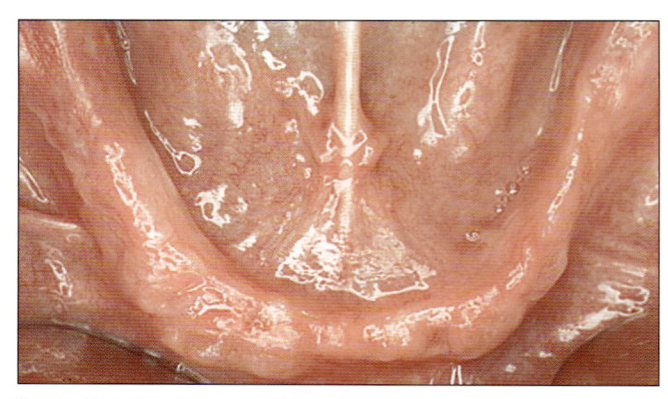

**Fig 10-3b** Edentulous mandible before surgery.

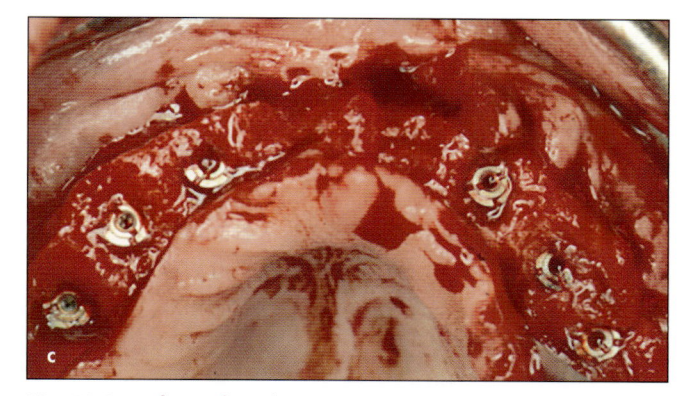

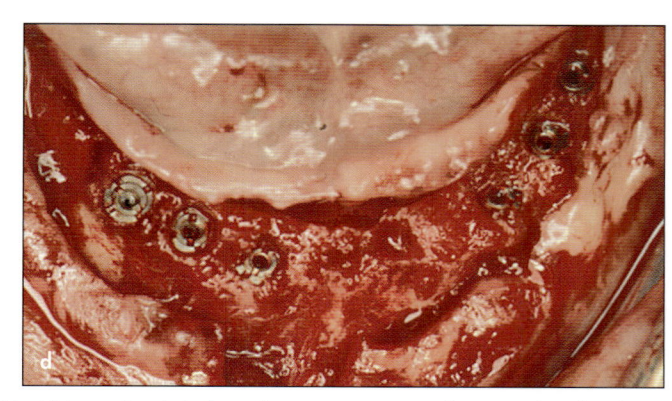

**Figs 10-3c and 10-3d** Implants in place in the maxilla (c) and in the mandible (d) immediately before abutment connection for immediate loading.

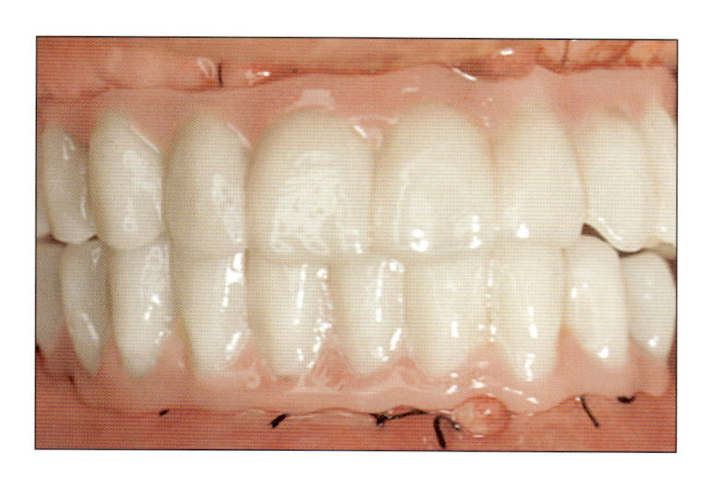

**Fig 10-3e** Provisional restorations in occlusion immediately after implant placement and loading.

tained (Fig 10-3e). A soft/liquid diet was recommended for the first 6 to 8 weeks of healing.

The definitive metal-ceramic implant-supported fixed restorations were placed and cemented temporarily 4 months after loading (Figs 10-3f to 10-3k). Because of functional, esthetic, and phonetic considerations, two distal cantilevers were used on each side in the mandible, and one distal cantilever was incorporated on each side in the maxilla. Seven months after loading, the patient was re-examined because the prosthetic reconstruction had loosened. At this time she was hospitalized due to severe lung cancer. The peri-implant tissues were examined clinically and radiographically, and the clinical measurements were evaluated. All implants were stable, the soft tissues were in excellent condition, and no crestal bone loss was observed radiographically (Fig 10-3l).

The patient died 2 weeks later. She had agreed to donate the implants and surrounding tissues. Autopsy of the implants, including the surrounding tissues, were performed and examined histologically and histomorphometrically (Figs 10-3m to 10-3p). An interface without any epithelial migration was found in all of the implants. A high number of bone-implant contacts were also presented after histomorphometric evaluation. A more detailed analysis of the histologic findings of this clinical case has been presented elsewhere.[22]

Heavy Smokers

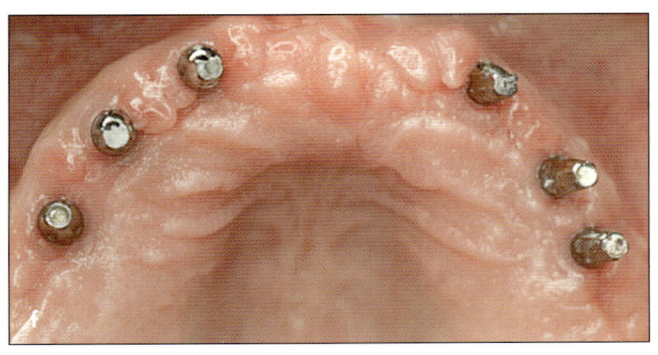

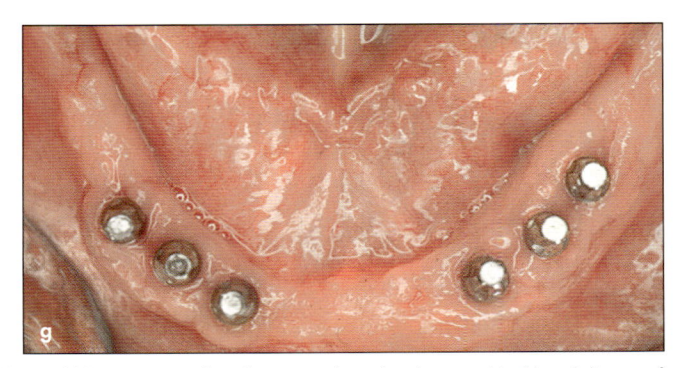

**Figs 10-3f and 10-3g** Excellent peri-implant soft tissues in the maxilla (f) and mandible (g) 4 months after immediate loading and before delivery of the definitive prostheses.

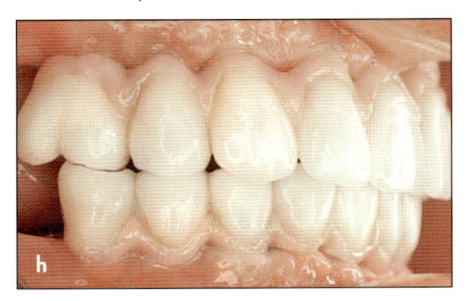

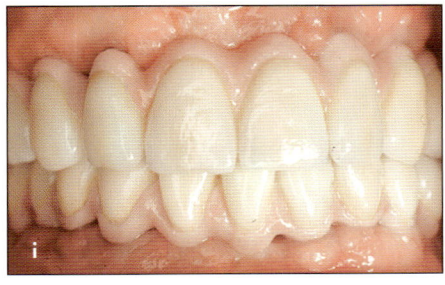

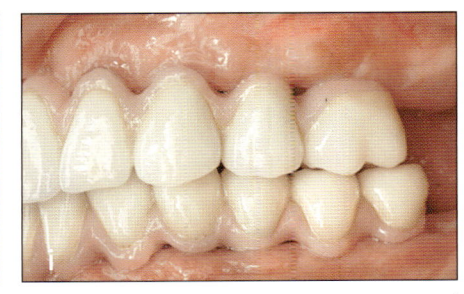

**Fig 10-3h to 10-3-j** Definitive restorations 7 months after immediate loading. Metal-ceramic fixed implant-supported restorations were cemented temporarily. At this point in treatment, the patient was undergoing chemotherapy because of a bronchial carcinoma.

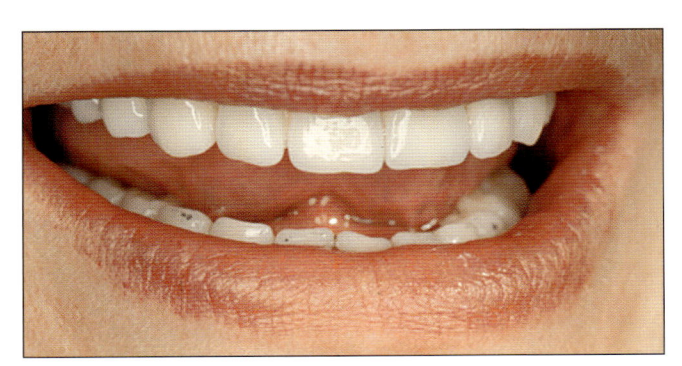

**Fig 10-3k** Excellent esthetic result with the final restorations. (Dental technician: Mike Funk, Reichelsheim, Germany.)

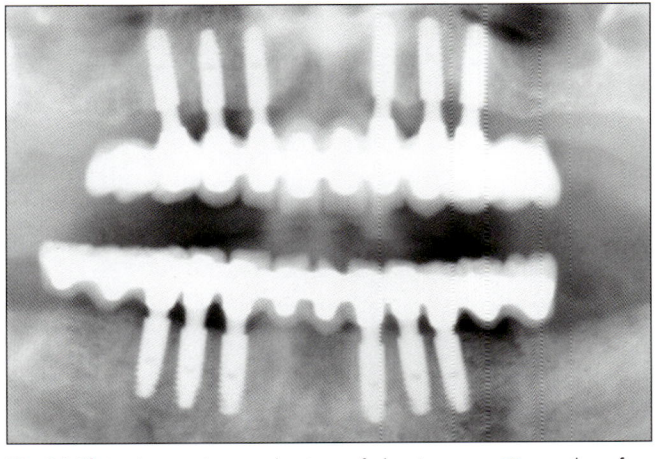

**Fig 10-3l** Radiographic evaluation of the implants 7 months after loading in a heavy smoker. Note the excellent bone condition.

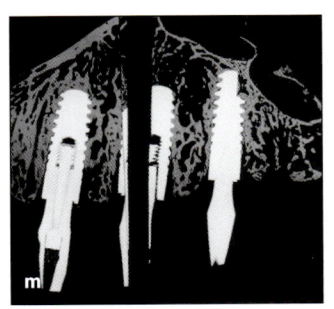

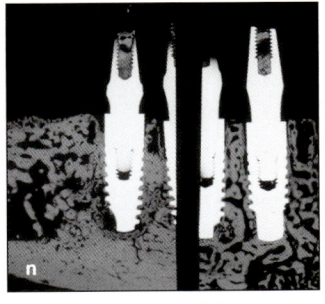

**Figs 10-3m and 10-3n** Microradiographic examination of the autopsy specimens of the maxillary (m) and mandibular (n) implants showing an excellent bone quality at the interface 7.5 months after immediate loading.

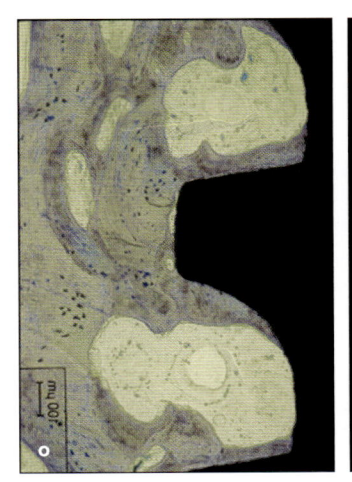

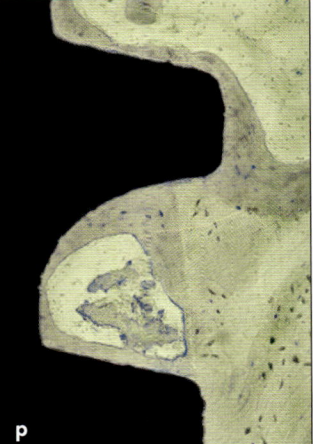

**Figs 10-3o and 10-3p** Histologic evaluation of the interface of maxillary (o) and mandibular (p) implants after immediate loading in a heavy smoker. Note the excellent bone contact with the implant surface without fibrous encapsulation. (See also Romanos and Johansson.[22])

113

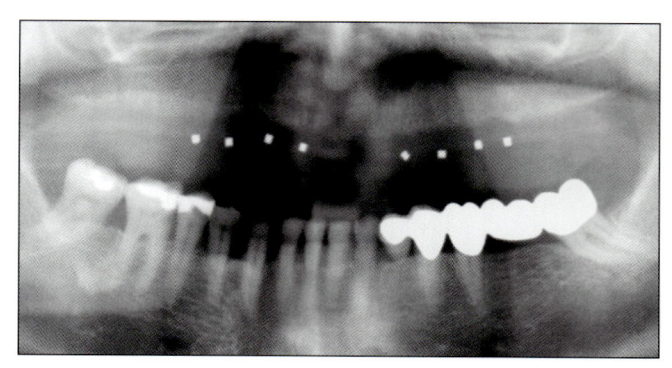

# 10 Immediate Loading in Immunocompromised Patients

**Fig 10-4a** Presurgical radiographic examination of a heavy smoker. Metal pins represent the planned position of the implants.

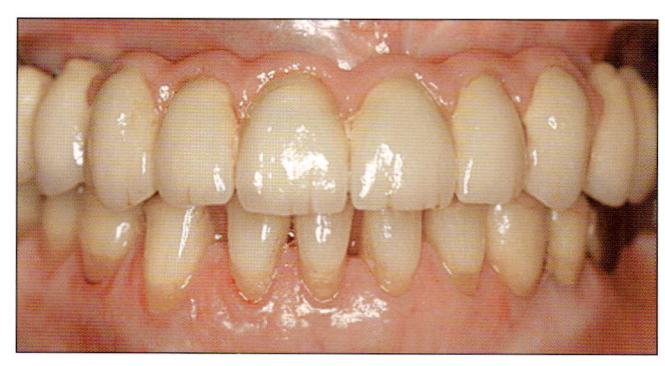

**Fig 10-4b** Definitive implant-supported maxillary prosthesis with pink porcelain shown 2 years after immediate loading in a heavy smoker.

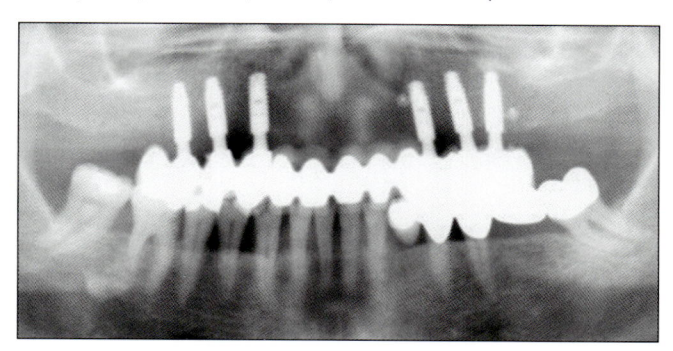

**Fig 10-4c** No bone loss is evident on the panoramic radiograph 2 years after immediate loading.

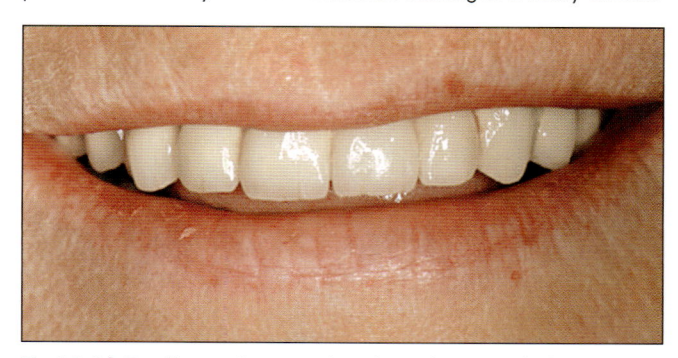

**Fig 10-4d** Excellent esthetic result with moderate smile line and the definitive prosthesis 3 years after immediate loading.

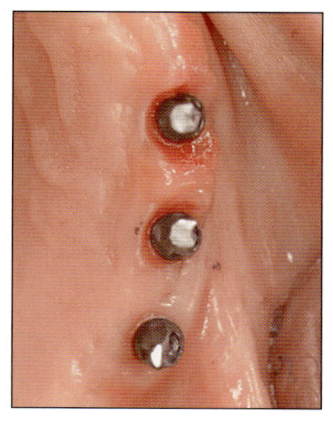

**Fig 10-4e** Healthy peri-implant soft tissues after 3 years of loading in a heavy smoker.

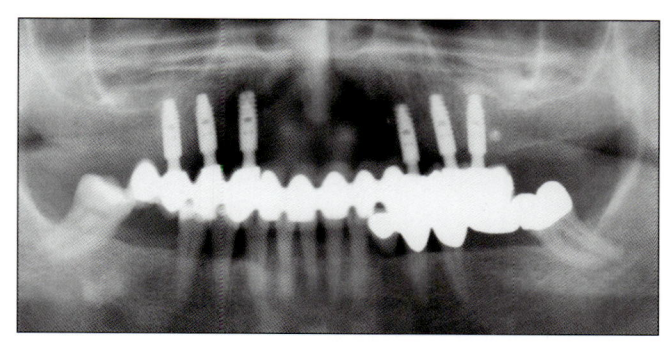

**Fig 10-4f** Radiographic examination 8 years after immediate loading presenting minimal crestal bone loss (less than 2 mm). The abutments were never removed from the implants after the implant surgery.

## Case 4: Immediate loading with simultaneous bone grafting in a heavy smoker

The following clinical case presents the maxillary implant-supported rehabilitation of a 54-year-old woman with a heavy smoking habit. Treatment included the placement of six implants in the narrow alveolar ridge (expanded using the bone spreading technique), lateral augmentation with autogenous bone from the left tuberosity and an internal sinus elevation procedure (osteotome technique) at the maxillary left second premolar site, and immediate functional loading.

To accurately plan the implant surgery, a panoramic radiograph was taken with the surgical template in place. In the template, small (2 × 2–mm thick) metal pins were placed in the center of the planned crowns to represent the position of the implants (Fig 10-4a). In this way, the implants could be placed at the correct positions (middle fossae of the teeth) according to prosthetic considerations. After implant placement, the abutments were connected to the provisional prosthesis, which was fabricated chairside based on the immediate loading protocol presented previously (see chapter 7).

The definitive restoration was fabricated after 3 to 4 months and fixed temporarily with TempBond. The soft tissues showed excellent healing, and the metal-ceramic fixed implant-supported prosthesis had pink porcelain at the cervical margins of the anterior teeth to improve esthetics (Fig 10-4b). No implant failures occurred, and the peri-implant soft tissue condition was excellent.

At the 2-year follow-up, the bone level was found to be stable (Fig 10-4c). Three years after loading, the esthetic result was very satisfactory (Fig 10-4d) and the soft tissues were healthy (Fig 10-4e). In the last follow-up visit after 8 years of immediate loading, the implants presented a very small marginal bone loss (Fig 10-4f).

# HIV-Positive Patients

The use of implant therapy in HIV-positive patients is a treatment option that has not been described extensively in the literature, even though there is a need for implant rehabilitation in this population. Recent publications have shown that the placement of dental implants in HIV-positive patients is a reasonable treatment option, regardless of patients' viral load levels, cluster of differentiation 4 (CD4) cell count, and type of antiretroviral therapy. However, the predictability and long-term success of dental implant restoration used in HIV-positive patients has yet to be evaluated in long-term studies.[23] The following presents one case demonstrating the long-term effects of the immediate loading concept for dental implants placed in an HIV-positive patient.

## Case 5: Immediate loading in an HIV-positive patient

A 43-year-old HIV-positive man presented as fully edentulous. He had been completely edentulous for 4 years. According to the patient history, most teeth were lost due to deep carious lesions despite undergoing multiple dental procedures in an to attempt to save his remaining teeth. The patient's chief complaint was that he could not smile and eat like he did when he had teeth.

According to the medical history, the patient had been HIV seropositive (asymptomatic) for 15 years. He had been undergoing treatment with a regimen of medications including a combination of antiretroviral therapies. Extraoral examination revealed no asymmetry, no swellings, and no tender or palpable cervical or submandibular lymph nodes. The intraoral examination revealed well-healed, fully edentulous ridges in the maxilla and mandible that presented healthy U-shaped anatomy with adequate attached and keratinized soft tissue (Figs 10-5a and 10-5b). The radiographic examination (Fig 10-5c) revealed very limited bone resorption in the maxilla and mandible with sufficient bone for anterior and posterior implant placement.

The initial treatment included a complete set of maxillary and mandibular dentures. The patient insisted that the prosthesis mimic a diastema between the maxillary central incisors that existed in his natural dentition. The patient was pleased with the prostheses and the improvements in esthetics and function. At a later follow-up he decided he wanted implant-supported prostheses. After clinical and radiographic evaluation, the patient was accepted for treatment with immediately loaded implant prostheses in the maxilla and mandible. The patient elected to have both arches treated on the same day.

The recently fabricated dentures were duplicated in clear acrylic resin, and an Omnivac shell was made over the entire occlusal surface and flanges. The Omnivac shell was used as a prosthetic guide by cutting 2-mm holes in the teeth positions for the maxillary left and right canines, first and second premolars, and first molars. Before the surgical procedure commenced, a vertical dimension measurement was taken, which was maintained throughout the procedures. In addition, interocclusal records were made with the maxillary denture in place against the mandibular denture with the Omnivac shell in place as well as the mandibular denture in place against the maxillary denture with the Omnivac shell in place. Therefore, the Omnivac shell could be used for provisional restorations at the proper vertical dimension against the existing prostheses (see chapter 9).

A record of the previous blood tests showed a stable CD4 count at more than 200 for several years, and the current CD4 count was 479 with a ratio of T-lymphocyte helper/suppressor cells (T4/T8) of 0.99. All of the other blood cell counts tested within normal limits, and no neutropenia or thrombocytopenia was detected. To prevent infection, penicillin was prescribed to start with 2.0 g 1 hour before surgery and then 500 mg taken three times a day for 1 week.

Following the administration of local anesthesia, a crestal incision was performed in the edentulous ridges and a mucoperiosteal flap was elevated. Placement of 16 Ankylos implants followed in accordance with the prosthetic guide. Because the bone quality in the maxilla was extremely poor, eight implants were placed in the left and right canine to the first molar sites without tapping. In the mandible, alveolar bone was also very poor quality in the left and right first molar sites; therefore, two implants were placed without tapping. In the other mandibular sites, osteotomies were performed in the left and right canine to second premolar sites using tapping before placing six implants. Given the amount of bone at the osteotomy sites, 3.5-mm-diameter implants were selected; 12 implants had a 14-mm length, while the 4 implants placed in the first molar sites had an 11-mm length. All implants had excellent primary stability, and no bone augmentation was necessary (Figs 10-5d and 10-5e).

Sixteen abutments (eight straight in the mandible and eight angulated in the maxilla) of 6.0 mm in height, 3.5 mm in diameter, and 3.0 mm of sulcus height were fixed with angulation to create parallel positions to accommodate the arch-shaped fixed prosthetic restorations delivered immediately after implant placement. Periotest values were evaluated to record implant stability. Temporary caps were placed on the final abutments prior to fabricating a provisional restoration, and the mucoperiosteal flaps were closed with 4-0 silk sutures.

The provisional prostheses were made chairside using ProTemp resin material in the Omnivac templates and were cemented with temporary cement (Figs 10-5f and 10-5g). Immediately after the cementation, a panoramic radiograph was taken to evaluate the peri-implant crestal bone levels (Fig 10-5h).

The patient was advised to maintain a soft/liquid diet for the first 4 to 6 weeks and to rinse the oral cavity with 0.2% chlorhexidine digluconate solution for chemical plaque control until the sutures were removed. The interdental spaces of the temporary prostheses were also kept open to improve the hygiene access. In addition, 300 mg of clindamycin was prescribed three times a day for the first 10 days. Ten days after surgery the sutures were removed.

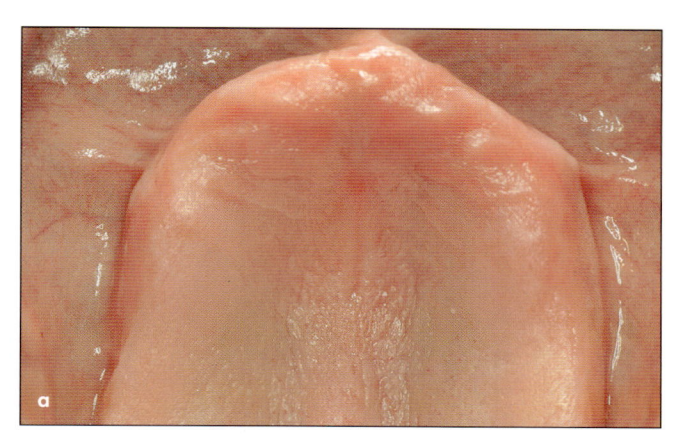

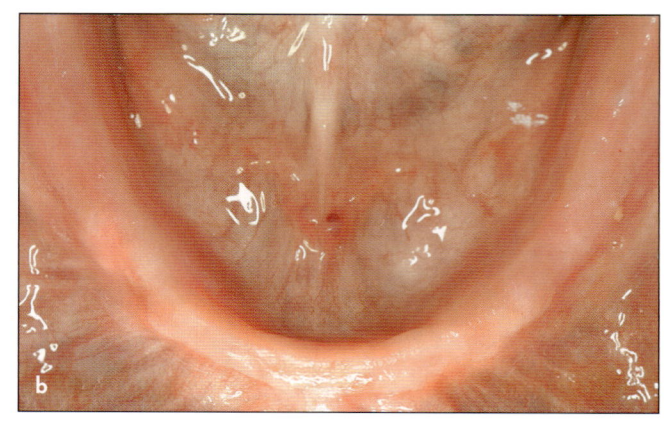

**Figs 10-5a and 10-5b** Preoperative views of the maxilla (a) and mandible (b) in an HIV-positive patient.

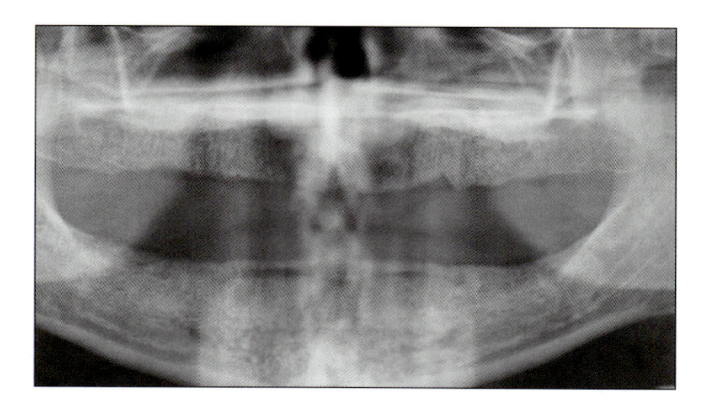

**Fig 10-5c** Preoperative radiologic examination demonstrating sufficient height in the residual ridges for implant placement.

After 10 weeks, final abutment-level impressions were made using Impregum impression material (Espe); the abutments were not removed. New interocclusal wax rims were fabricated on the abutment-level casts. Centric relation records were made using the adjusted rims, and an artificial tooth arrangement was prepared for the maxillary and mandibular arches. Once esthetics and phonetics were deemed acceptable, indices of the artificial tooth arrangements were made, and the records were sent to the laboratory.

The final prostheses were designed with pink porcelain to mimic the gingival architecture and tooth-colored porcelain for the dental components. The diastema was maintained. Prior to final cementation of the prostheses, clinical peri-implant indices were evaluated, including a radiologic examination to determine the peri-implant crestal bone level.

The patient was re-evaluated every 3 months for professional oral hygiene control. Within 6 months, maxillary and mandibular nightguards were fabricated for the patient following the fracture of the porcelain incisal edge on the maxillary right central incisor. Repair was performed using mechanical surface preparation, hydrofluoric acid etching, silane, bonding agent, a layer of flowable composite, and packable composite. The occlusion was carefully checked in all excursive movements. No further fractures or complications were noted. Possible reasons for the fracture include framework flexure, occlusion, or bruxing habits.

Two years after surgery, the clinical and radiologic examinations showed an optimal soft tissue condition (Figs 10-5i to 10-5p). No pain or infection was noted during the entire observation period. Periotest values measured in all implants after removal of the restorations showed normal values (Table 10-2) representing implant stability as well as healthy and stable peri-implant mucosa. Peri-implant bone loss was not observed; however, some crestal bone loss was noted around the mandibular left second premolar site without any pathologic soft tissue changes (ie, pocket formation, suppuration). The crestal bone level was stable 4 years after loading (Fig 10-5q).

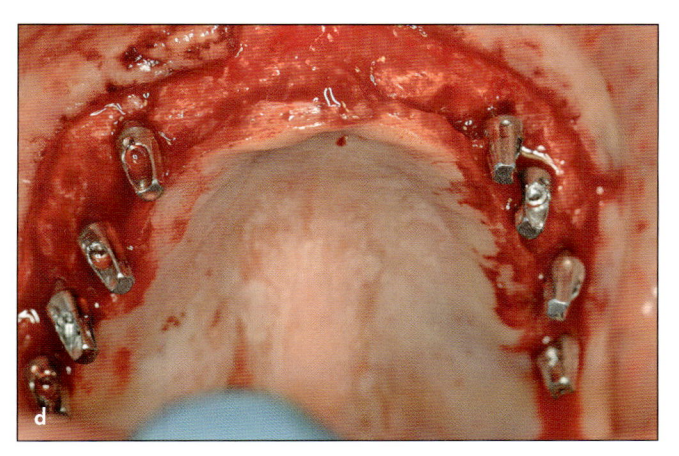

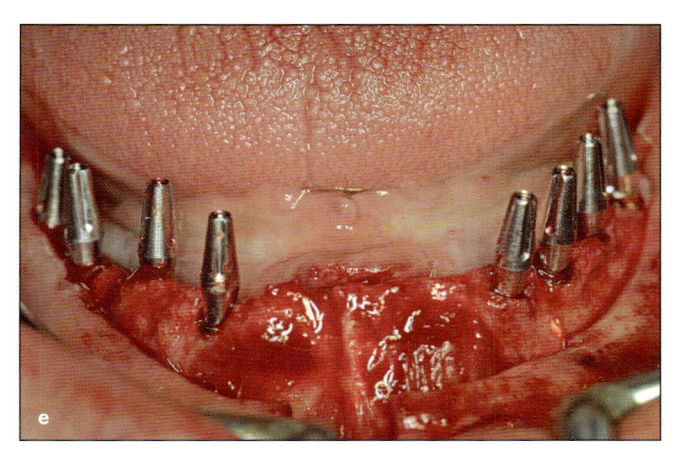

**Figs 10-5d and 10-5e** Implant placement and final abutment connection for immediate functional (occlusal) loading in the maxilla *(d)* and mandible *(e)*.

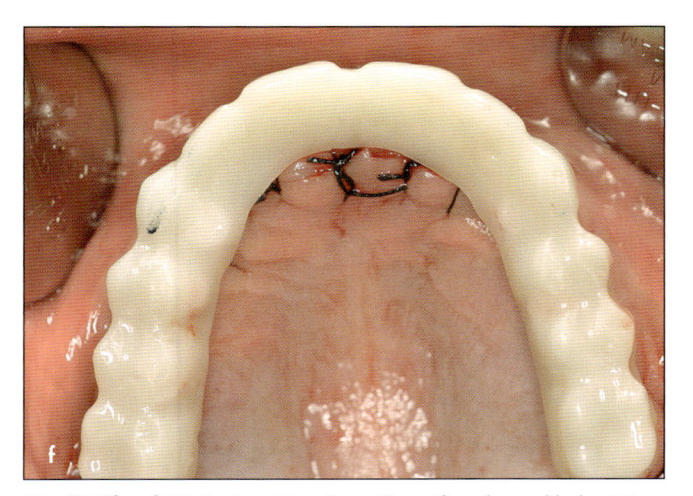

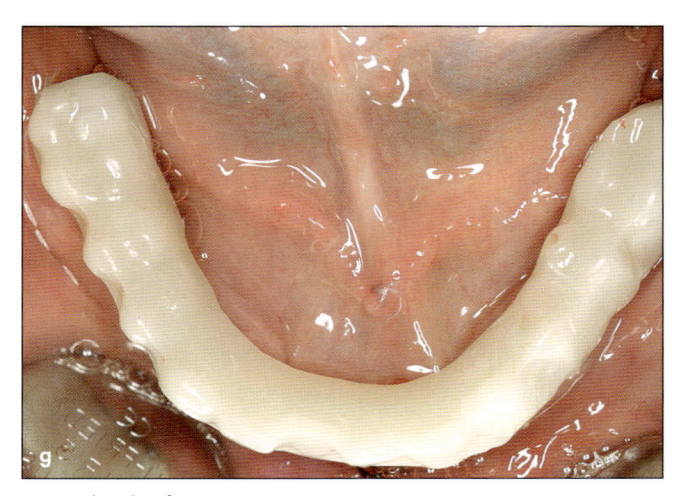

**Figs 10-5f and 10-5g** Provisional maxillary *(f)* and mandibular *(g)* restorations immediately after surgery.

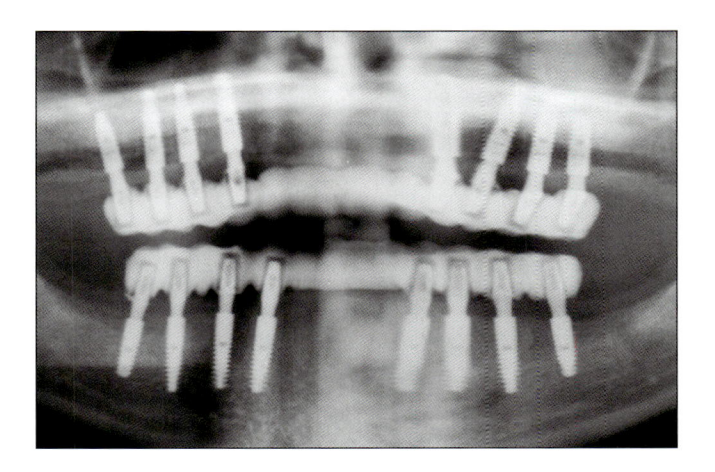

**Fig 10-5h** Radiographic examination following surgery and placement of the provisional restorations for immediate functional loading.

## 10 Immediate Loading in Immunocompromised Patients

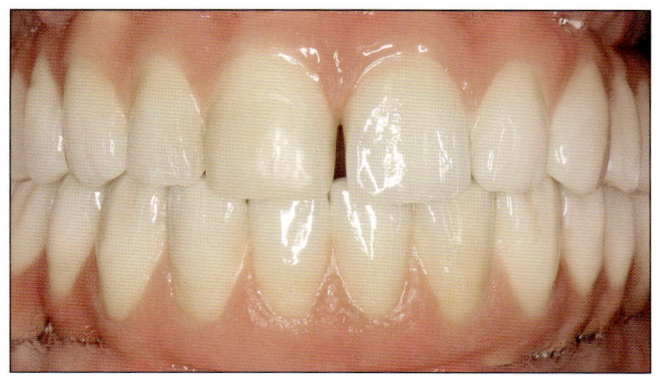

**Fig 10-5i** Final prostheses in occlusion 2 years after immediate loading. Note the anterior diastema and the pink porcelain at the gingival level to improve the esthetic result.

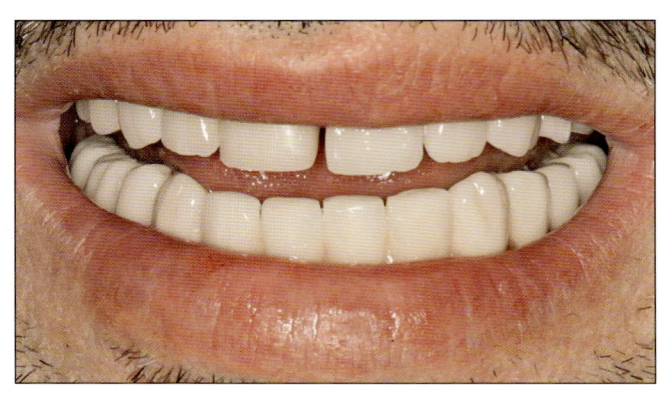

**Fig 10-5j** The patient's smile presents an excellent esthetic result with the full-arch metal-ceramic restorations.

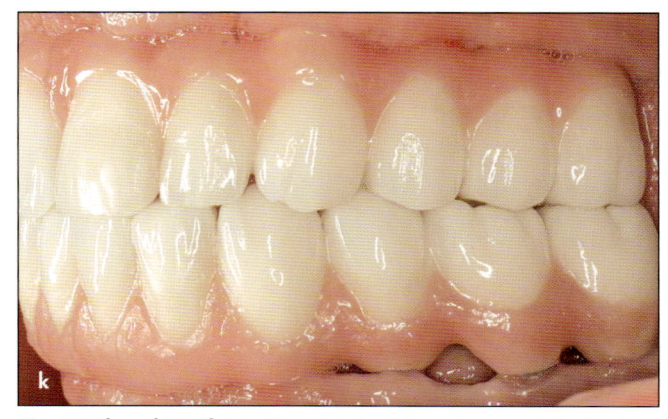

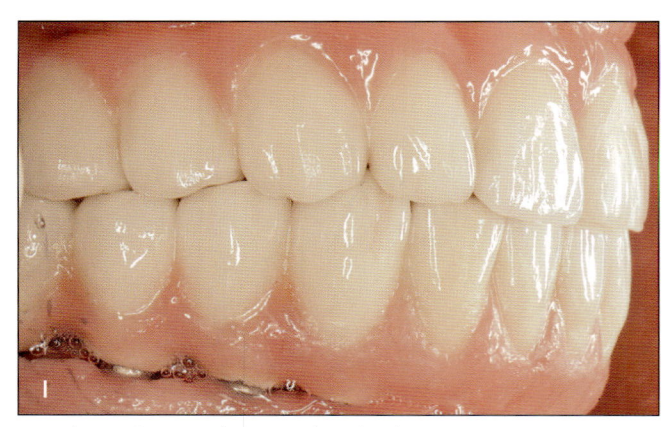

**Figs 10-5k and 10-5l** Left (k) and right (l) lateral views of the final prostheses in occlusion 2 years after immediate loading.

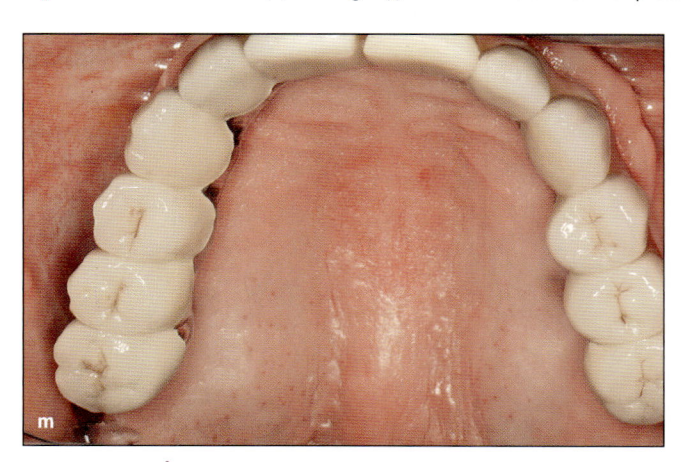

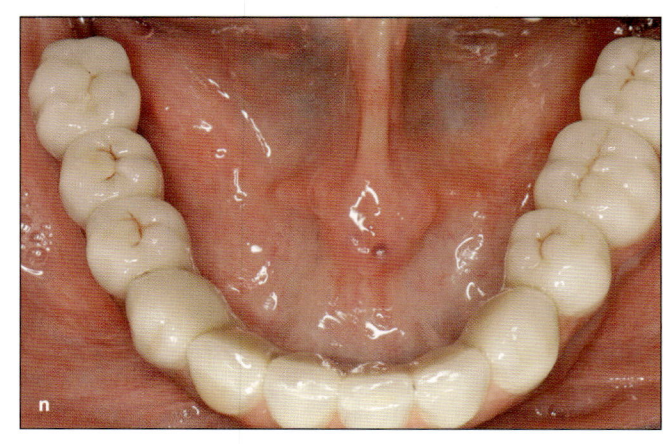

**Figs 10-5m and 10-5n** Occlusal views of the maxillary (m) and mandibular (n) restorations 2 years after immediate loading.

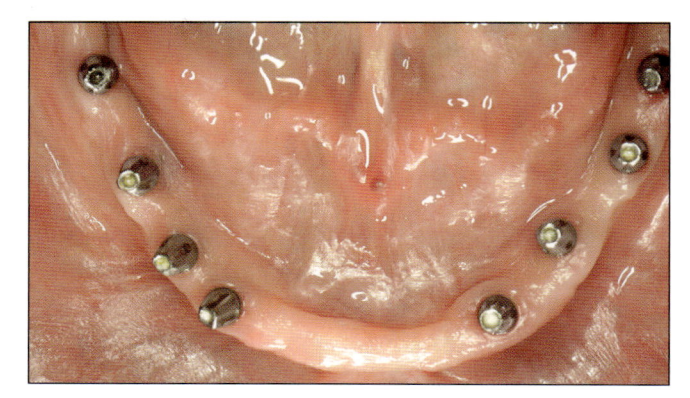

**Fig 10-5o** Excellent peri-implant soft tissues in the mandible 2 years after immediate loading.

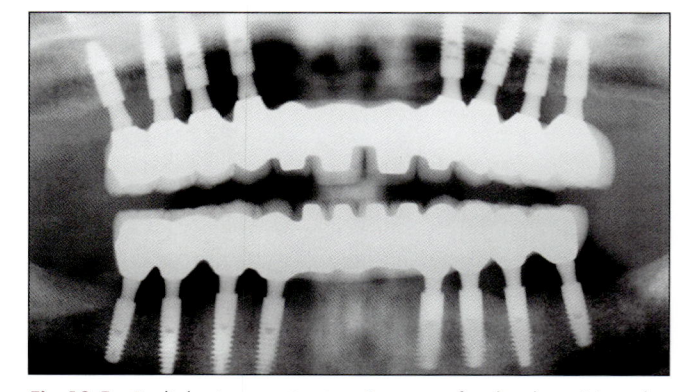

**Fig 10-5p** Radiologic examination 2 years after loading. Note that only minimal crestal bone resorption is observed around the mandibular left second premolar. No soft tissue inflammatory reaction was observed.

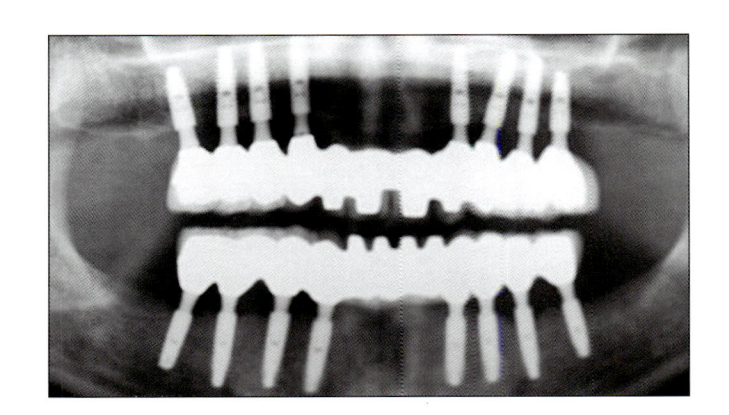

**Fig 10-5q** Radiologic examination 4 years after loading presenting crestal bone stability. (Prosthodontics by E. Goldin and dental technician L. Marotta, New York, NY.)

**Table 10-2** Peri-implant clinical values around immediately loaded implants in an HIV-positive patient

| Implant area | T0 | T1 | T2 | T3 | T4 | T5 |
|---|---|---|---|---|---|---|
| Maxillary right first molar | 2 | 4 | 3 | 5 | 0 | 0 |
| Maxillary right second premolar | 2 | 4 | 4 | 4 | 0 | 1 |
| Maxillary right first premolar | 2 | 2 | 2 | 3 | 0 | 0 |
| Maxillary right canine | 2 | 2 | 2 | 3 | 0 | 0 |
| Maxillary left canine | 2 |  | 2 | 2 | 0 | 0 |
| Maxillary left first premolar | 2 | 2 | 2 | 2 | 0 | 0 |
| Maxillary left second premolar | 2 | 1 | 2 | 2 | 0 | −1 |
| Maxillary left first molar | 4 | 2 | 2 | 2 | 0 | 0 |
| Mandibular left first molar | −2 | −2 | −1 | −3 | 0 | 0 |
| Mandibular left second premolar | −3 | −2 | −1 | −2 | 0 | −1 |
| Mandibular left first premolar | −3 | −2 | −1 | −2 | 0 | 0 |
| Mandibular left canine | −3 | −2 | −2 | −2 | 0 | 0 |
| Mandibular right canine | −2 | −2 | −2 | −2 | 0 | 0 |
| Mandibular right first premolar | −3 | −2 | −2 | −2 | −1 | −1 |
| Mandibular right second premolar | −3 | −3 | −2 | −2 | −1 | −1 |
| Mandibular right first molar | −2 | −3 | −1 | −3 | – | 1 |
| Mean values | −2.06 | −2.5 | 1.09 | 0.53 | 1.07 | −0.12 |
| Standard deviation | 0.63 | −0.62 | 1.09 | −0.28 | −0.73 | 0.57 |

T0, baseline; T1, 5 weeks; T2, 10 weeks; T3, 18 months; T4, 24 months; T5, 4 years.

# Conclusion

Based on the case reports presented here, immediate functional loading in edentulous arches of immunocompromised patients (ie, heavy smokers and HIV-positive patients) appears to be successful and to have long-term predictability. The main factors contributing to the long-term success of this technique include the following:

- Excellent primary implant stability that implements good implant design and thread geometry as well as gentle osteotomy preparation.
- Splinting (immobilization) immediately after surgery.
- Control of the magnitude and direction of the initial masticatory (occlusal) forces by creating narrow occlusal surfaces in the provisional prosthesis and by encouraging patients to adhere to a soft or liquid diet.
- Encouraging the biologic seal in the soft tissue area by connecting the abutments to the implants the day of surgery and never removing them. This area was not manipulated for the entire observation period of loading and may be one of the reasons for the high success rates of immediately loaded implants in heavy smokers. Because impressions were taken with the abutments in place, nicotine could not influence the soft tissues during the impression. In addition, the biologic soft tissue seal allowed blood from the surgery to fill the wound area around the abutment neck (platform switching) and to promote connective tissue formation.

# References

1. Rivera-Hidalgo F. Smoking and periodontal disease. Periodontol 2000 2003;32:50–58.
2. Widmark G, Andersson B, Carlsson GE, Lindvall AM, Ivanoff CJ. Rehabilitation of patients with severely resorbed maxillae by means of implants with or without bone grafts: A 3- to 5-year follow-up clinical report. Int J Oral Maxillofac Implants 2001;16:73–79.
3. Bain CA, Moy PK. The association between failure of dental implants and cigarette smoking. Int J Oral Maxillofac Implants 1993;8:609–615.
4. Bain CA, Moy PK. The influence of smoking on bone quality and implant failure [abstract]. Int J Oral Maxillofac Implants 1994;9:123.
5. De Bruyn H, Collaert B. The effect of smoking on early implant failure. Clin Oral Implants Res 1994;5:260–264.
6. Lemons JE, Laskin DM, Roberts WE, Tarnow DP. Changes in patient screening for a clinical study of dental implants after increased awareness of tobacco use as a risk factor. J Oral Maxillofac Surg 1997;55(suppl 5):72–75.
7. Wallace RH. The relationship between cigarette smoking and dental implant failure. Eur J Prosthodont Restor Dent 2000;8:103–106.
8. Lindquist LW, Carlsson GE, Jemt T. Association between marginal bone loss around osseointegrated mandibular implants and smoking habits: A 10-year follow-up study. J Dent Res 1997;76:1667–1674.
9. Haas R, Haimböck W, Mailath G, Watzek G. The relationship of smoking on peri-implant tissue: A retrospective study. J Prosthet Dent 1996;76:592–596.
10. Bergström J, Eliasson S, Dock J. A 10-year prospective study of tobacco smoking and periodontal health. J Periodontol 2000;71:1338–1347.
11. Larcos G. Predicting clinical discordance of bone mineral density. Mayo Clin Proc 1998;73:824–828.
12. Wilson TG Jr, Nunn M. The relationship between the interleukin-1 periodontal genotype and implant loss. Initial data. J Periodontol 1999;70:724–729.
13. Meechan JG, MacGregor DM, Rogers SM, Hobson RS. The effect of smoking on immediate post-extraction socket filling with blood and on the incidence of painful sockets. Br J Oral Maxillofac Surg 1988;26:402–409.
14. Kan JYK, Rungcharassaeng K, Lozada JL, Goodacre CJ. Effects of smoking on implant success in grafted maxillary sinuses. J Prosthet Dent 1999;82:307–311.
15. Keller EE, Tolman DE, Eckert SE. Maxillary antral-nasal inlay autogenous bone graft reconstruction of compromised maxilla: A 12-year retrospective study. Int J Oral Maxillofac Implants 1999;14:707–721.
16. Chiapasco M, Gatti C, Rossi E, Haefliger W, Markwalder TH. Implant-retained mandibular overdentures with immediate loading. A retrospective multicenter study on 226 consecutive cases. Clin Oral Implants Res 1997;8:48–57.
17. Randow K, Ericsson I, Nilner K, Petersson A, Glantz PO. Immediate functional loading of Brånemark dental implants. An 18-month clinical follow-up study. Clin Oral Implants Res 1999;10:8–15.
18. Degidi M, Piattelli A. Immediate functional and non-functional loading of dental implants: A 2- to 60-month follow-up study of 646 titanium implants. J Periodontol 2003;74:225–241.
19. Testori T, Del Fabbro M, Szmukler-Moncler S, Francetti L, Weinstein RL. Immediate occlusal loading of Osseotite implants in the completely edentulous mandible. Int J Oral Maxillofac Implants 2003;18:544–551.
20. Testori T, Meltzer A, Del Fabbro M, et al. Immediate occlusal loading of Osseotite implants in the lower edentulous jaw. A multicenter prospective study. Clin Oral Implants Res 2004;15:278–284.
21. Romanos GE, Nentwig GH. Immediate loading using cross-arch fixed restorations in heavy smokers: Nine consecutive case reports for edentulous arches. Int J Oral Maxillofac Implants 2008;23:513–519.
22. Romanos GE, Johansson C. Immediate loading with complete implant-supported restorations in an edentulous heavy smoker: Histologic and histomorphometric analyses. Int J Oral Maxillofac Implants 2005;20:282–290.
23. Oliveira MA, Gallottini M, Pallos D, Maluf PS, Jablonka F, Ortega KL. The success of endosseous implants in human immunodeficiency virus–positive patients receiving antiretroviral therapy: A pilot study. J Am Dent Assoc 2011;142:1010–1016.

# Immediate Loading with Simultaneous Sinus Elevation

11

The use of the immediate occlusal loading treatment concept and simultaneous sinus elevation procedures has not yet been studied. There are no data in the literature regarding this treatment approach, and it should be avoided if primary stability and absence of micromotions cannot be absolutely assured. As was discussed earlier in this book (see chapters 2 to 4), the threshold level of micromotions is dependent on the characteristics of the implant design and surface properties. This chapter presents data from a case series using an implant system with a progressive thread design and sand-blasted, acid-etched surface. The design of the implant allows for better condensation of the bone and higher compressive forces in the apical compared with the cervical part of the implant during implant placement.[1,2]

Compression of bone and tension lead to new bone formation.[3] The bone-implant contact percentages are higher around immediately loaded versus nonloaded implants,[4,5] and the bone density around immediately loaded implants is higher than that around delayed loaded implants.[5,6] Based on these facts, the author used the concept of immediate loading in selected case series and presents here the related protocol and clinical experience.

In previous publications, the author has presented the advanced surgical and prosthetic concept of immediate loading in the maxilla with simultaneous bone grafting.[7]

In cases with residual maxillary height of at least 4 mm, implants can be placed with simultaneous sinus augmentation and can be loaded after healing with a new height of 5 to 6 mm. When primary stability is achieved and micromovements are absent (via splinting), implant placement with simultaneous sinus elevation and immediate functional loading can be used successfully.

The sinus membrane is elevated and augmentation is performed using autogenous bone (harvested from the tuberosity, adjacent areas in the maxilla, or donor sites of the mandible), xenografts (eg, Bio-Oss, Geistlich), or allografts (eg, Puros, Zimmer). Excellent condensation of the particulated bone grafting material in contact with the implant surface is necessary, especially around the apical part of the implant.

The osteotomy should be performed very gently and without tapping to improve the primary stability; the use of tapered rather than cylindric implants is also recommended. After implant placement, immobilization (splinting) is essential, as it is in any case of immediate (occlusal) loading in sites with poor bone quality or in combination with simultaneous augmentation of dehiscences or fenestrations (see chapters 7 and 8). In such clinical situations, both the implant system and especially the surgical and prosthetic experience of the clinician are also of great importance. Overloading and excessive eccentric contacts should be eliminated. The provisional restoration must not have distal cantilevers, and a soft or liquid diet is mandatory for the first 3 to 4 months. The impression for the final prosthesis should be performed after completion of the healing stages confirmed by radiographic evaluation of the bone-implant interface. This avoids excessive pull-out forces, which are deleterious for osseointegration. Alternatives to immediate occlusal loading are immediate nonocclusal loading and the use of cross-arch stabilization in edentulous arches, both of which decrease the biomechanical risks.

The following general parameters are important and should be considered for the success of implants placed simultaneously with a sinus elevation procedure and immediately (occlusally) loaded after surgery:

# Immediate Loading with Simultaneous Sinus Elevation

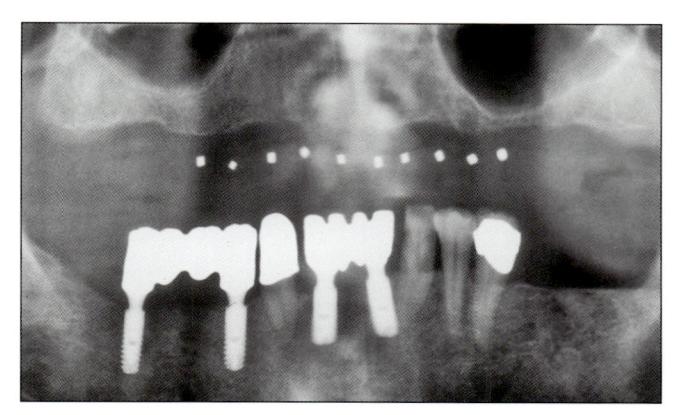

**Fig 11-1a** Radiographic examination immediately prior to surgery representing the pneumatization of the sinus.

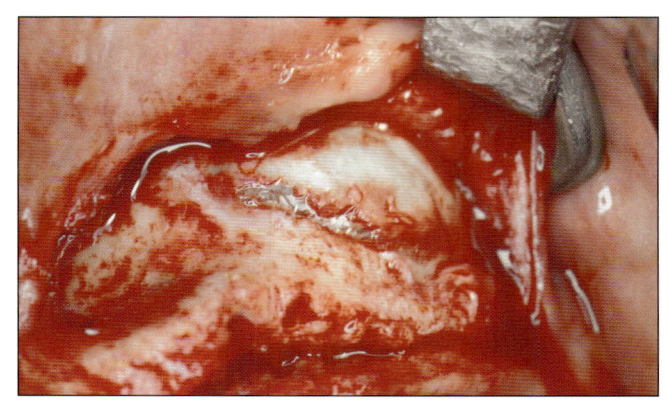

**Fig 11-1b** Lateral window preparation for sinus elevation and implant placement.

- Sufficient (at least 4 to 6 mm) vertical height of residual bone in the posterior maxilla to secure the primary stability of the implants
- Rigid immobilization (splinting) of adjacent implants through metal reinforcement of the provisional prosthesis
- Maintenance of a soft or liquid diet for the entire healing period of 3 to 4 months
- Elimination of excessive occlusal contacts in the provisional prostheses

The following clinical cases demonstrate the step-by-step treatment protocol for immediate functional loading in conjunction with simultaneous sinus elevation.

## Case Reports

### Case 1: Immediate loading with simulaneous sinus augmentation using an autograft

A 54-year-old man presented for an implant-supported rehabilitation of the maxilla. Based on the clinical and radiographic examination (Fig 11-1a), the left posterior maxilla was sufficient in width but not in height. After local anesthetic was provided, a mucoperiosteal flap was elevated. A window preparation and sinus floor elevation was performed on the left side (Fig 11-1b). The bone grafting material was autogenous bone harvested using a bone scraper from the tuberosity and adjacent sites of the maxilla. Six Ankylos implants (Dentsply Friadent) with a progressive thread design were placed (Fig 11-1c), two of them in conjunction with sinus augmentation.

The implants had excellent primary stability, as evidenced by the fact that the implant stability did not change when the cover screws were removed. All angulated abutments were connected with the final torque of 15 Ncm and covered with plastic resin caps (Fig 11-1d). The flap was closed with 4-0 silk suture material. The provisional restoration was fabricated chairside according to the predetermined vertical dimension and using a duplicate of the denture as a template in the Omnivac shell technique (Figs 11-1e and 11-1f). The resin material used for the provisional restoration was ProTemp (Espe).

Finally, the provisional restoration was polished in the lab, pink-colored resin was added for esthetic reasons in the crestal area to represent the soft tissues, and metal (wire) reinforcement was used to connect and stabilize the implants. This method of the provisional restoration has been used extensively for many years and was first published about in 2003[8] (see chapter 9). The occlusion was checked to ensure that there were sufficient occlusal contacts in intercuspal position and group contacts in the lateral movements of the mandible. A radiograph was taken immediately after surgery (Fig 11-1g) to evaluate the crestal bone levels. Observe the apical portion of the implants at the left canine and first premolar sites where there is a lack of radiopacity because of the decreased density of the grafting material. The implants were checked for stability using the Periotest device (Medizintechnik Gulden) on the day of surgery. A soft or liquid diet was necessary for the first 3 to 4 months of healing in order to avoid overloading the implants (see diet protocol described in chapter 7). Three months after surgery, the radiographic examination presented an increase in the bone density in the augmented area. The clinical evaluation presented excellent peri-implant soft tissue healing as well as implant stability after the removal of the provisional prosthesis (Figs 11-1h).

Impressions for the final restorations were performed and the implant-supported restoration was placed almost 6 months after surgery (Fig 11-1i) and fixed with TempBond (Kerr). Clinical and radiographic examinations were performed every 6 months for the first 5 years of loading. Excellent peri-implant soft tissue conditions, clinical stability measured by Periotest values, and no bone loss were observed. Of great biologic and clinical importance is the increased bone density of the grafting material, which indicates excellent remodeling in the left sinus area according to the radiographic and clinical evaluation at the 6-month, 2-year, 5-year, and 9-year follow-ups (Figs 11-1j to 11-1m).

## Case Reports

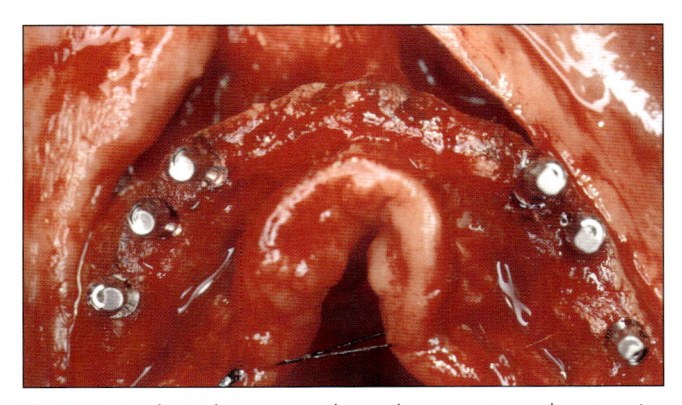

**Fig 11-1c** Implant placement with simultaneous sinus elevation. Implants are placed in the sinus cavity immediately before augmentation. Abutment connection immediately follows sinus elevation.

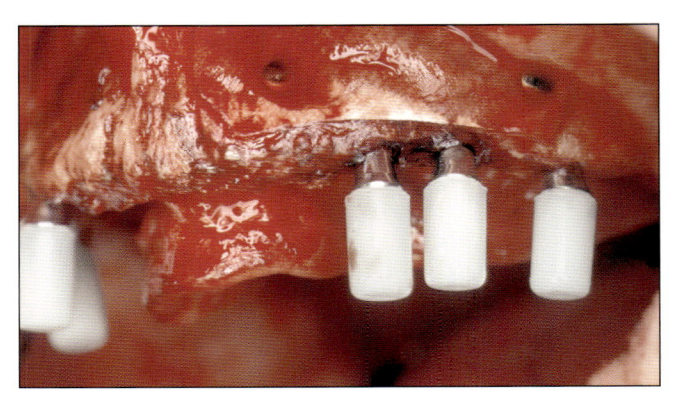

**Fig 11-1d** A collagen membrane is used to cover the lateral window. Resin caps are placed on the abutments for the fabrication of the temporary partial denture.

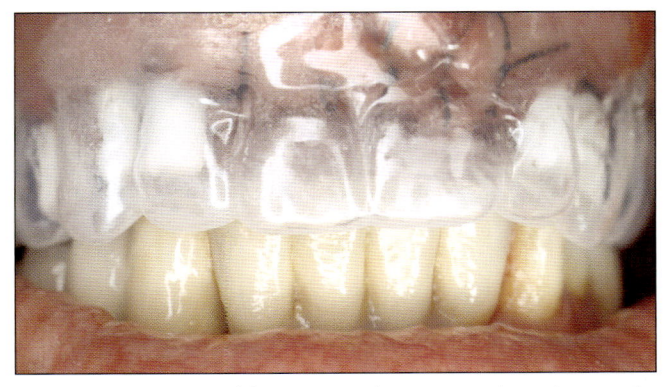

**Fig 11-1e** Fabrication of the provisional restoration chairside using the Omnivac shell technique.

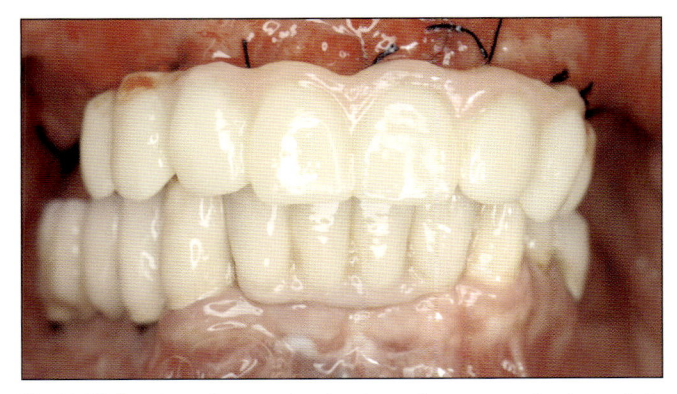

**Fig 11-1f** Provisional restoration in place after surgery (ie, immediate occlusal loading).

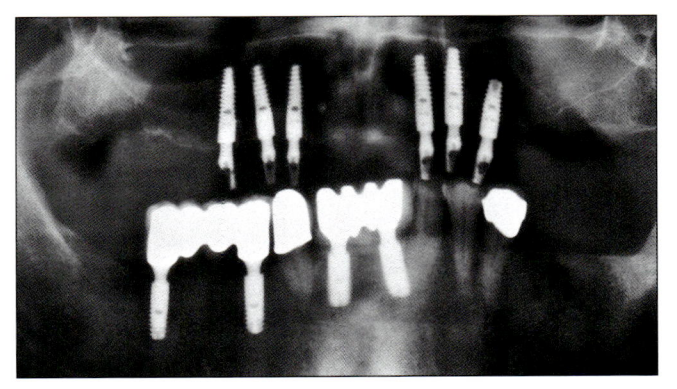

**Fig 11-1g** Radiographic examination immediately after implant placement with simultaneous sinus elevation.

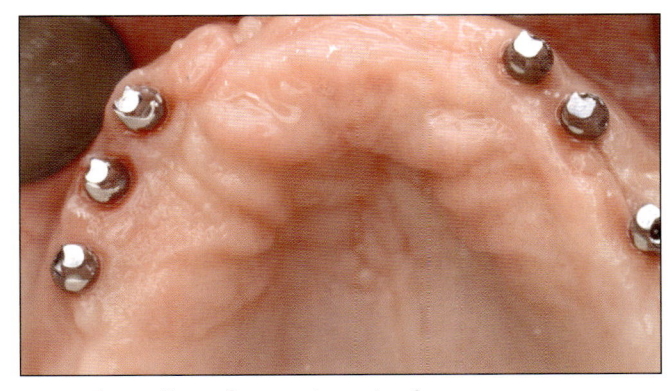

**Fig 11-1h** Excellent soft tissues 3 months after surgery.

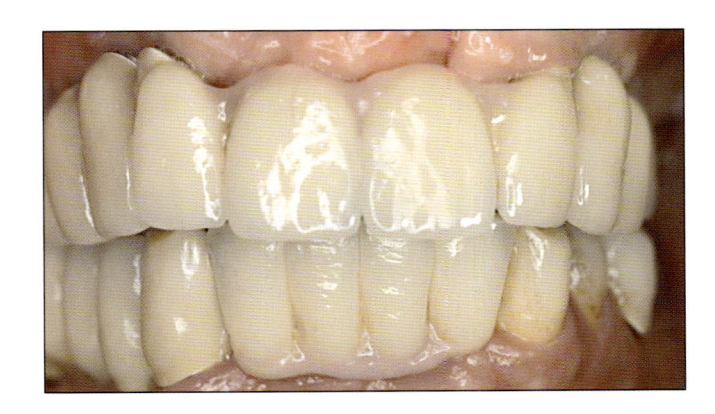

**Fig 11-1i** Final restoration in place.

123

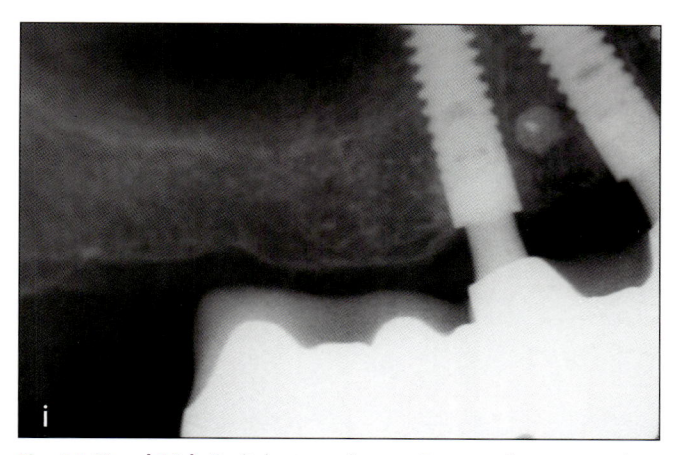

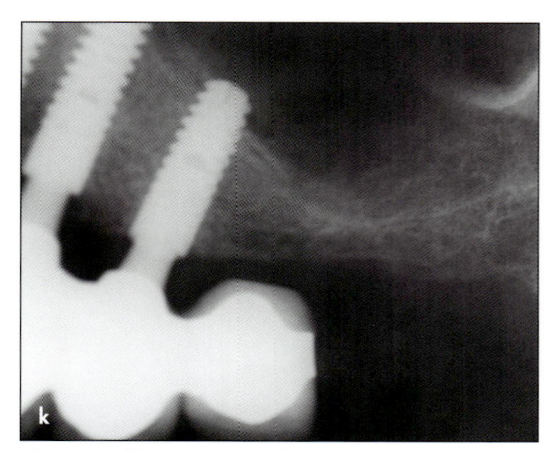

**Figs 11-1j and 11-k** Radiologic evaluation 5 years after surgery showing excellent crestal bone around all implants in the right *(j)* and left *(k)* sides. Note the new bone formation on the left side under immediate loading conditions.

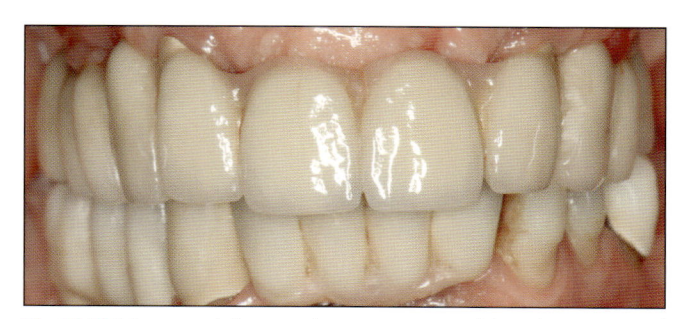

**Fig 11-1l** Nine-year follow-up showing a successful implant-supported maxillary restoration.

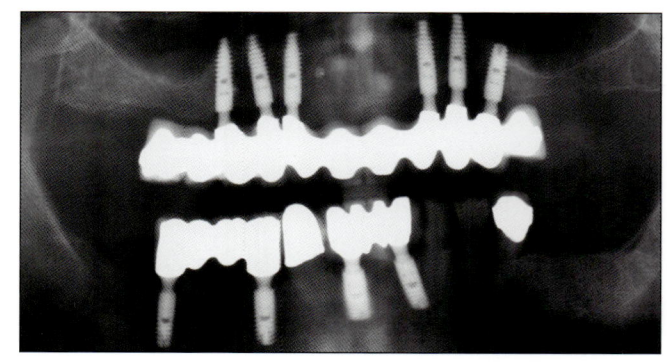

**Fig 11-1m** Radiographic evaluation after 9 years of excellent healing. No crestal bone loss was observed. No abutments were removed during the entire observation period. (Dental technician: S. Roth, Frankfurt, Germany.)

## Case 2: Immediate loading in the maxilla with a cross-arch implant-supported prosthesis and simultaneous bilateral sinus elevation

The treatment was provided for a woman who presented with an edentulous maxilla (Fig 11-2a). Eight Ankylos implants were placed symmetrically in the maxilla in the areas of the canines, first and second premolars, and first molars. The posterior implants were placed in conjunction with simultaneous bilateral sinus elevation procedures. The grafting material was composed of Bio-Oss and autogenous bone from the tuberosity (Figs 11-2b to 11-2d). Collagen membranes were used to cover the lateral window and were fixed in place with Frios titanium membrane tacks (Friadent) (Fig 11-2e). The implants were stabilized in the residual maxillary bone at a height between 4 and 5 mm. The distalmost implant on the left side was stabilized in the residual maxilla at only 3 mm. The implants were splinted together after abutment connection using 15-Ncm final torque (Fig 11-2f). This treatment concept can be used with implants having Morse taper implant-abutment connections because the final torque can be lower than that required for traditional implant-abutment connections.

The provisional restoration was fabricated chairside with ProTemp resin material and cemented using TempBond (Figs 11-2g and 11-2h). The occlusion was checked to have group function with symmetric occlusal contacts. A panoramic radiograph was taken immediately after surgery to evaluate both the positioning of the implants and the crestal bone levels (Fig 11-2i). A soft or liquid diet was necessary for the first 3 to 4 months of healing.

The patient was examined weekly to check for the stability of the provisional restoration, potential occlusal discrepancies, and fractures of the restoration. After 4 weeks of healing, the provisional restoration was removed carefully using a needle holder and gentle pull-out forces. The implants were evaluated for stability and soft tissue healing (Figs 11-2j and 11-2k).

The provisional restoration was replaced 9 months later because of difficulties in patient compliance and follow-up. For that reason, the new provisional restoration was reinforced with metal to securely splint the implants. This provisional restoration was in use for almost 2 years (Figs 11-2l and 11-2m). The final restorations were completed after 4 years of immediate loading because of financial reasons (Figs 11-2n and 11-2o).

Case Reports

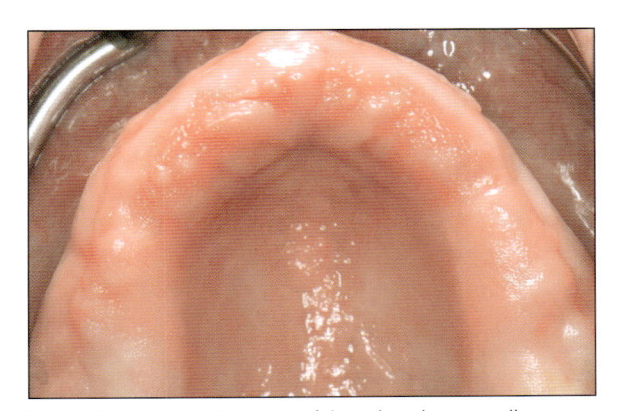

**Fig 11-2a** Preoperative view of the edentulous maxilla.

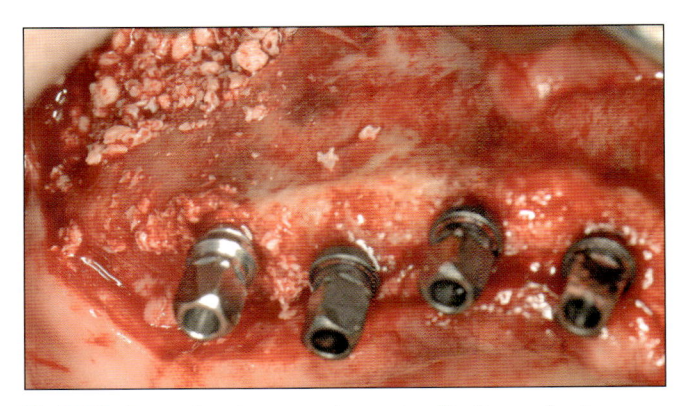

**Fig 11-2b** Sinus elevation procedure, using Bio-Oss and autogenous bone, and implant placement have been performed on the right side.

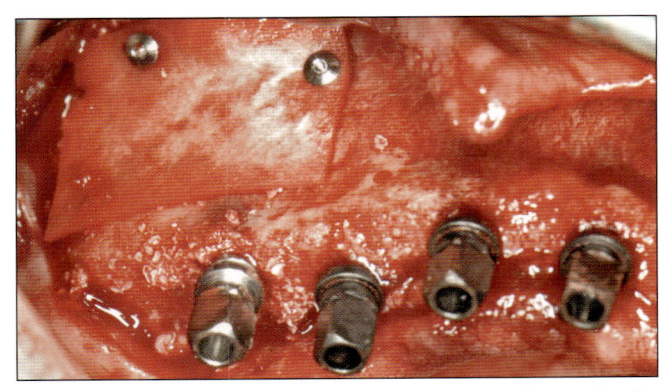

**Fig 11-2c** Right window area covered with a Biomend Extend collagen membrane (Zimmer) fixed with Frios titanium tacks.

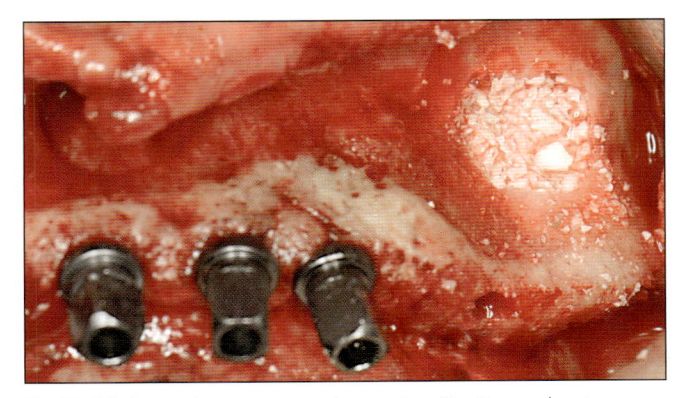

**Fig 11-2d** Sinus elevation procedure, using Bio-Oss and autogenous bone, and implant placement have been performed on the left side.

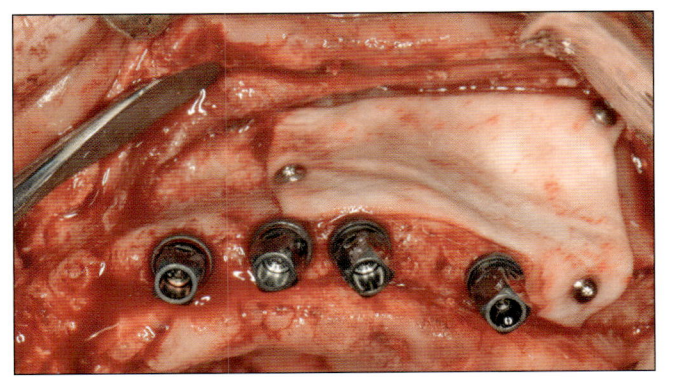

**Fig 11-2e** Window area covered with a Bio-Gide collagen membrane (Geistlich) fixed with Frios titanium tacks.

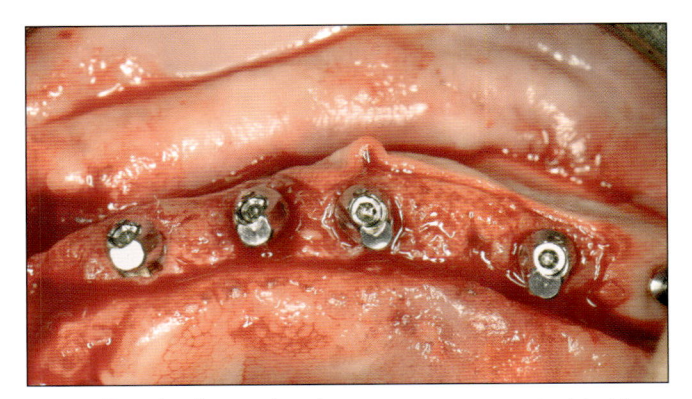

**Fig 11-2f** Occlusal view after abutment connection on the left side.

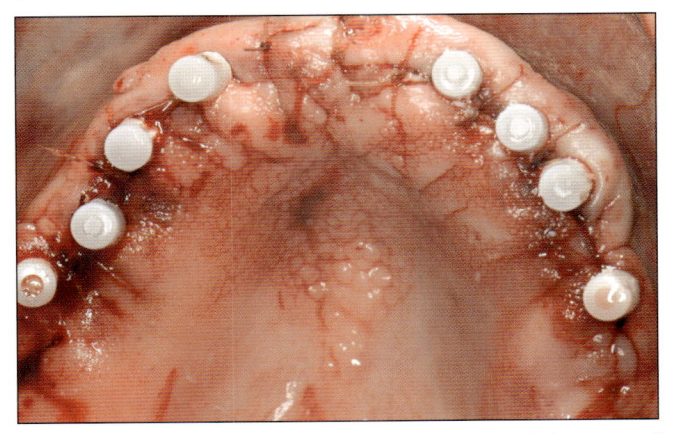

**Fig 11-2g** Occlusal view after abutment connection and placement of resin caps for the chairside fabrication of the provisional prosthesis.

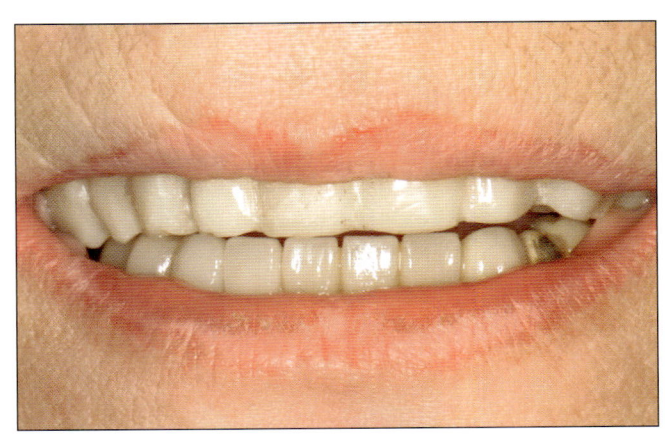

**Fig 11-2h** Smile line immediately after surgery presenting an acceptable result.

# 11 | Immediate Loading with Simultaneous Sinus Elevation

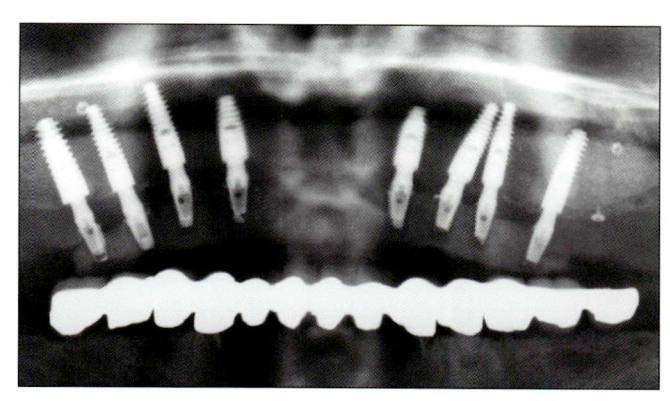

**Fig 11-2i** Baseline radiographic examination immediately after bilateral sinus elevation procedures and implant placement for immediate loading.

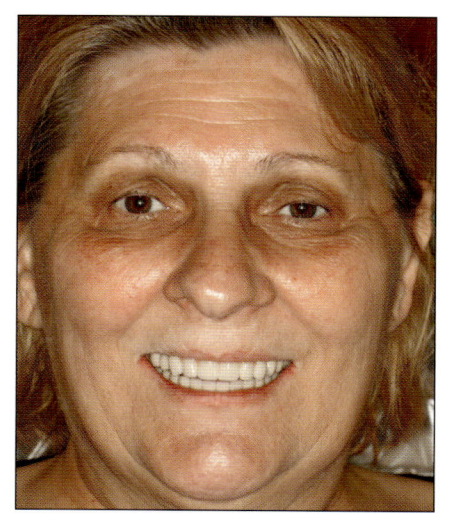

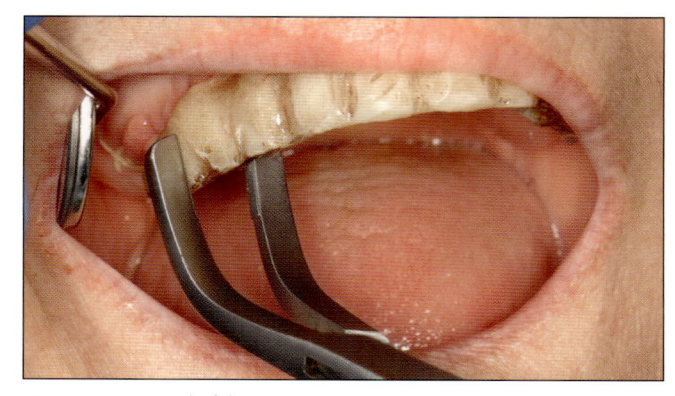

**Fig 11-2j** Removal of the provisional restoration 4 weeks after surgery for suture removal and evaluation of the implant stability. The use of a conventional crown removal instrument is contraindicated because of the uncontrolled, high pull-out forces.

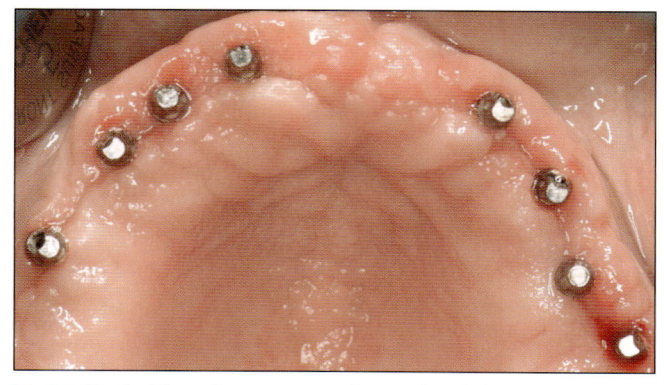

**Fig 11-2k** Healthy soft tissue around immediately loaded implants 4 weeks after surgery.

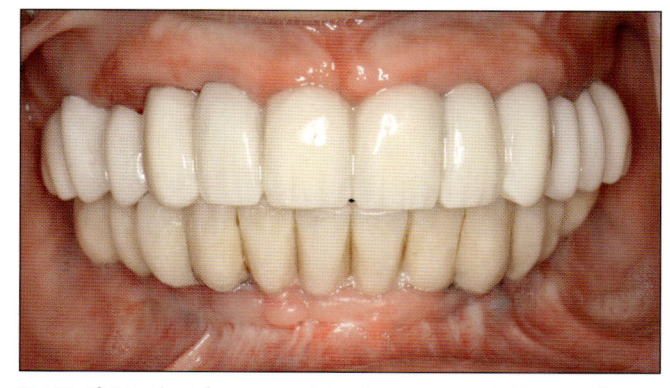

**Fig 11-2l** Metal-reinforced provisional restorations 1.5 years after implant placement and immediate loading in the maxilla and mandible.

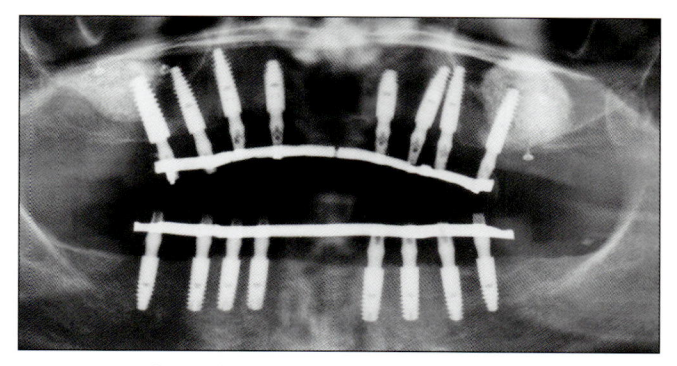

**Fig 11-2m** Radiographic examination 1.5 years after surgery presenting excellent bone stability around all implants. Note that there is no crestal bone loss.

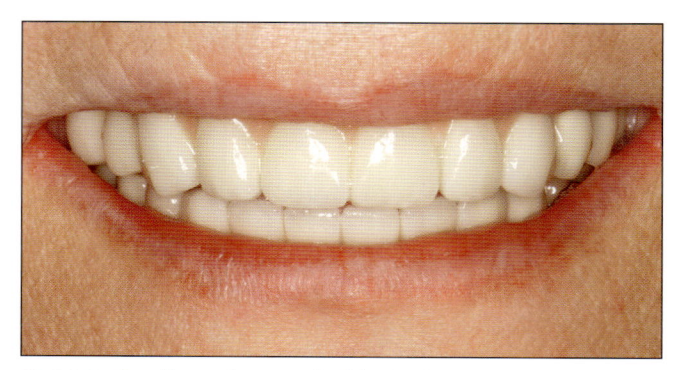

**Fig 11-2n** Excellent esthetic result of the final restorations 4 years after immediate loading.

**Fig 11-2o** Harmony of the restoration in association with the patient's face 4 years after surgery. (Surgery by G.E. Romanos and A. Basha Hijazi, New York, NY. Dental technician: L. Marotta, New York, NY. Restorations by W. Oweity and P. Barientos, New York, NY.)

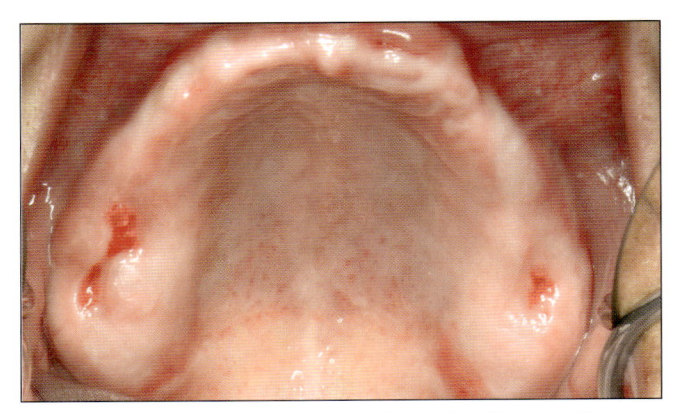

**Fig 11-3a** Preoperative occlusal view of the edentulous maxilla

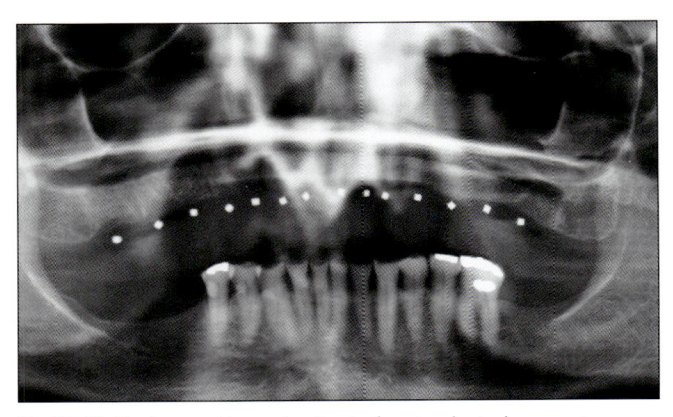

**Fig 11-3b** Radiographic evaluation before implant placement.

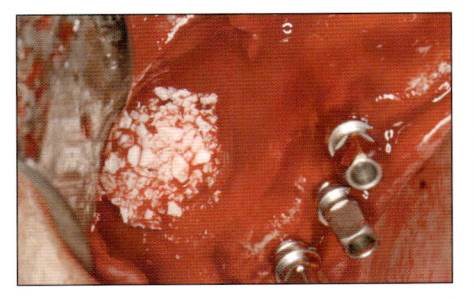

**Fig 11-3c** Sinus elevation using Bio-Oss and autogenous bone in conjunction with implant (Ankylos Plus) placement on the right side.

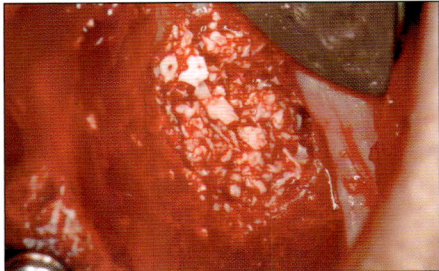

**Fig 11-3d** Sinus elevation using Bio-Oss and autogenous bone in conjunction with implant (Ankylos Plus) placement on the left side.

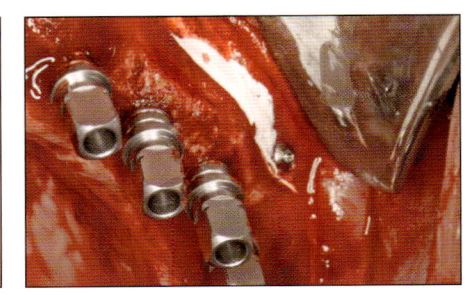

**Fig 11-3e** Left sinus window area covered with a Bio-Gide collagen membrane fixed with Osteo-Med titanium tacks.

## Case 3: Immediate loading in the maxilla with a cross-arch implant-supported prosthesis and simultaneous bilateral sinus elevation

This case presents the prosthetic rehabilitation of an edentulous atrophic maxilla of a woman with simultaneous bilateral sinus elevation and in conjunction with implant placement and immediate loading. A new full-arch denture was fabricated for the edentulous maxilla (Fig 11-3a), which was used as a prosthetic guide for implant placement. A panoramic radiograph was taken to evaluate the height of the residual bone in the posterior maxilla (Fig 11-3b). The sinus elevation procedures were performed using the traditional lateral window technique. After elevation of the sinus membrane, augmentation was completed using autogenous bone from the tuberosity and Bio-Oss cancellous bone grafting material.

Eight Ankylos Plus implants (Dentsply Friadent) were placed in the maxilla, five of which in the area of the sinus elevation and augmentation, and final abutments were connected using the final torque recommended by manufacturer guidelines (Figs 11-3c and 11-3d). The lateral windows were covered with Bio-Gide collagen membranes fixed with titanium tacks (Fig 11-3e).

Immediately after flap closure, a provisional restoration was made using a template and cemented in place with TempBond (Fig 11-3f). The patient was satisfied with the fixed restoration (Fig 11-3g). The implant positions were evaluated with a postoperative radiograph (Fig 11-3h). During evaluation a couple of weeks later, the implants demonstrated clinical stability, and the soft tissues were healthy. Three months after surgery, an impression was taken over the final abutments without their removal in preparation for fabrication of the final restoration (Figs 11-3i and 11-3j). The final prosthesis was cemented temporarily 5 months after surgery (Fig 11-3k). Over the 2-year observation period, the implants showed an excellent stability with no crestal bone loss (Fig 11-3l).

# 11 | Immediate Loading with Simultaneous Sinus Elevation

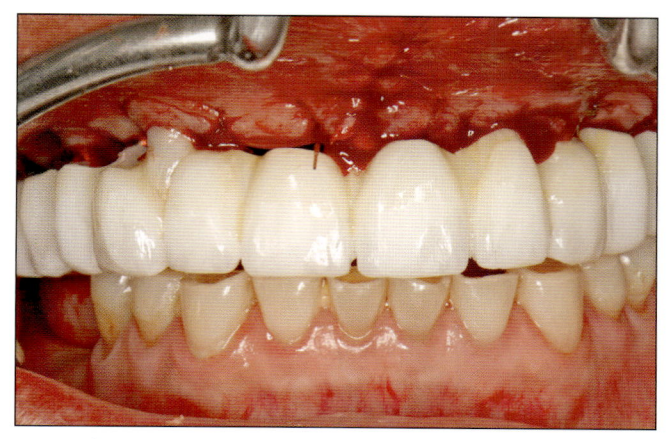

**Fig 11-3f** Provisional restoration in occlusion immediately after surgery.

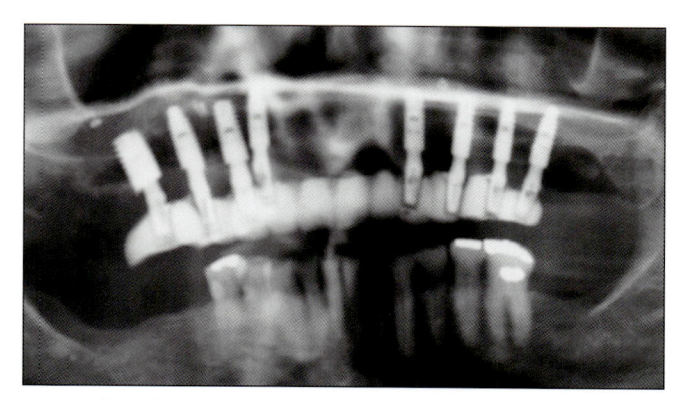

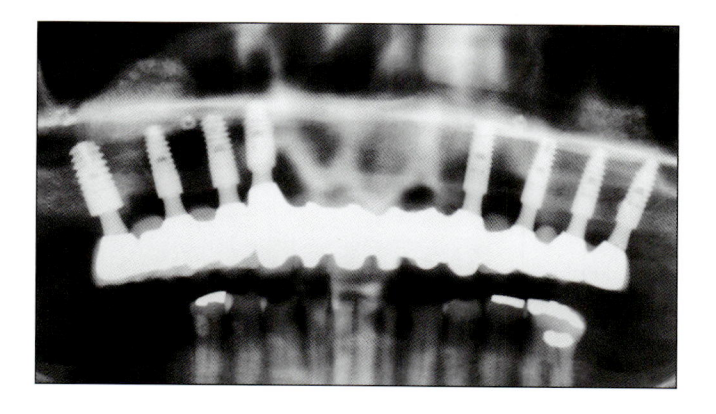

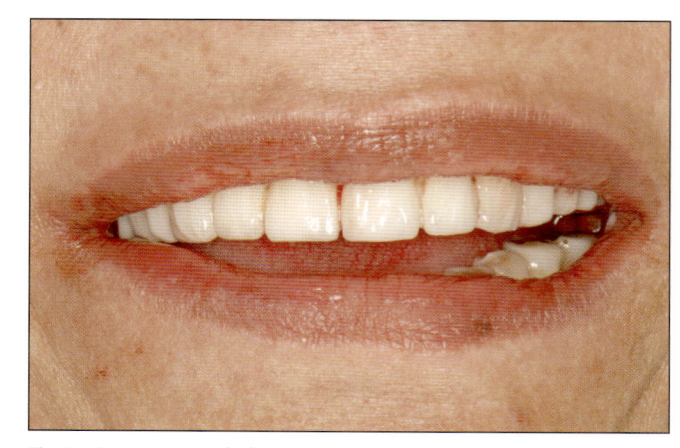

**Fig 11-3g** Patient smile line immediately after surgery.

**Fig 11-3h** Radiographic examination immediately after surgery with the provisional cross-arch implant-supported prosthesis in place.

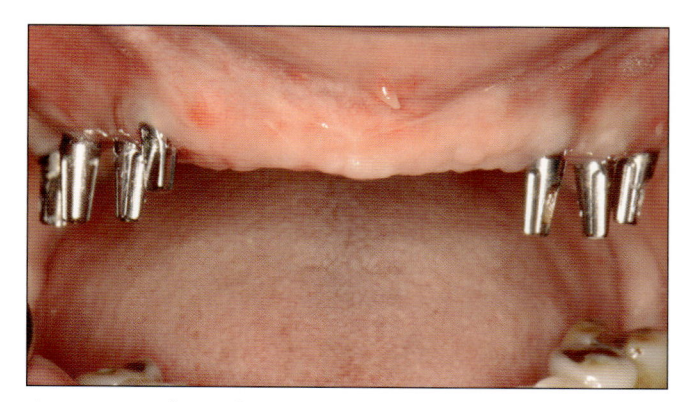

**Fig 11-3i** Excellent soft tissues around the immediately loaded implants 3 months after placement (at time of final impression).

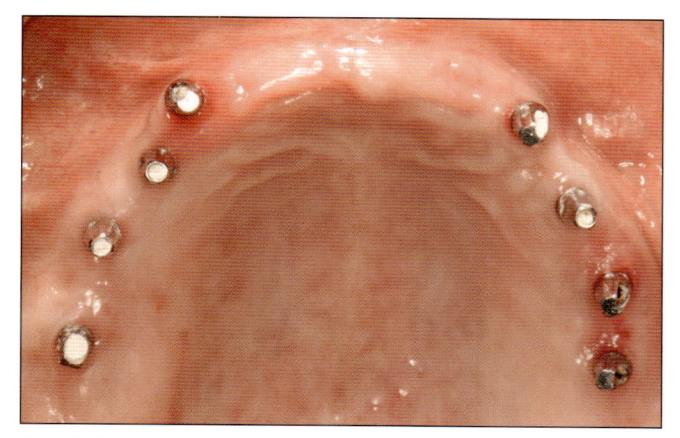

**Fig 11-3j** Excellent soft tissue condition around immediately loaded implants 3 months after loading.

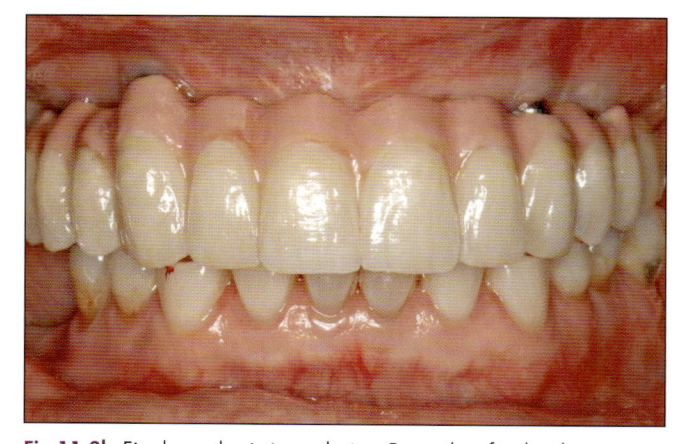

**Fig 11-3k** Final prosthesis in occlusion 5 months after loading.

**Fig 11-3l** Panoramic radiograph 2 years after immediate loading presenting excellent implant conditions and consolidation of the bone grafting materials bilaterally. (Surgical and restorative team: G. E. Romanos and Chih-Han Tai, New York, NY.)

# Case Reports

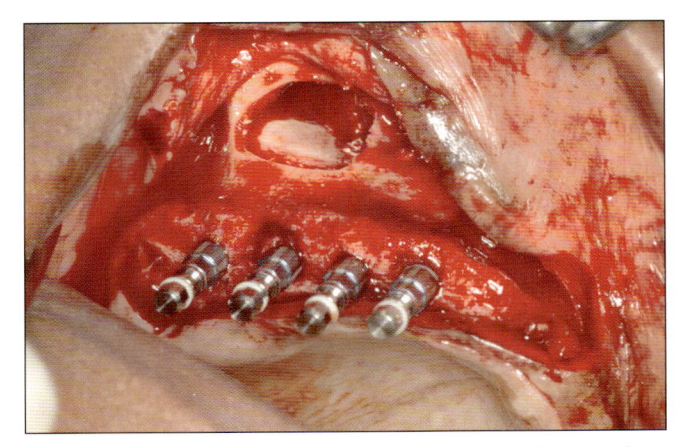

**Fig 11-4a** Sinus elevation procedure with simultaneous implant placement in the right side of the maxilla.

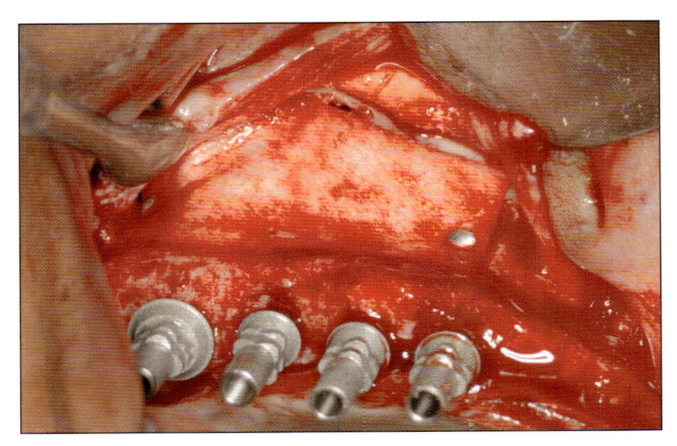

**Fig 11-4b** Coverage of the lateral window with a collagen membrane. The temporary cylinders were connected with multibase abutments for a screw-retained restoration.

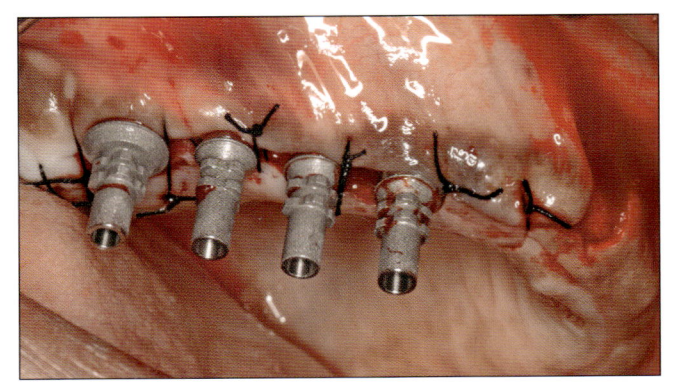

**Fig 11-4c** Flap closure showing temporary cylinders in place.

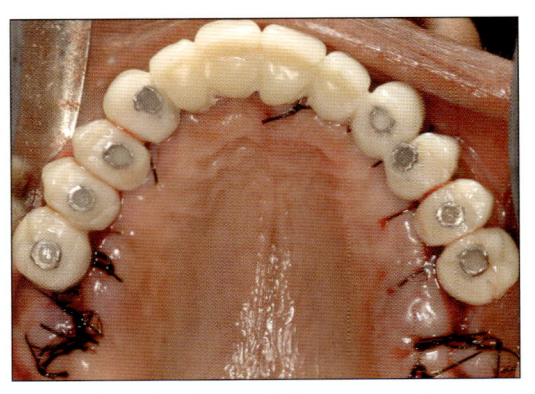

**Fig 11-4d** Occlusal view of the provisional restoration immediately after surgery.

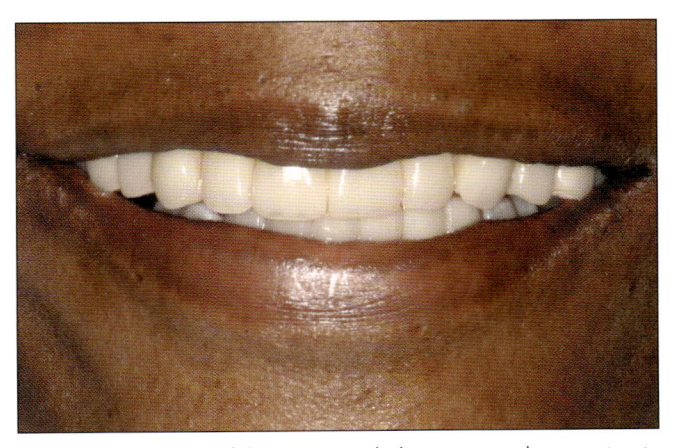

**Fig 11-4e** Smile line of the patient with the provisional restoration in place immediately after surgery. The patient was satisfied with the restoration and postponed the final rehabilitation.

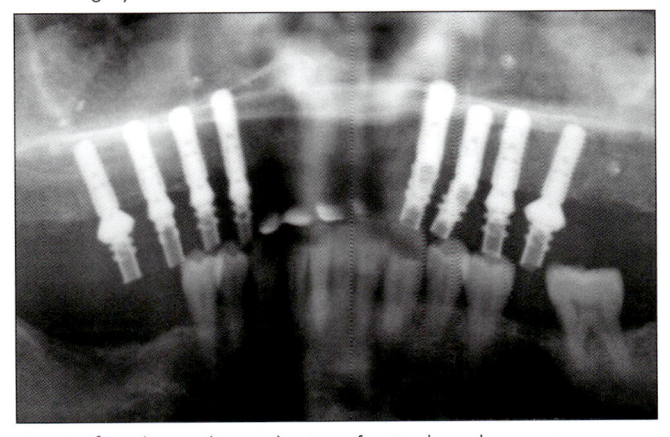

**Fig 11-4f** Radiographic evaluation after implant placement.

## Case 4: Immediate loading in the maxilla with simultaneous bilateral sinus elevation

The present case report presents the treatment of a 45-year-old woman with an edentulous maxilla involving simultaneous bilateral sinus elevation procedures in conjunction with implant placement and immediate functional loading. Straumann Bone Level implants were used with a screw-retained implant-supported restoration (Figs 11-4a to 11-4c).

Immediately after implant placement and evaluation of the primary stability, multibase abutments were placed and connected with final torque. Temporary cylinders were screwed over the multibase abutments. The flaps were closed with sutures, and the provisional restoration was fabricated chairside and placed immediately to secure the implants and splint them together (Figs 11-4d to 11-4f). A soft or liquid diet protocol was recommended for the first 3 to 4 months of healing to ensure the best healing of the implants.

During the implant healing, follow-up was completed every 2 weeks (Figs 11-4g and 11-4h). The patient was very satisfied with the temporary restoration and was not eager to return for the final prosthetic rehabilitation.

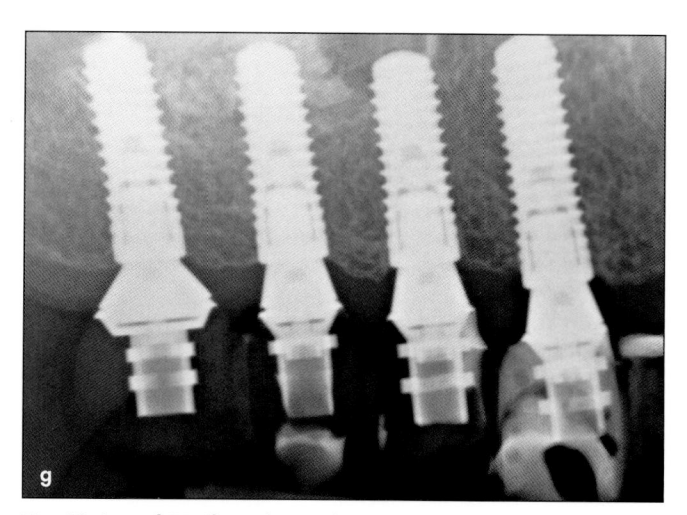

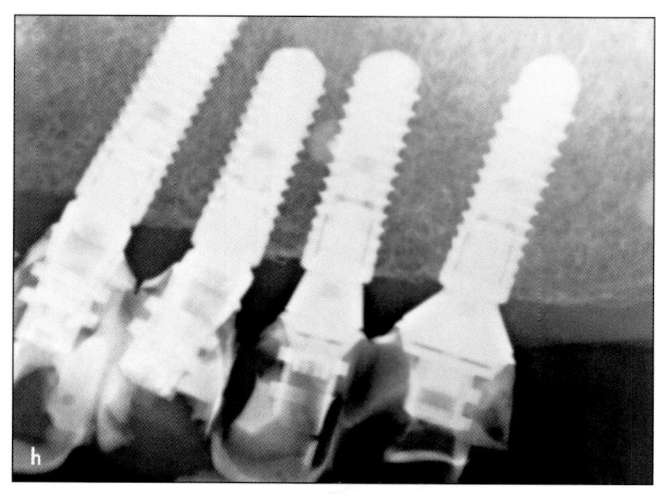

**Figs 11-4g and 11-4h** Radiographic evaluation on the right *(g)* and left *(h)* sides 28 months after surgery presenting excellent crestal bone stability. (Surgery by G. E. Romanos and G. Ciornei; restoration by P. Cortes, Rochester, NY.)

# References

1. Nentwig GH, Moser W, Knefel T, Ficker E. Dreidimensionale spannungsoptische Untersuchungen der NM-Implantatgewindeform im Vergleich mit herkömmlichen Implantatgewinden. Z Zahnärztl Implantol 1992;8:130–135.
2. Nentwig GH, Moser W, Mairgünther R. Das Ankylos-Implantatsystem. Konzept, Klinik, Ergebnisse. Implantologie 1993;3:225–237.
3. Oda J, Sakamoto J, Aoyama K, Sueyoshi Y, Tomita K, Sawaguchi T. Mechanical stresses and bone formation. In: Hayashi K, Kamiya A, Ono K (eds). Biomechanics: Functional Adaptation and Remodeling. Tokyo: Springer, 1996:123–140.
4. Piattelli A, Corigliano M, Scarano A, Costigliola G, Paolantonio M. Immediate loading of titanium plasma-sprayed implants: An histologic analysis in monkeys. J Periodontol 1998;69:321–327.
5. Romanos GE, Toh CG, Siar CH, Wicht H, Yaacob H, Nentwig GH. Bone-implant interface around titanium implants under different loading conditions: A histomorphometrical analysis in the *Macaca fascicularis* monkey. J Periodontol 2003;74:1483–1490.
6. Romanos GE, Toh CG, Siar CH, Swaminathan D. Histologic and histomorphometric implant bone subjected to immediate loading: An experimental study with *Macaca fascicularis*. Int J Oral Maxillofac Implants 2002;17:44–51.
7. Romanos GE. Surgical and prosthetic concepts for predictable immediate loading of oral implants. J Calif Dent Assoc 2004;32:991–1001.
8. Romanos GE. Treatment of advanced periodontal destruction with immediately loaded implants and simultaneous bone augmentation: A case report. J Periodontol 2003;74:255–261.

# Immediate Loading of Single-Tooth Implants 12

The single-tooth implant is the main clinical indication in daily implant practice, and the promising therapeutic results have convinced many clinicians to attempt modified surgical and loading protocols, such as immediate implant placement and immediate functional and nonfunctional loading, with the single-tooth implant.

Clinical studies have presented high survival and success rates related to single-tooth implants with immediate provisionalization in the anterior[1-11] and posterior[3,12-15] regions. In addition, different implant systems with various designs, diameters, and surfaces have been used in the anterior and posterior regions and the implant prognosis evaluated. Degidi et al[16] showed high success rates in immediate restoration of single-tooth implants independent of the bone quality and implant system. However, there is limited long-term documentation[17] focused on the peri-implant soft tissues and changes in the buccal margin, such as gingival recession around single-tooth implants.

The survival rate of immediately loaded implants seems to be quite high based on bone levels and implant stability over the period of loading (Table 12-1). However, in order to consider an outcome a success and satisfy the patient, the additional considerations of the prosthetic restoration as well as soft tissue conditions are very important. Further studies should be done with a focus on these concerns in order to make implant therapy with immediate loading concepts more predictable, especially for single-tooth implant restoration. When there is a new concept in therapy, the long-term soft and hard tissue stability is important, especially in the highly demanding cases. For example, the use of implant systems with platform switching seems to provide peri-implant soft tissue stability and papilla preservation in association with immediate loading.[17] It has been proven that the soft tissues around immediately versus delayed loaded implants with platform switching do not have significant histologic and histomorphometric differences.[22]

Important parameters in the placement of single-tooth implants in the esthetic zone include minimally invasive surgery with papilla preservation, flapless or advanced flap elevation, augmentation (dependent on the thickness of the buccal plate and the presence of a fenestration or dehiscence), proper augmentation and membrane materials, the distance between the implant and the surrounding hard tissue, flap advancement, and suturing technique. These parameters may be even more critical when using a wide-body implant system to enable a prosthetic approach that will improve esthetics. Very often the soft tissue thickness is of importance, and soft tissue management is one of the significant milestones in implant therapy. In addition, the dental technician and ceramist play a significant role in meeting esthetic demands.

From a scientific standpoint, many animal and clinical studies have been performed to document hard tissue stability in the socket after immediate implant placement. Dependent on the surgical technique (ie, flap or flapless approach),[10,23] the type of augmentation material and membrane,[24,25] the advancement of the flap,[23] the papilla preservation, and the animal model,[26] different levels of bone remodeling or resorption have been documented. In addition, the distance between the implant surface and the surrounding bone has been evaluated in various studies using implant systems with different types of implant surface.[26] In some studies, if the distance was greater than 1 mm, the gap was filled with a mixture of bovine bone matrix (Bio-Oss, Geistlich) and blood.[17,27,28]

The author believes in the healing power of blood clot stabilization in the socket at the time of the implant

**Table 12-1** Clinical studies on immediate loading of single-tooth implants

| Authors | System | N | Region | Loading period | Survival rate (%) |
|---|---|---|---|---|---|
| Chaushu et al 2001[3] | AlphaBio, SteriOss | 28 | A/P | Up to 2 y | 82.4–100 |
| Ericsson et al 2001[4] | Brånemark (Nobel Biocare) | 14 | A | 1.5 y | 85.7 |
| Hui et al 2001[5] | Brånemark | 24 | A (maxilla) | Up to 1.5 y | 100 |
| Kan et al 2003[7] | Replace Select (Nobel Biocare) | 35 | A (maxilla) | 1–3.5 y | 100 |
| Lorenzoni et al 2003[8] | Frialit-2 (Dentsply Friadent) | 20 | A (maxilla) | 1 y | 100 |
| Malo et al 2003[2] | Brånemark | 63 | A | 1 y | 93.7 |
| Norton 2004[9] | Astra Tech | 44 | A (maxilla) | 1.5–2.25 y | 96.4 |
| Abboud et al 2005[14] | Ankylos (Dentsply Friadent) | 20 | P | 1 y | 100 |
| Cornelini et al 2005[18] | Straumann | 19 | A (maxilla) | 1 y | 100 |
| Barone et al 2006[10] | Premium (Sweden and Martina) | 18 | Incisors, canines, premolars | 1 y | 94.44 |
| Degidi et al 2006[16] | Ankylos, Frialit-2, XiVE (Dentsply Friadent), Restore (Lifecore), Maestro (BioHorizons), Brånemark | 111 | Incisors, canines, premolars | 5 y | 97.2 |
| Ferrara et al 2006[19] | Frialit-2 | 33 | A | 4 y | 93.94 |
| Canullo and Rasperini 2007[17] | Defcon (Impladent) | 10 | A (maxilla) | 21.9 mo | 100 |
| Schincaglia et al 2008[15] | MK III WP (Brånemark) | 30 | P (mandible) | 1 y | 100 |
| Siddiqui et al 2008[20] | Tapered Screw-Vent (Zimmer) | 69 | A/P | 1 y | 98.55 |
| Nissan et al 2008[21] | 3i, Zimmer | 12 | A (maxilla) | 18 mo | 100 |
| Mijiritsky et al 2009[11] | XiVE, Frialit-2, MIS | 24 | A (maxilla) | 24–72 mo | 95.8 |

A, anterior; P, posterior.

placement, which is significantly different in animal models than in humans and may contribute to hard and soft tissue stability (see chapter 13). Long-term results in different clinical cases have been emphasized. Similar concepts of therapy have been introduced in protocols for placement of implants in fresh extraction sockets, with or without simultaneous augmentations, by various clinicians.[29]

There are limited human histologic studies evaluating bone around immediate implants placed in fresh extraction sockets simultaneously with immediate functional (occlusal) loading. Dense bone has been shown with a high number of osteons and remodeling compared with unloaded immediate implants, which are characteristically surrounded by thin bone trabeculae.[30]

Several implant manufacturers have introduced new scalloped implants designed to stabilize the bone crest using microthreads in the cervical part of the implants, platform switching, and the exclusion of the microgap to form a better biologic width. Further studies with histologic evaluation are necessary to increase the scientific data and support the clinical evidence.

From a biologic standpoint, it is not necessary to have occlusal contacts (functional loading) immediately after implant placement in single-tooth restorations. Clinical studies used immediate provisionalization without occlusal contact,[11,19,31,32] with only slight contact,[3] and with complete occlusal contact.[12,20,33–35] Full occlusal contact is only safe for single-tooth restorations when primary implant stability, the appropriate occlusal load, and the correct case selection are achieved. Successful results have been documented in the anterior maxilla when augmentations have been performed with freeze-dried block allografts, and after healing, implants were placed and restored provisionally without occlusal contacts.[21]

In addition, minimal crestal bone loss (mesial and distal) around immediately loaded implants placed in fresh extraction sites with fully preserved walls was observed after 12 and 18 months in a study in which the implants were placed 1 mm subcrestally at the buccal wall.[35]

Therefore, the author strongly recommends subcrestal placement (3 mm deeper than the midfacial bone crest) to decrease bone resorption due to surgical trauma, flap

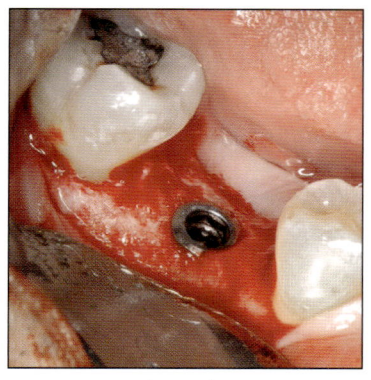

# Case Reports

**Fig 12-1a** Implant placement in the site of the mandibular right first molar.

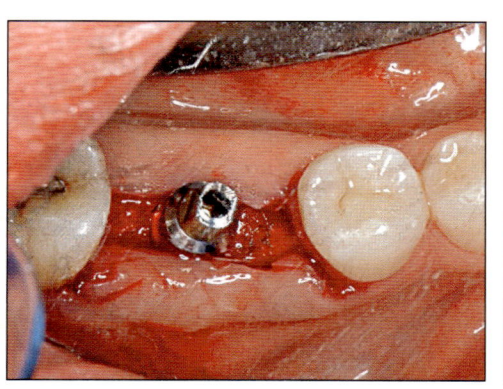

**Fig 12-1b** Platform switching abutment connection with final torque for immediate provisionalization.

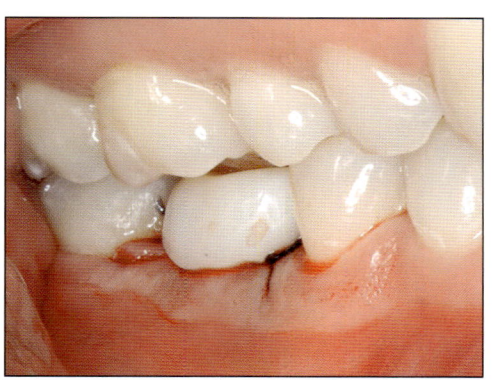

**Fig 12-1c** Provisional crown after surgery.

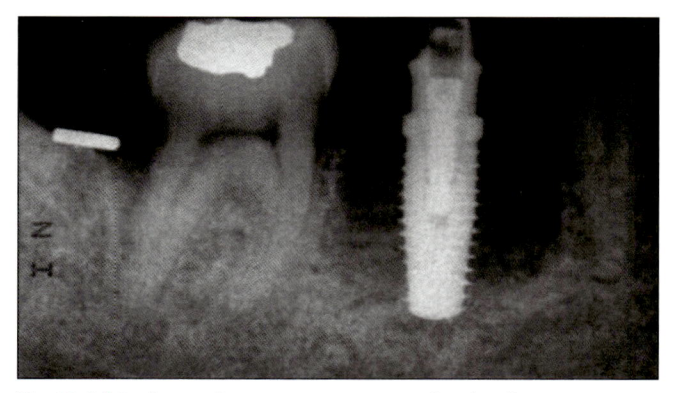

**Fig 12-1d** Radiographic examination immediately after surgery presenting the alveolar bone level related to the placed implant.

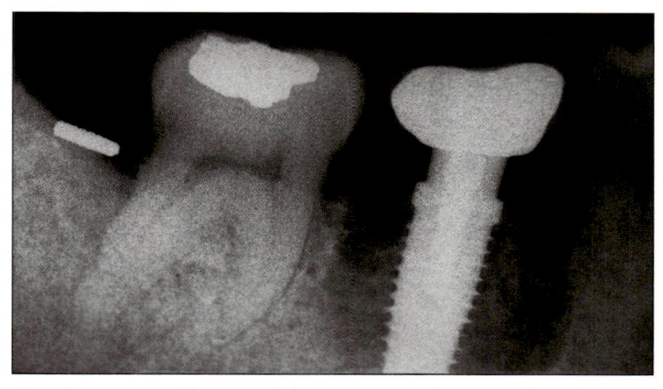

**Fig 12-1e** Crestal bone stability 3 years after immediate loading. There is no bone loss at the crestal bone because the abutment was never removed. Note the increased bone density. (Restoration by J. Lim, Rochester, NY.)

elevation, and augmentation procedures. This is essential in cases with thin tissue biotype or high cortical bone content, especially in the esthetic zone. In addition, the use of an implant system with platform switching and without removal of the abutment may stabilize the bone crest over a period of time. Prospective randomized clinical trials are needed to evaluate bone levels according to the vertical position of the implant platform, the soft tissue thickness, the surgical technique, and the loading protocols in order to substantiate the predictability of such protocols with evidence.

# Case Reports

The following clinical cases present the protocol for immediate (functional) loading of single-tooth implants. Various implant designs are used in healed ridges and fresh extraction sites with and without augmentation. Each clinical case has a different chief complaint and primary goal. In some cases, the primary goal is functional success and long-term stability and not primarily esthetic improvement in cases with a low or moderate smile line; in other cases, the best esthetic result was sought in association with acceleration of the biologic processes of wound healing.

## Case 1: Immediate loading in the posterior to improve bone quality

This case presents the treatment of a patient requiring a single-tooth restoration for an extracted mandibular right first molar. The first molar socket was filled with a bone grafting material (DynaBlast, Keystone Dental) immediately after tooth extraction. One year later, the patient decided to proceed with implant placement. Because of the compromised bone quality in this area of the mandible, an Osseotite implant (Biomet 3i) with a tapered design (Prevail, Biomet 3i) and platform switching was selected to increase primary stability. The implant was placed subcrestally and had a straight, nonextended platform (Fig 12-1a). The implant was connected with a Provide abutment (Biomet 3i) using final torque (Fig 12-1b). A provisional restoration was made and placed in occlusion with the opposing dentition (Fig 12-1c). The abutment was never removed, and an abutment-level impression was made 3 months later using a plastic impression coping. After delivery and cementation of the final crown, the patient followed up every 6 months for evaluation of the peri-implant soft and hard tissues. Over time there was an increase in bone density at the bone-implant interface as well as in the crestal bone stability because the implant was loaded immediately after surgery and the abutment was never removed (Figs 12-1d and 12-1e).

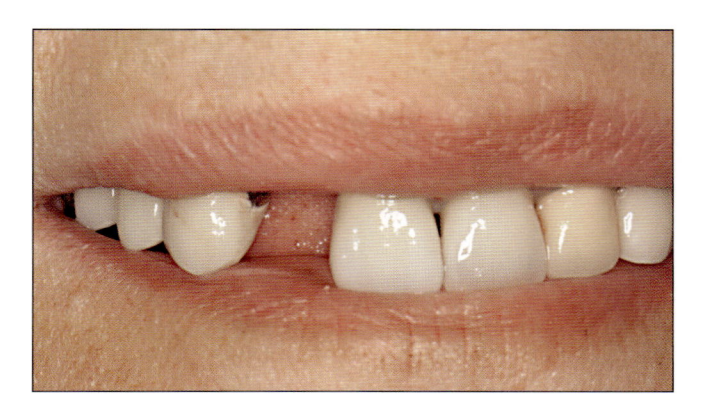

**Fig 12-2a** Smile line of the patient prior to surgery.

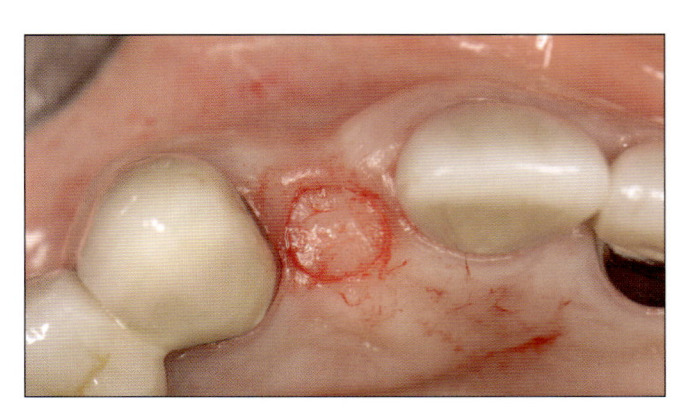

**Fig 12-2b** Soft tissue removed in preparation for implant placement.

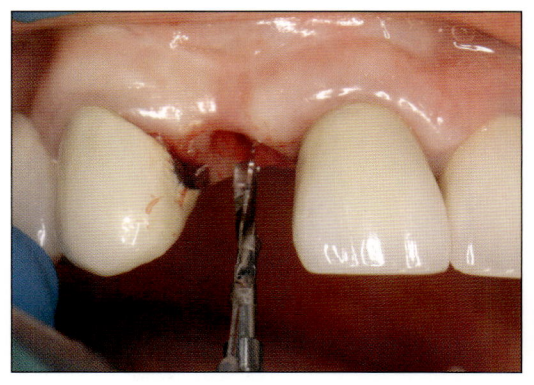

**Fig 12-2c** Pilot drill prior to use of osteotomes for bone spreading.

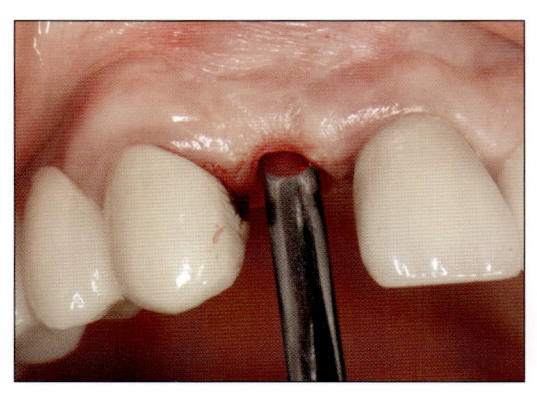

**Fig 12-2d** Bone-spreading technique to extend the width of the narrow alveolar ridge.

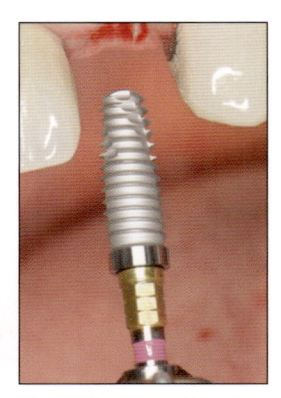

**Fig 12-2e** Tapered implant being placed for immediate loading.

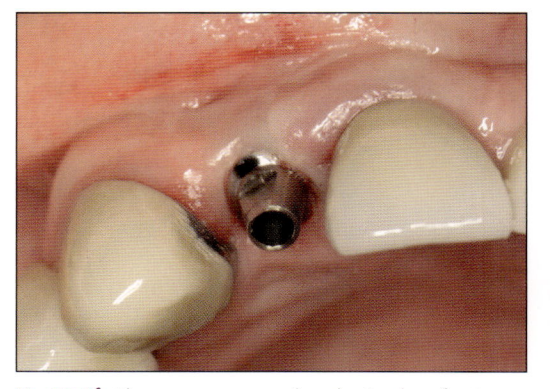

**Fig 12-2f** Abutment connected to the implant for immediate provisionalization.

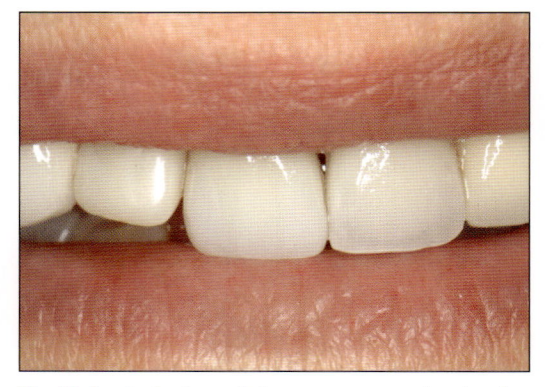

**Fig 12-2g** Smile line of the patient immediately after placement of the provisional crown.

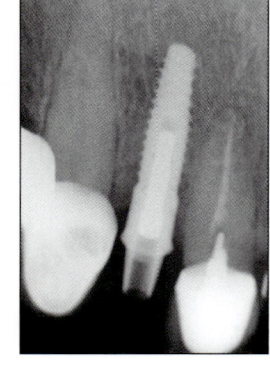

**Fig 12-2h** Radiographic examination following delivery of the provisional crown. (Restoration by M. Postol, New York, NY.)

## Case 2: Immediate loading without platform switching

This case presents a single-tooth implant placed in the site of a maxillary right lateral incisor for a patient with a moderate smile line (Fig 12-2a). Using a prosthetic template and a soft tissue punch, the soft tissue was removed in the right lateral incisor site (Fig 12-2b). An initial drill was used before the narrow alveolar ridge was extended with osteotomes (Ustomed) to increase the width (Figs 12-2c and 12-2d). This technique was used to avoid ridge augmentation. A tapered Osseotite implant was placed subcrestally with primary stability, and the abutment was connected using the final torque (Figs 12-2e and 12-2f). A provisional restoration was used as a template to fabricate a cement-retained resin crown (Fig 12-2g). A radiograph was taken at the end of the treatment to evaluate the bone levels (Fig 12-2h).

Case Reports

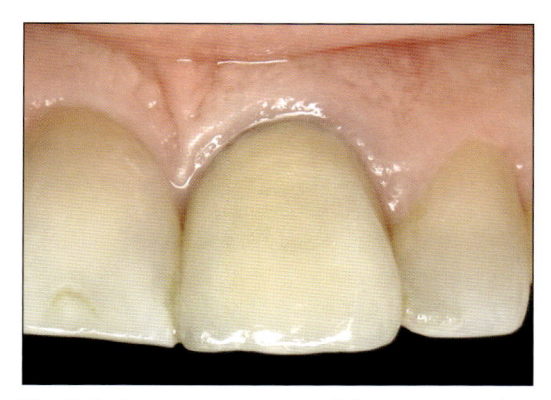

**Fig 12-3a** Preoperative situation following an incident in which the maxillary left central incisor was knocked.

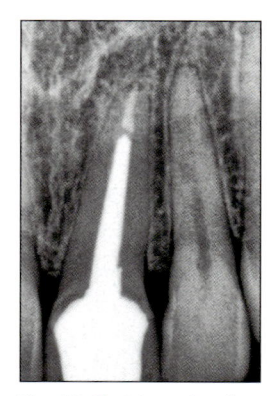

**Fig 12-3b** Note the fracture at the tip of the endodontic post.

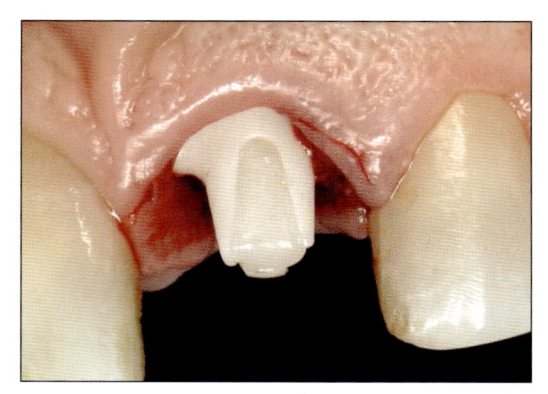

**Fig 12-3c** A Cercon ceramic abutment was connected to the immediate implant and fully torqued.

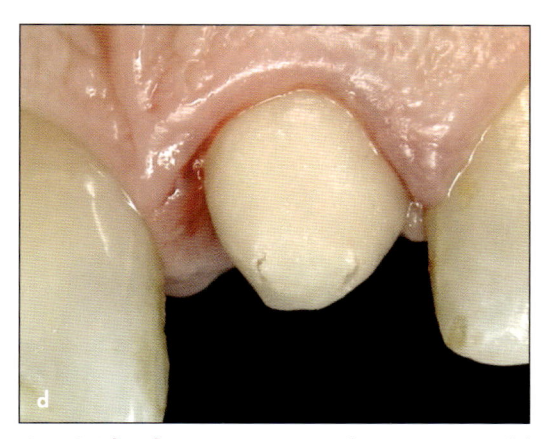

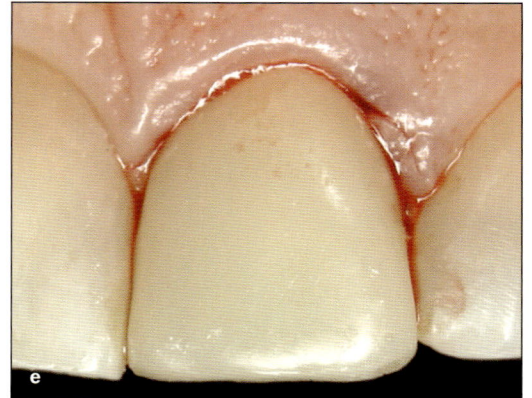

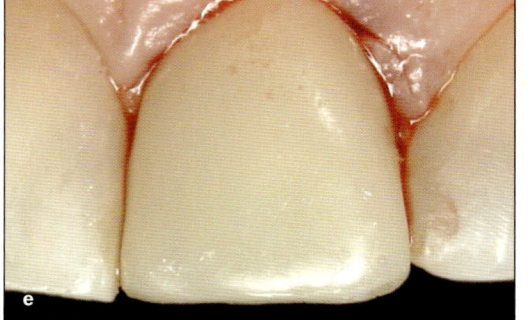

**Figs 12-3d and 12-3e** A provisional restoration was fabricated chairside and inserted on the same day.

**Fig 12-3f** Radiographic evaluation at baseline implant placement.

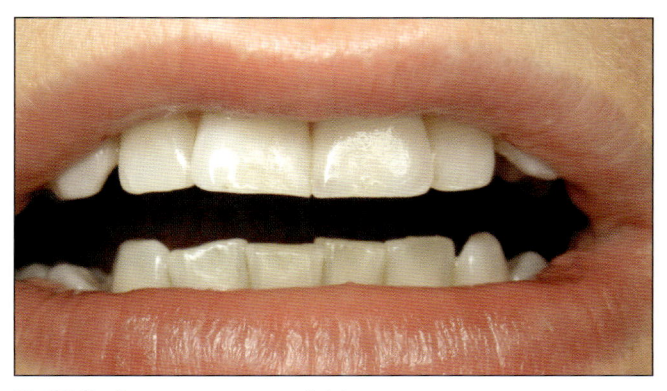

**Fig 12-3g** Restoration at time of delivery.

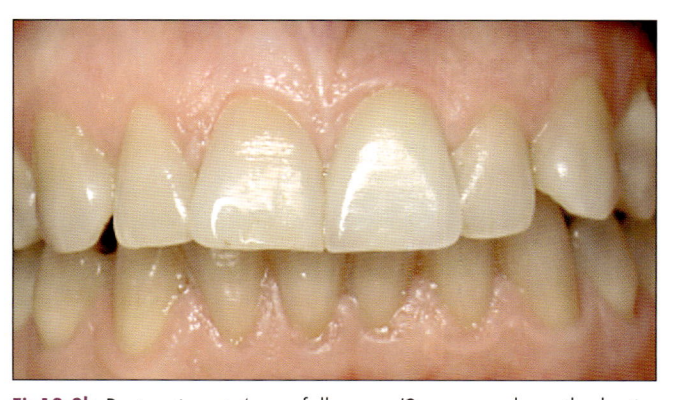

**Fig 12-3h** Restoration at 4-year follow-up. (Surgery and prosthodontics by N. Saynor, Manchester, UK.)

## Case 3: Esthetic immediate loading using a customized ceramic abutment and platform switching

A 38-year-old woman presented 2 days after trauma to her anterior maxilla. She experienced pain in the labial sulcus around her maxillary left central incisor as well as pain on biting (Fig 12-3a). Radiographic examination revealed a root fracture at the tip of the fabricated post (Fig 12-3b). The tooth was extracted atraumatically with periotomes. After socket debridement and osteotomy preparation with burs and osteotomes, an Ankylos implant (4.5-mm diameter and 14 mm long) was placed in the fresh extraction socket and torqued to 35 Ncm. Anorganic bovine bone (Bio-Oss) was placed facially. A Cercon ceramic abutment (Dentsply Friadent) was connected with a final torque and was never removed after this (Fig 12-3c). A provisional acrylic restoration was made at the time of extraction and implant placement and kept out of occlusal contact (Figs 12-3d to 12-3f). The final restoration was constructed 14 weeks after implant placement and presented an excellent long-term result (Figs 12-3g and 12-3h).

# 12 | Immediate Loading of Single-Tooth Implants

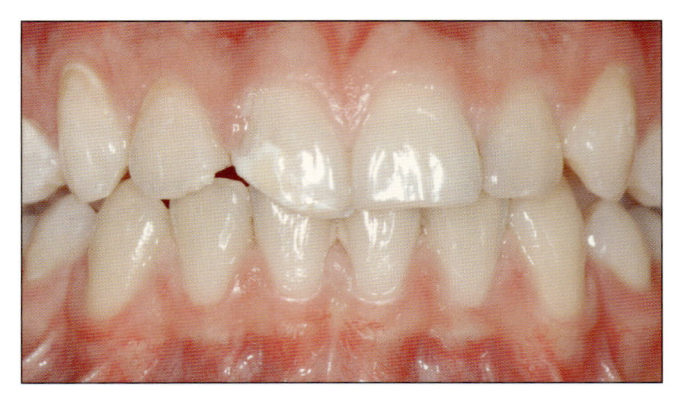

**Fig 12-4a** Intraoral view of fractured maxillary right central incisor.

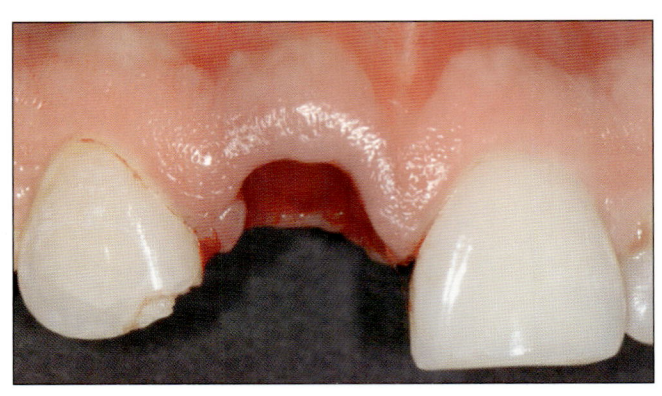

**Fig 12-4b** Clinical appearance following tooth extraction. No incision lines were made.

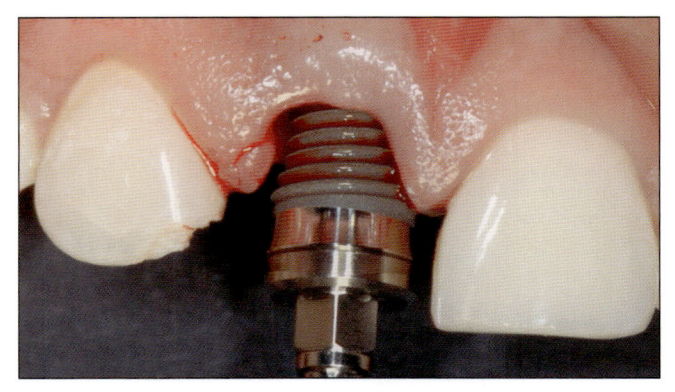

**Fig 12-4c** Immediate placement of a Straumann tapered implant.

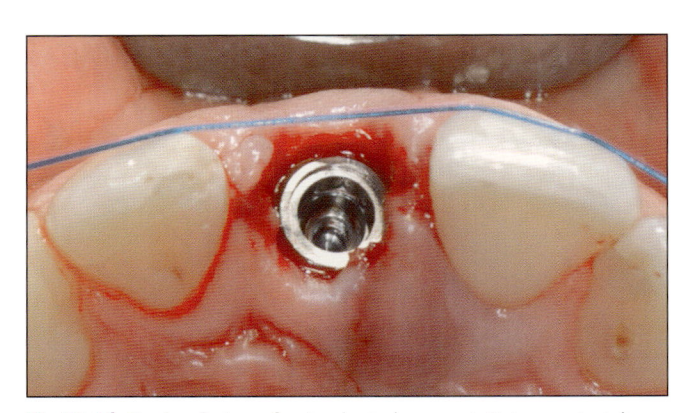

**Fig 12-4d** Occlusal view after implant placement. Suture material was used to determine the ideal buccolingual placement.

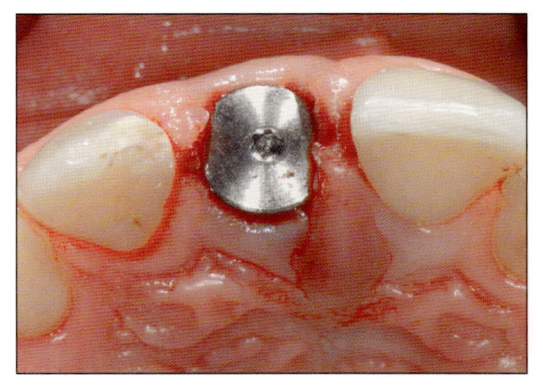

**Fig 12-4e** Occlusal view following impression and placement of a healing abutment.

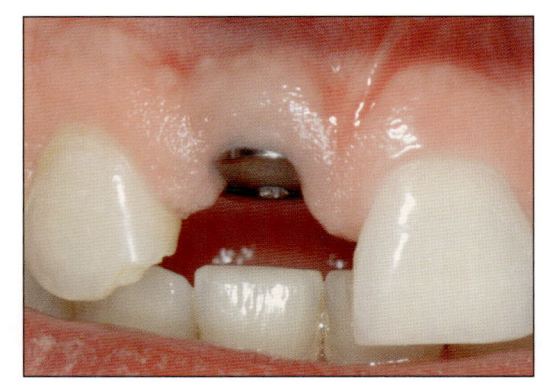

**Fig 12-4f** Frontal view with healing abutment in place.

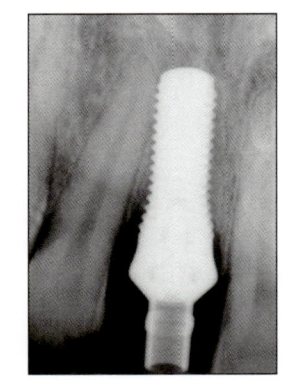

**Fig 12-4g** Radiograph taken immediately after implant placement.

## Case 4: Immediate loading with tapered implant design

The patient presented with a traumatic fracture of the maxillary right central incisor (Fig 12-4a). The fractured tooth was extracted (Fig 12-4b), and a Straumann tapered implant was immediately placed (Figs 12-4c to 12-4g). An impression was taken intraoperatively, and the following day the screw-retained provisional crown was delivered (Figs 12-4h and 12-4i). The final metal-ceramic crown was placed 6 weeks after the implant was placed (Figs 12-4j and 12-4k).

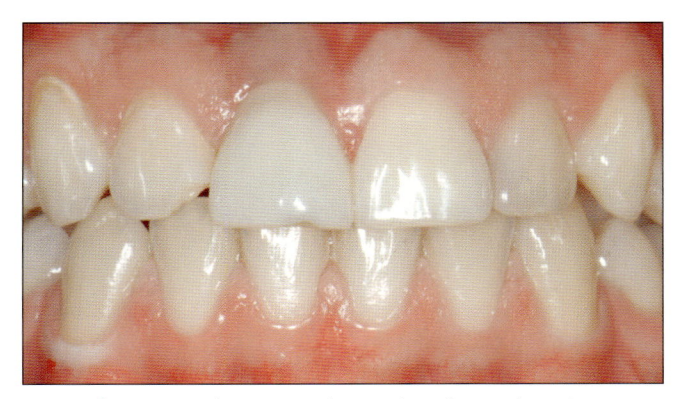

**Fig 12-4h** Provisional crown in place 1 day after implant placement.

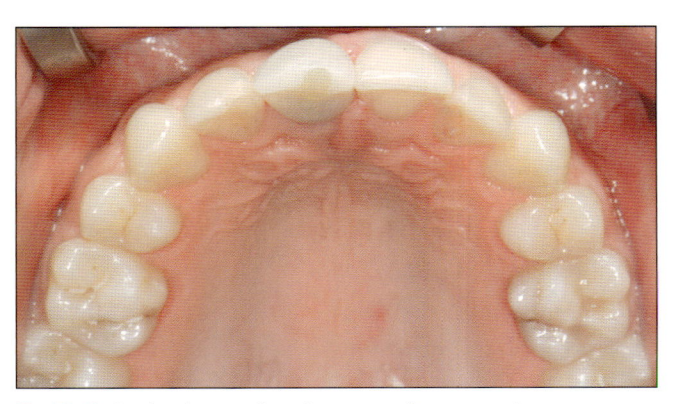

**Fig 12-4i** Occlusal view after placement of provisional crown.

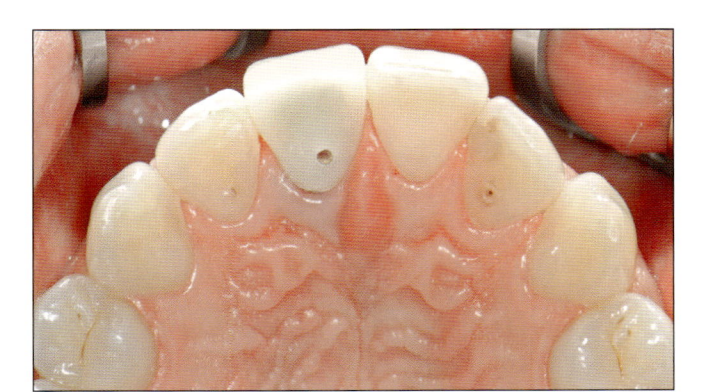

**Fig 12-4j** Occlusal view of final crown 6 weeks after implant placement.

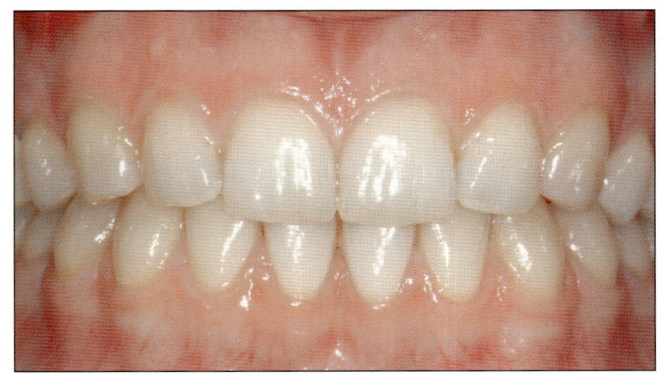

**Fig 12-4k** Frontal view of final crown 1 year after implant placement. (Surgery by K. A. Schlegel, University of Erlangen-Nürnberg, Germany; prosthodontics by W. Reinhardt, University of Jena, Germany.)

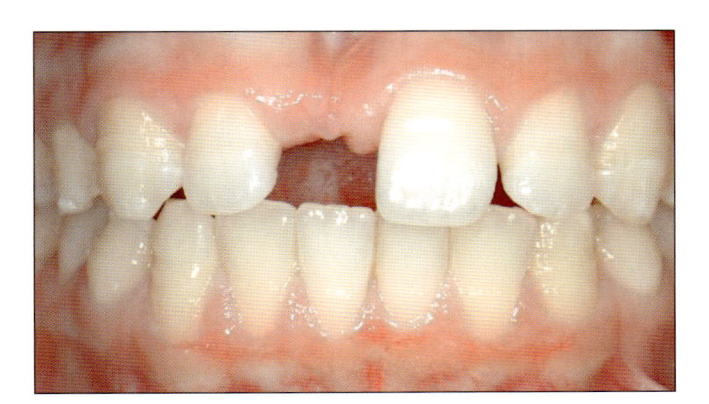

**Fig 12-5a** Frontal intraoral view of missing maxillary right central incisor.

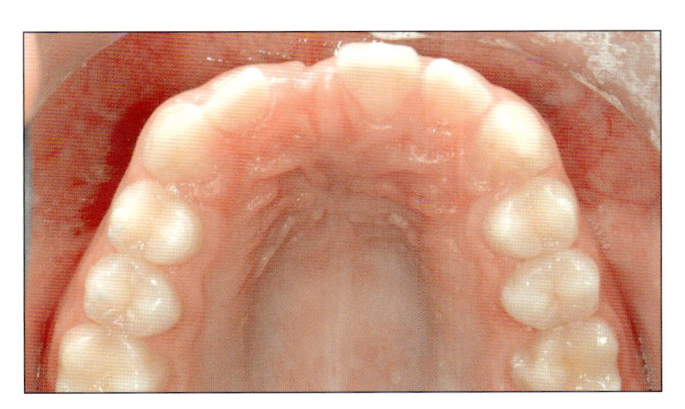

**Fig 12-5b** Occlusal view before treatment.

## Case 5: Immediate loading in augmented bone

The patient presented with traumatic loss of the maxillary right central incisor (Figs 12-5a and 12-5b). An orthodontic space holder was used during the growth period (Fig 12-5c). Augmentation using monocortical bone harvested from the retromolar area was performed (Figs 12-5d to 12-5i). After 4 months of healing, a Nobel Perfect (Nobel Biocare) implant was placed (Figs 12-5j to 12-5m), and an impression was taken intraoperatively. A provisional crown was placed the same day (Fig 12-5n). The soft tissues were contoured using the provisional crown (Figs 12-5o and 12-5p). A final metal-ceramic restoration was delivered 12 months after implant placement (Figs 12-5q to 12-5s).

137

## 12 · Immediate Loading of Single-Tooth Implants

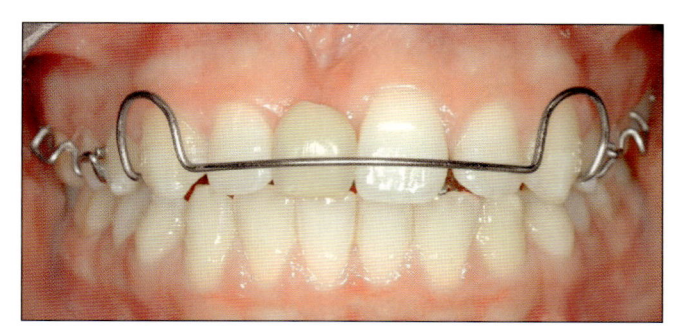

**Fig 12-5c** Orthodontic space holder in place.

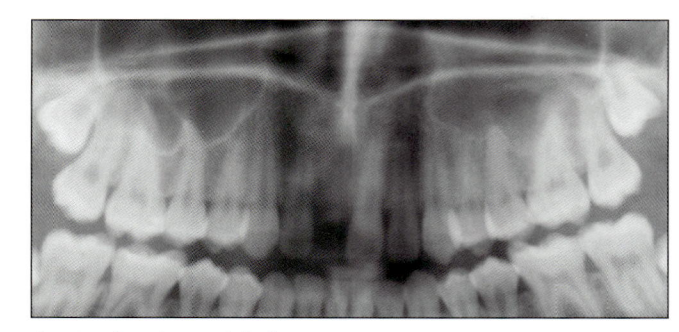

**Fig 12-5d** Radiograph before treatment.

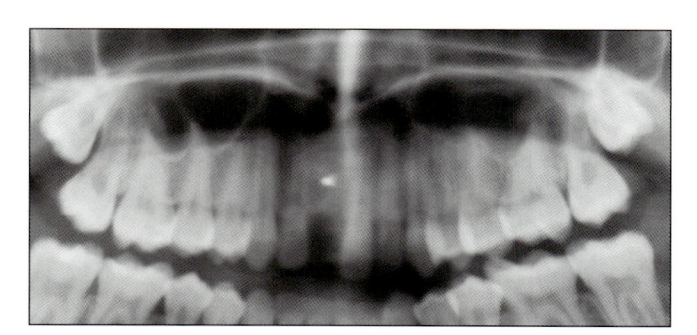

**Fig 12-5e** Radiograph taken after augmentation.

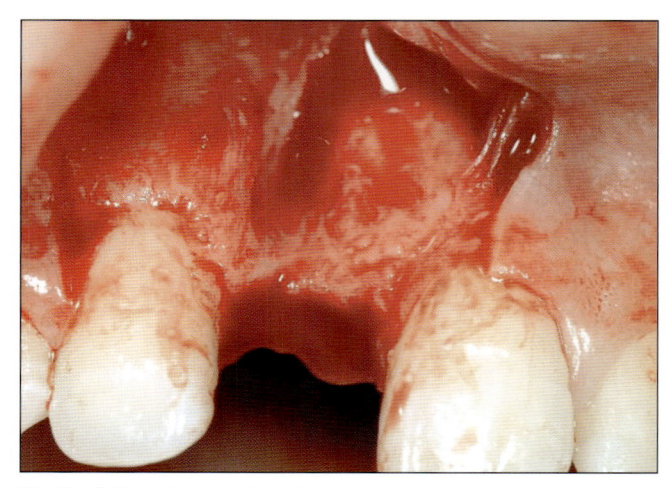

**Fig 12-5f** Flap elevation for ridge augmentation.

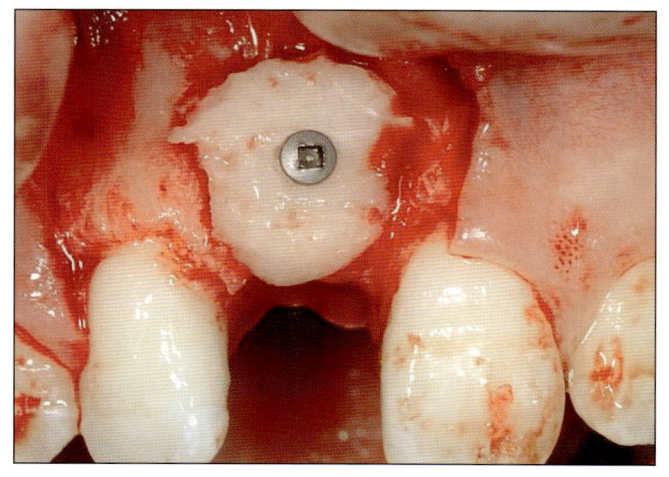

**Fig 12-5g** Monocortical block in place.

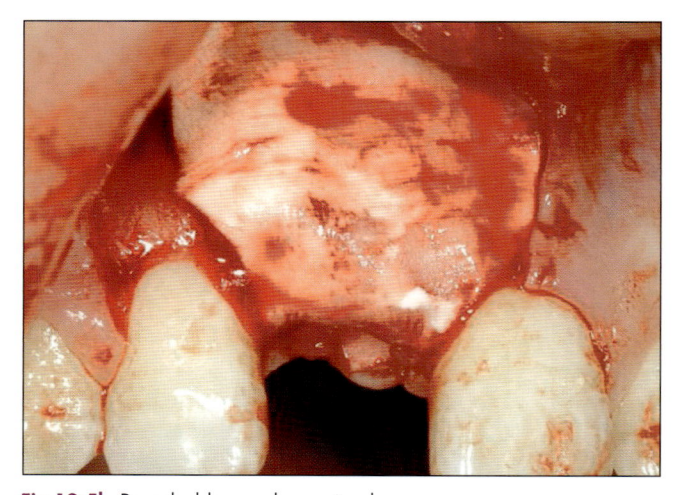

**Fig 12-5h** Resorbable membrane in place.

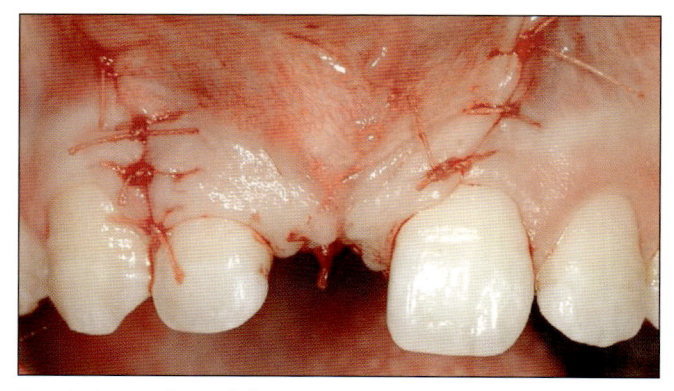

**Fig 12-5i** Frontal view following suturing.

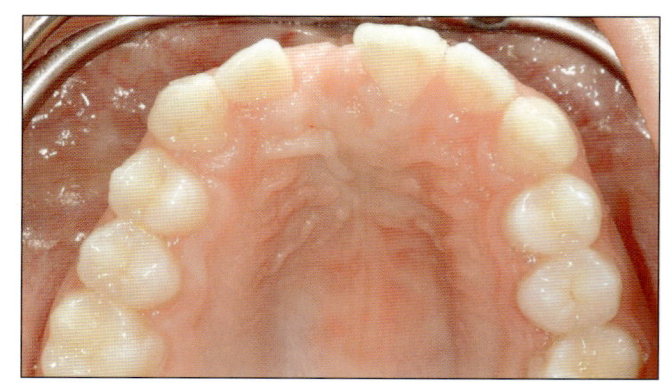

**Fig 12-5j** Occlusal view 4 months after augmentation, just before implant placement.

Case Reports

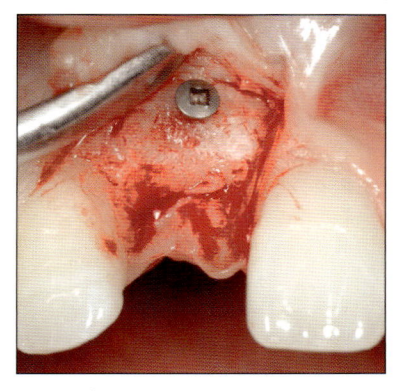

**Fig 12-5k** Reentry for implant placement.

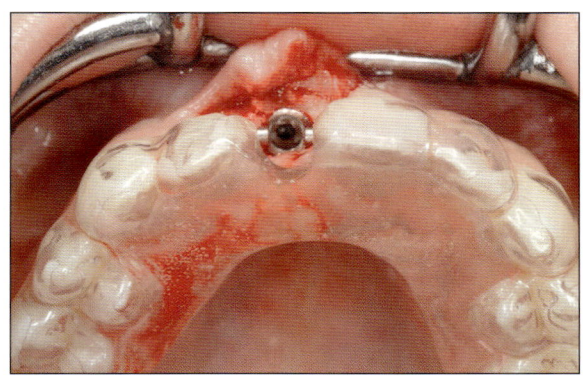

**Fig 12-5l** Occlusal view after implant placement showing ideal positioning of the implant using a prosthetic template.

**Fig 12-5m** Frontal view after implant placement.

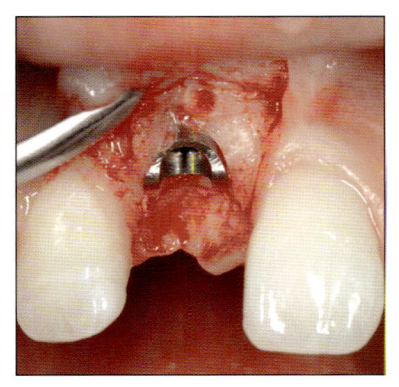

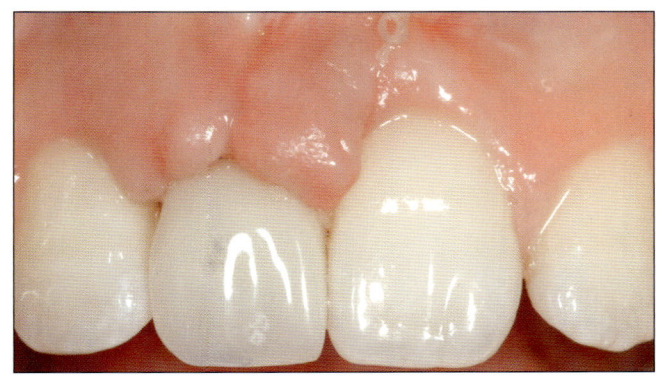

**Fig 12-5n** Provisional crown 10 days after placement.

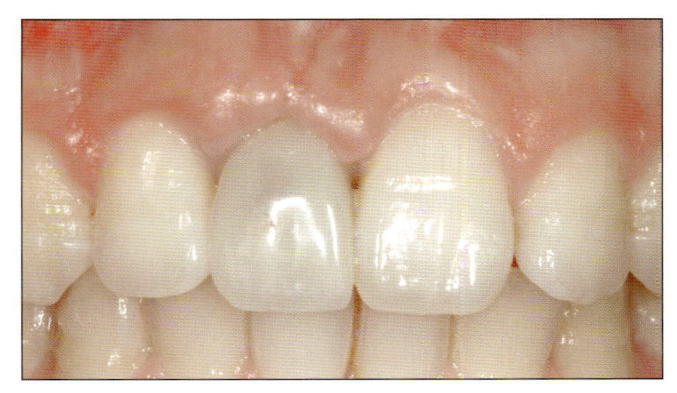

**Fig 12-5o** Provisional crown 3 months after placement.

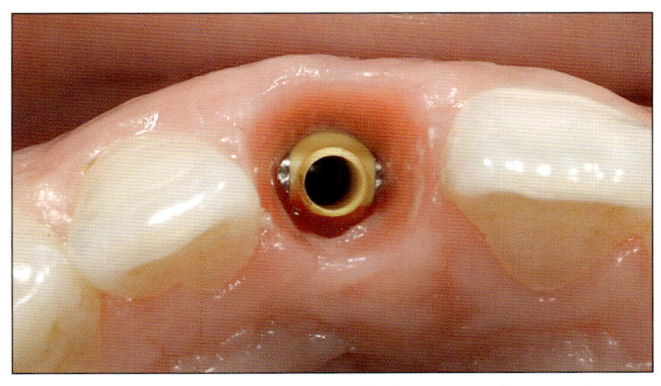

**Fig 12-5p** Occlusal view after removal of provisional crown showing healthy peri-implant soft tissues.

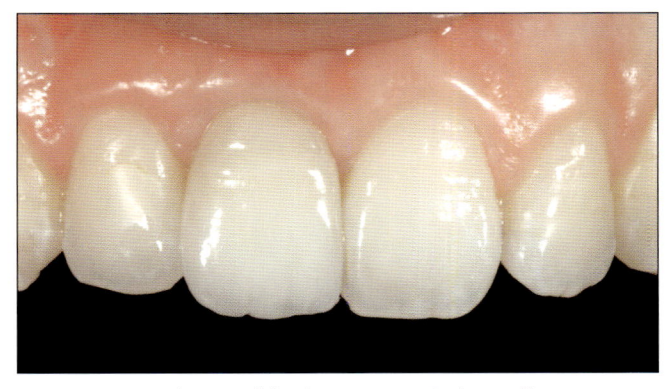

**Fig 12-5q** Frontal view of final restoration. Both papillae were reestablished.

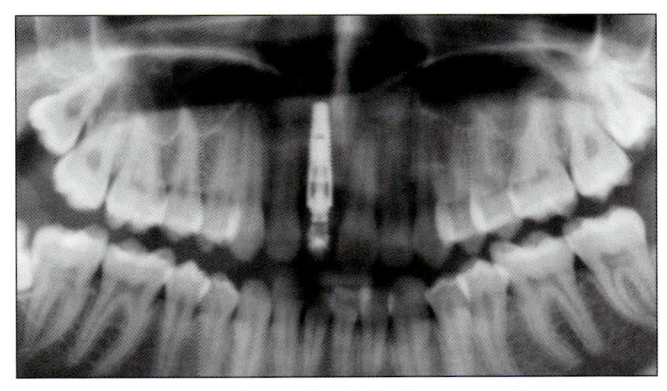

**Fig 12-5r** Panoramic radiograph with final crown in place.

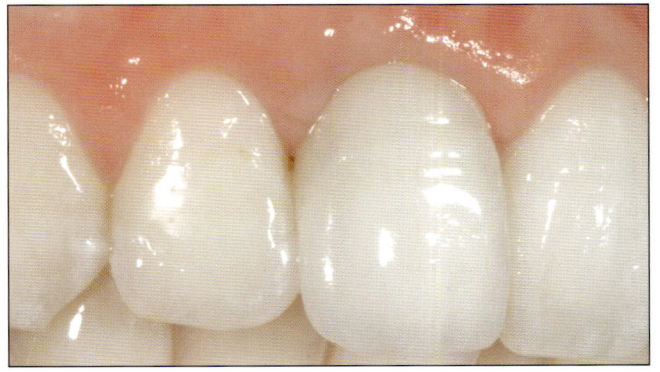

**Fig 12-5s** Close-up of the buccal aspect of the final crown. (Surgery by K. A. Schlegel and prosthodontics by S. Holst, University of Erlangen-Nürnberg, Germany.)

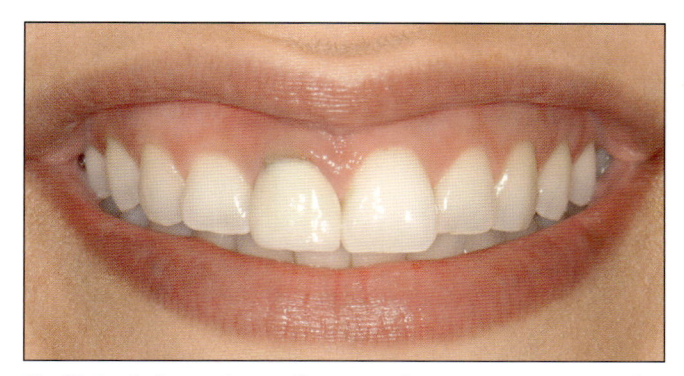

**Fig 12-6a** Failing right maxillary central incisor in a patient with a high smile line and medium biotype. Normal papilla heights mesial and distal to the central incisor with 1 to 2 mm of facial recession.

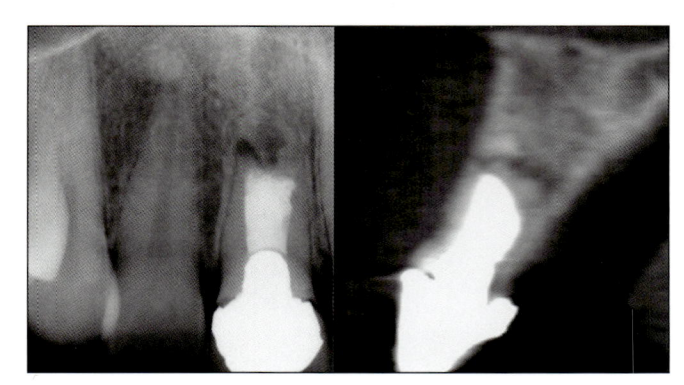

**Fig 12-6b** Preoperative radiographs illustrating apical resorption, ankylosis, and minimal buccal plate over the root surface.

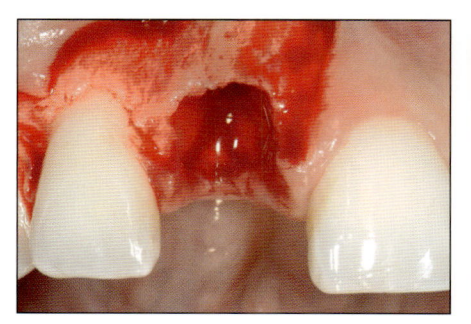

**Fig 12-6c** Minimally traumatic extraction of the maxillary right cental incisor after raising a buccal flap.

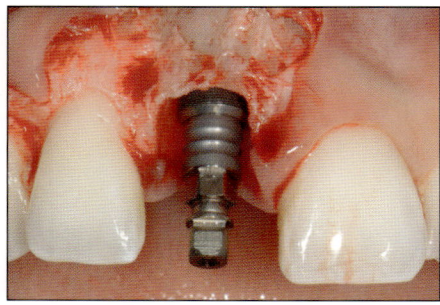

**Fig 12-6d** Implant placement centered mesiodistally. The coronal implant margin is level with the alveolar crest.

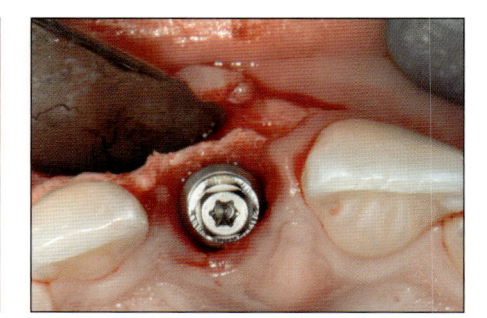

**Fig 12-6e** Palatal view illustrating implant placement against the palatal wall and the gap between the buccal alveolar bone and the facial surface of implant.

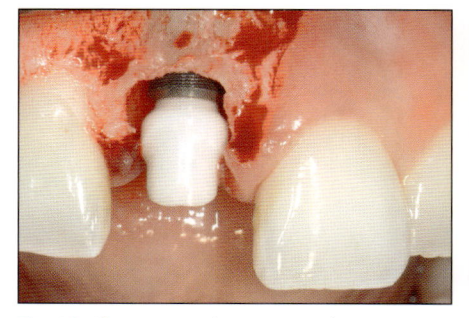

**Fig 12-6f** Provisional zirconia abutment contoured for the cement-retained provisional restoration.

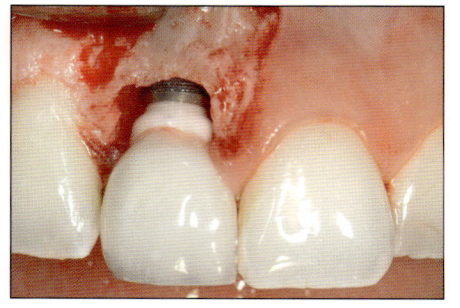

**Fig 12-6g** Acrylic provisional restoration cemented in place with excess cement removed. The emergence profile is deliberately undercontoured to promote coronal positioning of the flap and regeneration of abundant soft tissue.

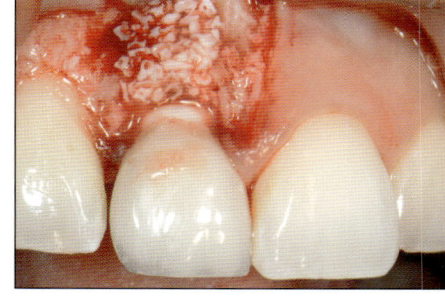

**Fig 12-6h** Grafting of the buccal gap and over-thin buccal plate with autogenous bone chips combined with anorganic bovine-derived bone mineral.

## Case 6: Esthetic immediate loading in conjunction with hard and soft tissue augmentation

A young woman presented with a hopeless right central incisor; she had a high smile line, a moderately thin biotype, and high esthetic demands (Figs 12-6a and 12-6b). After consultation and discussion of treatment options, it was decided to perform immediate placement and restoration of a dental implant to replace the hopeless tooth.

After raising a buccal flap, the tooth was extracted using a periotome to separate the ankylotic root from the alveolus (Fig 12-6c). An osteotomy was centered between the remaining teeth toward the palatal wall of the socket. This left an intentional gap between the implant and buccal plate. An Astra Tech implant was inserted with 35-Ncm torque to a point level with the alveolar crest (Figs 12-6d and 12-6e). The abutment and provisional restoration were contoured and inserted (Figs 12-6f). The subgingival shape of the provisional restoration was deliberately undercontoured to facilitate coronal tissue positioning during suturing and healing (Fig 12-6g). The provisional restoration was also shortened incisally and palatally to protect it from direct occlusal contact.

Hard and soft tissue grafting were accomplished to compensate for anticipated tissue shrinkage and resorption. A technique using autogenous bone chips against the implant and anorganic bovine bone peripherally

# Case Reports

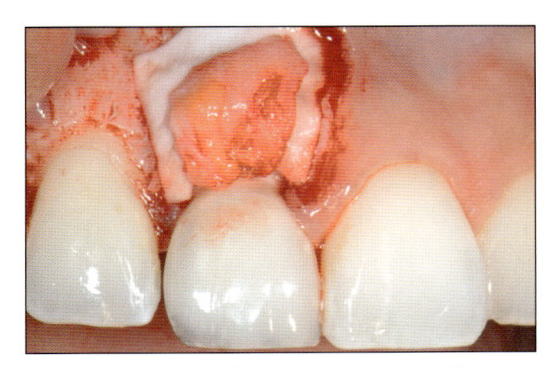

**Fig 12-6i** Hard and soft tissue grafts positioned facial to the implant to counteract anticipated buccal resorption of alveolar bone.

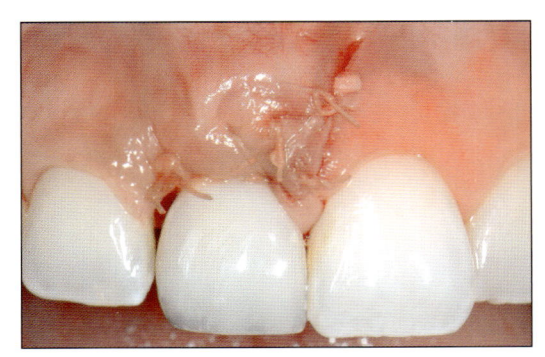

**Fig 12-6j** Coronally positioned flaps covering grafts are sutured in place.

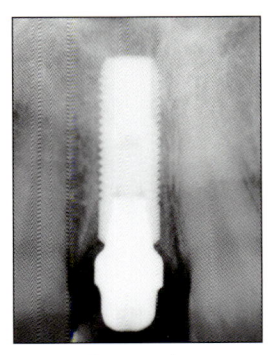

**Fig 12-6k** Immediate postoperative radiograph.

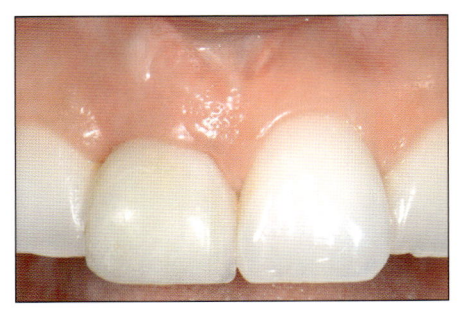

**Fig 12-6l** Three-month follow-up showing excellent healing. Note additional acrylic added previously to the provisional restoration to close the distal contact.

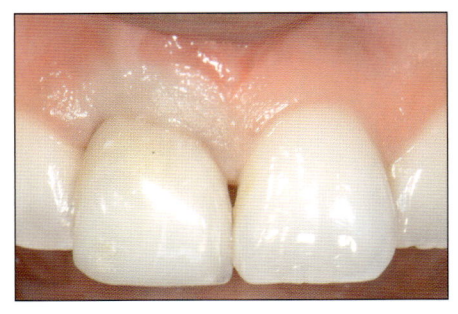

**Fig 12-6m** Modified provisional restoration causing blanching due to increased subgingival contour.

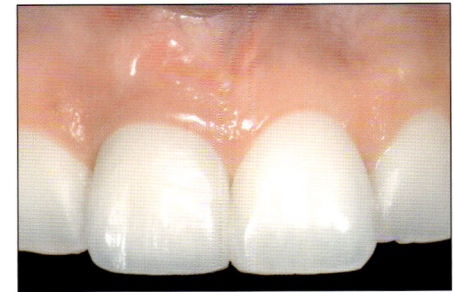

**Fig 12-6n** Final metal-ceramic restoration immediately following insertion. Papilla heights are similar to pretreatment levels. Simulated buccal root eminence is similar to adjacent central incisor.

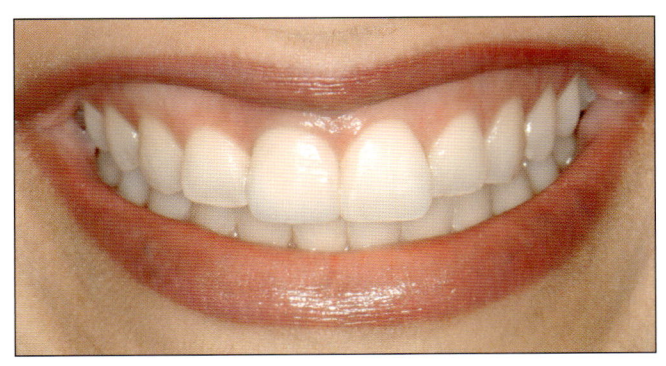

**Fig 12-6o** Full smile showing excellent esthetic result despite minor asymmetry in gingival contour.

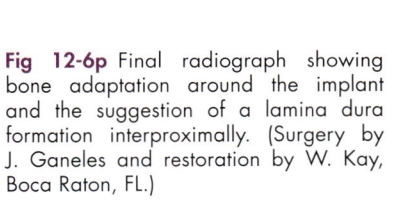

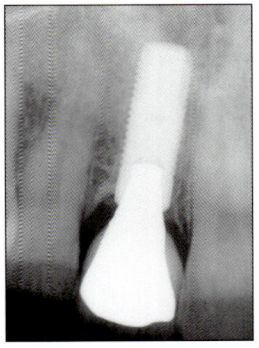

**Fig 12-6p** Final radiograph showing bone adaptation around the implant and the suggestion of a lamina dura formation interproximally. (Surgery by J. Ganeles and restoration by W. Kay, Boca Raton, FL.)

was used for hard tissue grafting (Fig 12-6h). A resorbable bovine collagen membrane was adapted over the particulate graft. Palatal gingival connective tissue was then harvested and adapted on top of the collagen membrane to augment gingival thickness (Fig 12-6i). Periosteal fenestrations were created in the facial flap to permit coronal positioning over the augmented site, which was sutured with slowly resorbing polyglactin sutures (Figs 12-6j and 12-6k).

After 3 months of healing, the gingival contours were altered by removing the provisional abutment and provisional restoration to add subgingival acrylic and increase the height of the gingival zenith to more closely simulate the left central incisor (Figs 12-6l and 12-6m). The final restoration, a screw-retained metal-ceramic crown, was placed with excellent esthetics and patient appreciation (Fig 12-6n). Despite minor asymmetry in the gingival zenith, full papillae and a simulated root eminence contribute to the natural appearance of the restoration (Figs 12-6o and 12-6p).

## 12 | Immediate Loading of Single-Tooth Implants

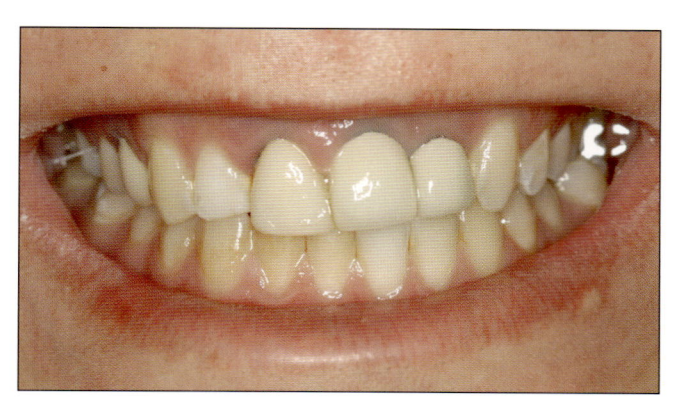

**Fig 12-7a** Smile line of the patient before treatment showing hopeless teeth due to deep caries.

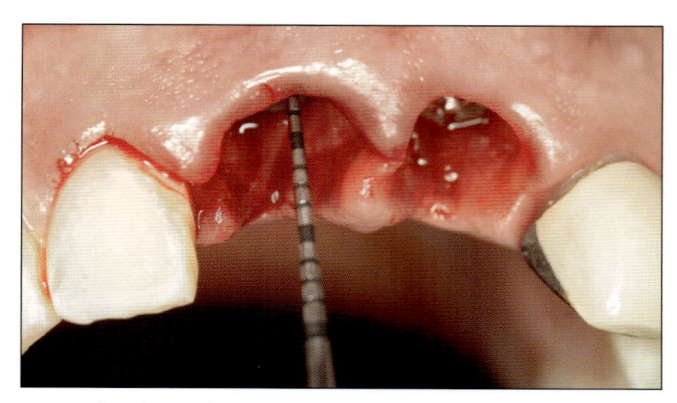

**Fig 12-7b** Subcrestal implant placement for immediate loading.

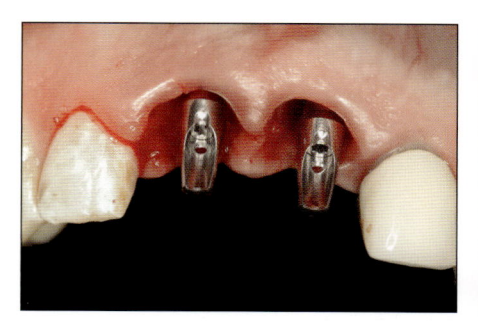

**Fig 12-7c** Abutment connection with the final torque.

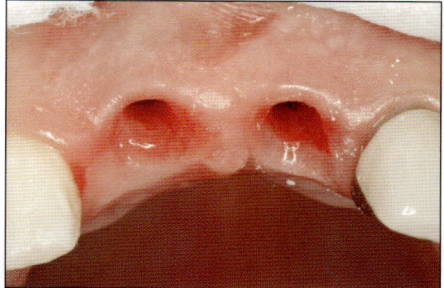

**Fig 12-7d** Excellent peri-implant soft tissues. Abutments were removed to take the final impression for customized abutments.

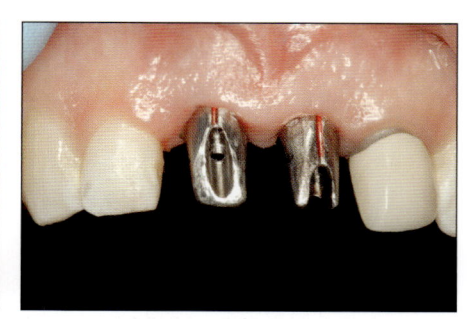

**Fig 12-7e** Customized abutments in place.

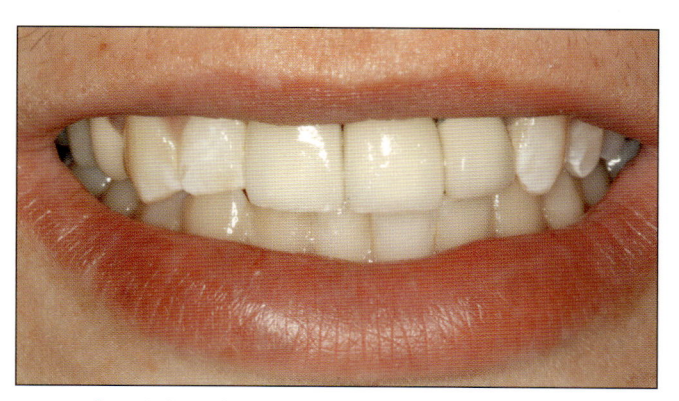

**Fig 12-7f** Smile line of the patient 16 months after treatment with the final restorations in place.

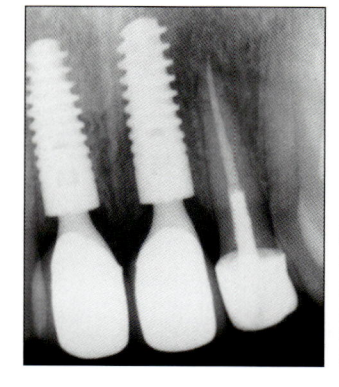

**Fig 12-7g** Radiograph 16 months after loading. Note the new bone covering the top of the implant. (Restoration by N. Melo, Rochester, NY; Arieno Dental Laboratory Spencerport, NY.)

## Case 7: Immediate loading in an adolescent patient

This case demonstrates the treatment of hopeless maxillary central incisors in an adolescent boy (Fig 12-7a). After tooth extraction, implants were placed subcrestally in fresh extraction sockets for immediate loading (Fig 12-7b). The abutments were connected immediately after surgery for loading with two resin provisional crowns (Fig 12-7c). After 3 to 4 months of healing that included a strict protocol of a soft or liquid diet, the abutments were removed and implant level impressions were taken for delivery of customized abutments and metal-ceramic crowns (Figs 12-7d and 12-7e). The final restorations showed a satisfactory result for the patient, and he was planning to undergo prosthetic rehabilitation of the adjacent left and right lateral incisors at a later time. The crestal bone level was stable over the entire observation period (Figs 12-7f and 12-7g).

Case Reports

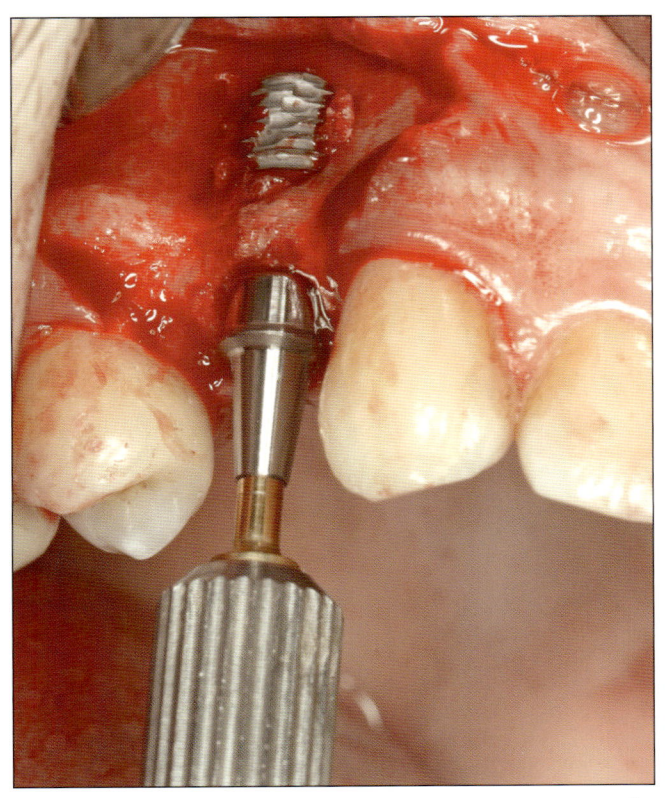

**Fig 12-8a** Implant placement and abutment connection in a premolar site presenting an excessive buccal deficiency.

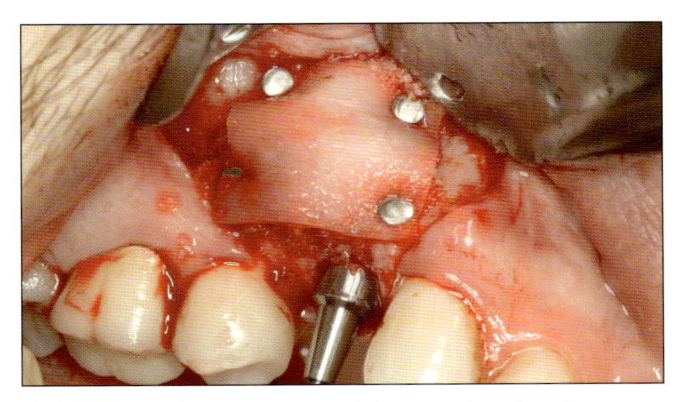

**Fig 12-8b** Lateral augmentation with human allograft and coverage with a collagen membrane to support the bone stability and increase the bone volume.

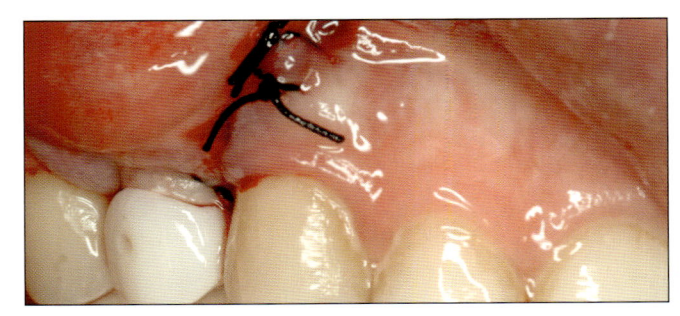

**Fig 12-8c** Provisional restoration in place for immediate loading while the patient followed a soft/liquid diet protocol.

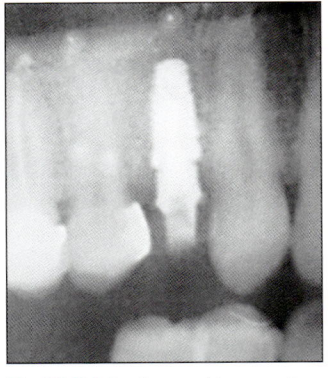

**Fig 12-8d** Radiographic examination illustrates the implant position and the crestal bone level at time of surgery.

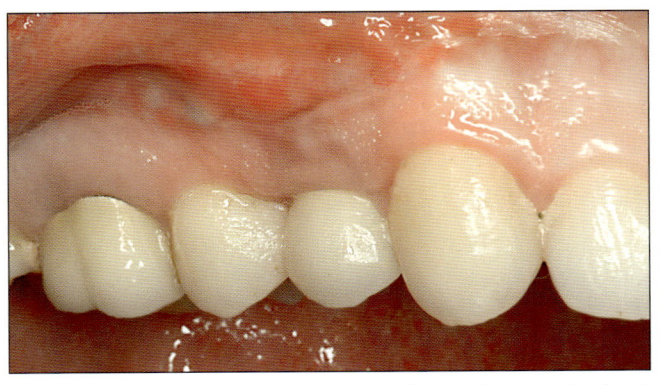

**Fig 12-8e** Final crown presenting an excellent esthetic result after 1 year.

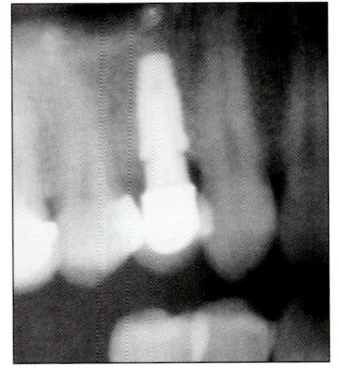

**Fig 12-8f** Radiographic examination 1 year after loading. Note the crestal bone stability. (Restoration by G. E. Romanos and B. Gruchalska, Rochester, NY; Arieno Dental Laboratory, Spencerport, NY.)

## Case 8: Immediate loading with bone grafting and platform switching

This case demonstrates the placement of a tapered implant in the alveolar ridge with an excessive undercut in the buccal aspect (Fig 12-8a). The implant system that was used has an internal polygonal connection and straight abutments (not angulated) for platform switching. The implant was connected with its abutment using final torque. The buccal fenestration was covered by cancellous human allograft (Endobon, Biomet 3i) and then covered by a collagen membrane (Osseoguard, Biomet 3i) (Fig 12-8b). After flap closure, the implant was loaded with a resin composite provisional crown (Fig 12-8c). The postoperative radiograph confirmed the implant position and the absence of a microgap at the implant-abutment interface under subcrestal placement conditions (Fig 12-8d). This is possible because the implant system used has platform switching, but it would be more difficult in a case with an abutment having the same diameter as the implant in a case of subcrestal placement (see also case 2).

The final restoration was delivered 5 months after implant placement (Fig 12-8e). The patient followed a strict soft/liquid diet protocol for the healing period. The abutment was never removed. The final clinical result was very satisfactory, and the bone condition was very stable for the entire observation period of 1 year (Fig 12-8f).

# References

1. Wöhrle PS. Single tooth replacement in the aesthetic zone with immediate provisionalization: Fourteen consecutive case reports. Pract Periodontics Aesthet Dent 1998;10:1107–1114.
2. Malo P, Friberg B, Polizzi G, Gualini F, Vighagen T, Rangert B. Immediate and early function of Brånemark System implants placed in the esthetic zone: A 1-year prospective clinical multicenter study. Clin Implant Dent Relat Res 2003;5(suppl):37–46.
3. Chaushu G, Chaushu S, Tzohar A, Dayan D. Immediate loading of single-tooth implants: Immediate versus non-immediate implantation. A clinical report. Int J Oral Maxillofac Implants 2001;16:267–272.
4. Ericsson I, Nilson H, Nilner K. Immediate functional loading of Brånemark single-tooth implant. A 5-year clinical follow-up. Appl Osseointegration Res 2001;2:12–17.
5. Hui E, Chow J, Li D, Liu J, Wat P, Law H. Immediate provisional for single-tooth implant replacement with Brånemark system: Preliminary report. Clin Implant Dent Relat Res 2001;3:79–86.
6. Andersen E, Haanaes HR, Knutsen BM. Immediate loading of single-tooth ITI implants in the anterior maxilla: A prospective 5-year pilot study. Clin Oral Implants Res 2002;13:281–287.
7. Kan JY, Rungcharassaeng K, Lozada J. Immediate placement and provisionalization of maxillary anterior single implants: 1-year prospective study. Int J Oral Maxillofac Implants 2003;19:855–860.
8. Lorenzoni M, Pertl C, Zhang K, Wimmer G, Wegscheider WA. Immediate loading of single-tooth implants in the anterior maxilla. Preliminary results after one year. Clin Oral Implants Res 2003;14:180–187.
9. Norton MR. A short-term clinical evaluation of immediately restored maxillary TiOblast single-tooth implants. Int J Oral Maxillofac Implants 2004;19:274–281.
10. Barone A, Rispoli L, Vozza I, Quaranta A, Covani U. Immediate restoration of single implants placed immediately after tooth extraction. J Periodontol 2006;77:1914–1920.
11. Mijiritsky E, Mardinger O, Mazor Z, Chaushu G. Immediate provisionalization of single-tooth implants in fresh-extraction sites at the maxillary esthetic zone: Up to 6 years of follow-up. Implant Dent 2009;18:326–333.
12. Calandriello R, Tomatis M, Vallone R, Rangert B, Gottlow J. Immediate occlusal loading of single lower molars using Brånemark System Wide-Platform TiUnite implants: An interim report of a prospective open-ended clinical multicenter study. Clin Implant Dent Relat Res 2003;5(suppl):74–80.
13. Cornelini R, Cangini F, Covani U, Barone A, Buser D. Immediate restoration of single-tooth implants in mandibular molar sites: A 12-month preliminary report. Int J Oral Maxillofac Implants 2004;19:855–860.
14. Abboud M, Koeck B, Stark H, Wahl G, Paillon R. Immediate loading of single-tooth implants in the posterior region. Int J Oral Maxillofac Implants 2005;20:61–68.
15. Schincaglia GP, Marzola R, Giovanni GF, Chiara CS, Scotti R. Replacement of mandibular molars with single-unit restorations supported by wide body implants: Immediate versus delayed loading. A randomized controlled study. Int J Oral Maxillofac Implants 2008;23:474–480.
16. Degidi M, Piattelli A, Gehrke P, Felice P, Carinci F. Five-year outcome of 111 immediate nonfunctional single restorations. J Oral Implantol 2006;32:277–285.
17. Canullo L, Rasperini G. Preservation of peri-implant soft and hard tissues using platform switching of implants placed in immediate extraction sockets: A proof-of-concept study with 12- to 36-month follow-up. Int J Oral Maxillofac Implants 2007;22:995–1000.
18. Cornelini R, Cangini F, Covani U, Wilson TG Jr. Immediate restoration of implants placed into fresh extraction sockets for single-tooth replacement: A prospective clinical study. Int J Periodontics Restorative Dent 2005;25:439–447.
19. Ferrara A, Galli C, Mauro G, Macaluso GM. Immediate provisional restoration of postextraction implants for maxillary single-tooth replacement. Int J Periodontics Restorative Dent 2006; 26:371–377.
20. Siddiqui AA, O'Neal R, Nummikoski P, et al. Immediate loading of single-tooth restorations: One year prospective results. J Oral Implantol 2008;34:208–218.
21. Nissan J, Romanos GE, Mardinger O, Chaushu G. Immediate nonfunctional loading of single-tooth implants in the anterior maxilla following augmentation with freeze-dried cancellous block allograft: A case series. Int J Oral Maxillofac Implants 2008;23:709–716.
22. Siar CH, Toh CG, Romanos G, Swaminathan D, Ong AH, Yaacob H, Nentwig GH. Peri-implant soft tissue integration of immediately loaded implants in the posterior macaque mandible: a histomorphometric study. J Periodontol 2003;74:571–578.
23. Covani U, Cornelini R, Barone A. Bucco-lingual bone remodeling around implants placed into immediate extraction sockets: A case series. J Periodontol 2003;74:268–273.
24. Lekovic V, Camargo PM, Klokkevold PR, et al. Preservation of alveolar bone in extraction sockets using bioabsorbable membranes. J Periodontol 1998;69:1044–1049.
25. Iasella JM, Greenwell H, Miller RL, et al. Ridge preservation with freeze-dried bone allograft and a collagen membrane compared to extraction alone for implant site development: A clinical and histologic study in humans. J Periodontol 2003;72:990–999.
26. Botticelli D, Berglundh T, Buser D, Lindhe J. The jumping distance revisited: An experimental study in the dog. Clin Oral Implants Res 2003;14:35–42.
27. Carmagnola D, Adriaens P, Berglundh T. Healing of human extraction sockets filled with Bio-Oss. Clin Oral Implants Res 2003;14:137–143.
28. Vance GS, Greenwell H, Miller RL, Hill M, Johnston H, Scheetz JP. Comparison of an allograft in an experimental putty carrier and a bovine-derived xenograft used in ridge preservation: A clinical and histologic study in humans. Int J Oral Maxillofac Implants 2004;19:491–497.
29. Dawson A, Chen S (eds.). The SAC Classification in Implant Dentistry. Berlin: Quintessence, 2009.
30. Guida L, Iezzi G, Annunziata M, Salierno A, Iuorio G, Costigliola G, Piattelli A. Immediate placement and loading of dental implants: A human histologic case report. J Periodontol 2008; 79:575–581.
31. Lindeboom JA, Frenken JW, Dubois L, Frank M, Abbink I, Kroon FH. Immediate loading versus immediate provisionalization of maxillary single tooth replacements: A prospective randomized study with BioComp implants. J Oral Maxillofac Surg 2006;64:936–942.
32. Schwartz-Arad D, Laviv A, Levin L. Survival of immediately provisionalized dental implants placed immediately into fresh extraction sockets. J Periodontol 2007;78:219–223.
33. Glauser R, Rée A, Lundgren AK, Gottlow J, Hämmerle CH, Schärer P. Immediate occlusal loading of Brånemark implants applied in various jawbone regions: A prospective, 1-year clinical study. Clin Implant Dent Relat Res 2001;3:204–213.
34. Quinlan P, Nummikoski P, Schenk R, et al. Immediate and early loading of SLA ITI single-tooth implants: An in vivo study. Int J Oral Maxillofac Implants 2005;20:360–370.
35. Crespi R, Cappare P, Gherlone E, Romanos GE. Immediate occlusal loading of implants placed in fresh sockets after tooth extraction. Int J Oral Maxillofac Implants 2007;22:955–962.

# Immediate Loading of Implants Placed in Fresh Extraction Sockets

## Extraction Socket Healing and Tissue Preservation

The biology of the alveolar socket is a topic that has been studied in humans and animals for many years. As wound healing takes place, different mechanisms are involved in achieving new bone formation.

The first studies in humans included only autopsy material from humans[1,2] and demonstrated healing in extraction sockets. One of the first studies in animals was published in 1923 in the German literature by Euler,[3] who analyzed the histologic changes of the socket and found that thrombus formation in the deep part of the socket is important for achieving new blood vessel formation. At the same time, the coronal aspect of the socket resorbs; laterally, periosteum and mucous membrane grow over the granulation tissue; the periosteum forms compact bone; and within the granulation tissue, small particles of trabecular bone form.

The first study in humans presenting sequences of healing after tooth extractions was performed by Mangos in 1941,[4] who confirmed the continuous bone resorption in the socket using parallel histologic specimens and periapical radiographs at the same time intervals. He also found that until 15 weeks of healing the crest of bone was without any significant change in height, with limited exceptions in patients in whom the bone crest absorbed 1 to 2 mm. The first evidence of bone change due to osteoblastic and osteoclastic activities was seen in the 10-day-old specimens.

The transformation of the socket content from the perspective of structure and tissue remodeling was described by Amler et al in 1960.[5] They showed individual variations within the treatment groups; however, after 20 days, the contour of the lamina dura was less well defined; after about 40 days, it could no longer be defined clearly; and by 50 days, it had completely disappeared.

A study published by Amler in 1969[6] demonstrated tissue remodeling in the extraction socket in humans using time intervals from the day of tooth extraction to 40 days of healing. There is complete healing with new bone formation in 15 weeks, but with a loss of bone height compared with the height of the adjacent structures.

In general, sockets heal in humans significantly more slowly than in dogs and monkeys, and healing in persons more than 50 years of age is significantly slower than in younger individuals. The characteristics of wound healing were evaluated in 1977 by Amler.[7] Similarly, delayed wound healing takes place in infected and compromised wounds.

In addition, histologic studies from Sweden presented the dimensional changes of the sockets in humans after the use of a full denture that was placed immediately after tooth extraction compared with sockets without the use of a denture. There were no significant differences in healing between the two groups of patients in terms of resorption of the bone and new bone formation, but a greater tendency for reformation of a continuous labial bone plate was observed in the patients fitted with a denture.[8]

The modeling and remodeling of extraction sockets were more recently studied by Trombelli et al[9] in 27 human biopsies. The study showed a decrease of the vascular structures and macrophages in the early phase of healing (2 to 4 weeks). A great variability was observed between subjects with respect to hard tissue formation within extraction sockets.

A recent study by Araújo and Lindhe[10] extensively examined socket healing in dogs, presenting confirmation of the resorption of the buccal plate during the healing period. Cardaropoli et al[11] studied the dynamics of bone tissue formation in tooth extraction sites in dogs for a period of 180 days after tooth extraction. The initial blood clot was replaced by a provisional connective tissue matrix, woven bone, and lamellar bone with bone marrow. A final bridge of cortical bone closed the entire socket.

In another study, Cardaropoli et al[12] showed that whether or not periodontal ligament cells in the socket are removed after tooth extraction does not seem to have any influence on socket healing. In the same study, sockets were filled with collagen sponge or Bio-Oss collagen (Geistlich) in dogs, and healing was studied for 3 months.[12] The new bone formation in the sockets filled with collagen sponge was higher (62%) compared with the sockets filled with Bio-Oss (26%); a soft and hard tissue shrinkage of almost 0.5 mm in height was found in the collagen sponge sites compared with the Bio-Oss sockets. The tissue shrinkage was greater (0.7 mm) in the healed sockets without any augmentation. Araújo et al[13] concluded that the placement of a biomaterial in an extraction socket may promote bone modeling and compensate, at least temporarily, for marginal ridge contraction.

Alveolar ridge preservation has been studied using different grafting techniques after tooth extraction.[14–20] The results of these studies differ but show that complete ridge preservation is not achieved with any of the methods of treatment. Moreover, when implants were placed after socket healing, the early implant osseointegration was not influenced by the application of bone materials.[21]

Araújo and Lindhe[22] presented ridge alterations following tooth extractions in dogs and the effects of flap elevation on tissue healing. With or without flap elevation, the long-term (6-month) outcome of socket healing was similar. Specifically, in the apical and middle portions of the socket site, minor dimensional alterations occurred, while in the coronal portion of the ridge, the reduction of the hard tissue volume was substantial.

Critical results regarding current alveolar socket preservation techniques were also demonstrated by Fickl et al.[23] According to their studies in dogs, when different grafting techniques are used after tooth extraction, the dimensional alterations of the sockets seem unpredictable due to unexpected contour shrinkage.

It is uncertain which socket preservation technique is the most predictable. No studies have compared dimensional changes after different preservation techniques under standardized conditions. Although studies in dogs have provided significant information, there is still insufficient data about socket healing in humans. The main questions are the long-term clinical outcome and the three-dimensional changes in the ridge after healing. Implant placement with flap elevation after preservation of the ridge (ie, delayed placement) violates the alveolar ridge height. A flapless surgical approach may be associated with less bone resorption because there is no violation of the blood supply. There is no doubt that extensive pretreatment planning and advanced surgical experience are necessary in order to avoid intra- and postoperative complications.

## Implant Placement in Fresh Extraction Sockets

Is tissue remodeling improved if an implant is placed in the socket immediately after tooth extraction? What are the effects of functional loading of this implant after immediate placement?

The concept of immediate placement of an implant in the socket was first introduced and evaluated in clinical studies by Schulte et al.[24] Since then, there have been many studies in humans demonstrating the soft and hard tissue effects of immediate implant placement. Covani et al[25] showed complete bone healing after immediate implant placement in fresh sockets, using flap advancement for primary closure without grafting. The buccolingual dimension of the alveolar ridge was measured at the time of implant placement and at stage-two surgery. A narrowing of almost 3 mm was found at the coronal aspect of the socket. Using a similar therapeutic concept, the same authors evaluated the vertical crestal bone changes around immediate implants and showed a bone loss between 0 and 2 mm.[26]

Crespi et al[27] placed implants in periapical infected sites in humans and reported successful osseointegration and a 100% survival rate at the 4-month follow-up. In another study, these authors immediately restored a group of implants placed in fresh extraction sockets and compared them with a group of immediate implants that were loaded after osseointegration. The implants included in this study were placed in the anterior maxilla (esthetic zone) at the buccal level of the bone crest. The study showed no differences in terms of soft and hard tissues between the two loading groups.[28]

In a study on platform switching, the marginal bone levels around implants with and without platform switching were similar when implants were placed in extraction sockets and loaded immediately. The cumulative survival rate was 100% within the observation period of 2 years.[29] In another study, a mean gain of 0.2 mm of soft tissue at the buccal aspect and a mean gain of 0.25 mm of papilla were observed after 36 months of healing around implants with platform switching placed in fresh extraction sockets.[30] Recent studies with implants using the platform-switching concept showed marginal bone maintenance over a 21-month loading period.[31]

Grunder[32] reported long-term experience in private practice using protocols with implants placed in fresh extraction sockets without the use of any bone substitutes or barrier membranes for fixed complete-arch restorations successfully for a 2-year observation period. The author presented similar protocols and the requirements for long-term success with the use of simultaneous augmentation and immediate loading in different publications.[33,34] Limited human histologic reports show that immediate loading of implants placed in fresh extraction sockets does not have any negative effects on osseointegration compared with unloaded implants. The implants appeared radiographically osseointegrated and clinically stable at retrieval. The implant interface was well mineralized with almost 58% bone-implant contact after 6 months of loading. Specifically, the bone around the immediately loaded implants placed in the extraction sockets was mature, well organized, compact, and characterized by many areas of remodeling.[35]

## Considerations for Clinical Application of the Protocol

- An important selection criterion for this clinical protocol is the smile line of the patient. For patients with an extremely high smile line and thin tissue biotype, alveolar socket preservation may be considered an essential treatment step after tooth extraction.
- The use of an implant system with platform switching allows deeper implant placement and simultaneous abutment connection using the final insertion torque. This avoids the need for abutment removal, maintaining crestal bone stability over a long period of time.
- The author tries to avoid use of implants with a wide diameter because wider-diameter implants are associated with more long-term functional and esthetic complications.[36,37]

## Case Reports

The following clinical cases provide the reader with the step-by-step clinical protocol for immediate loading of implants placed in fresh extraction sockets that has been used by the author to achieve outcomes of soft and hard tissue stability over periods of nearly 10 years.

### Case 1: Advanced protocol for immediate loading of implants placed in fresh extraction sockets

A 43-year-old woman with a moderate smile line presented with generalized advanced periodontal disease (Fig 13-1a). She was a smoker, and all teeth demonstrated severe attachment loss and tooth mobility (Figs 13-1b to 13-1f). For esthetic and phonetic reasons, the patient had used a gingival mask to cover the interdental spaces. The radiographic examination showed advanced bone loss and insufficient width of the anterior maxilla (Fig 13-1g). Following discussion of a comprehensive treatment plan, the patient decided to quit smoking and to proceed with a protocol of tooth extraction, immediate implant placement, and simultaneous loading.

The maxillary and mandibular teeth were extracted (Figs 13-1h and 13-1i), and granulation tissue was removed from the sockets. Immediately after surgery, the implants were connected to their abutments using final torque. Buccal dehiscences were addressed with autogenous bone taken from the residual areas, in accordance with guided bone regeneration guidelines, and were covered with collagen membranes (Figs 13-1j to 13-1l). Provisional restorations were fabricated using the Omnivac shell technique (OST).

The patient followed the recommend soft/liquid diet during the uneventful first 3 months of healing. After 3 months, the implants were evaluated for stability and the soft tissues presented a healthy condition (Fig 13-1m). New provisional restorations were made with the help of a diagnostic wax-up to improve the esthetic result (Fig 13-1n). It was decided that the maxillary abutments would be removed in order to make implant-level impressions for customized abutments. This was the first time that the abutments were removed (and only in the maxilla). New abutments were customized in the dental laboratory and delivered a couple of weeks later (Fig 13-1o). The final prostheses were delivered and cemented with TempBond (Kerr), and the patient was very satisfied with the final clinical and esthetic outcome.

The stability of the implants was evaluated every 6 months, and 2 years after immediate loading, the clinical examination demonstrated good soft and hard tissue stability (Figs 13-1p to 13-1s). Radiographic examination showed crestal bone stability and bone growth over the implant platforms, especially in the mandible (Fig 13-1t).

After 3 years of loading, a soft tissue complication was observed at the buccal aspect of the maxillary left lateral incisor because of bone resorption; no signs of peri-implantitis were found (Fig 13-1u). A connective tissue graft was pouched underneath the soft tissue to cover the exposed implant surface. The peri-implant bone levels and the soft tissue condition were evaluated every year for 11 years.

As is usual in such cases, significant buccal bone resorption was seen in some areas despite use of augmentation (Fig 13-1v). The patient was not concerned because of her moderate smile line. The radiologic evaluation showed crestal bone stability.

Note that the bone gain is greater in the mandible, where the abutments were never removed (Fig 13-1w).

# 13 Immediate Loading of Implants Placed in Fresh Extraction Sockets

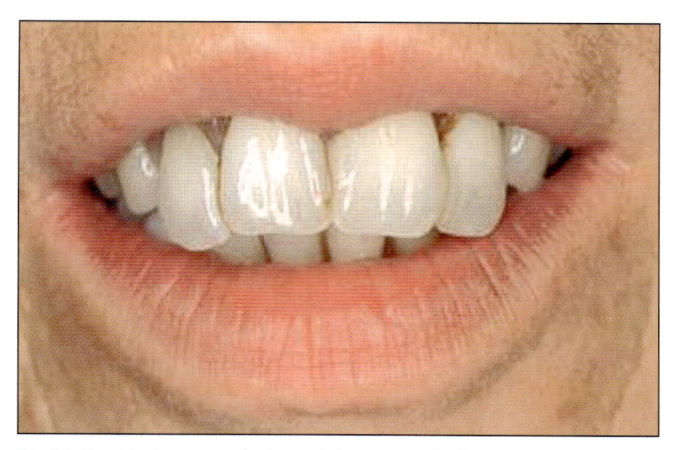

Fig 13-1a Moderate smile line of the patient before treatment.

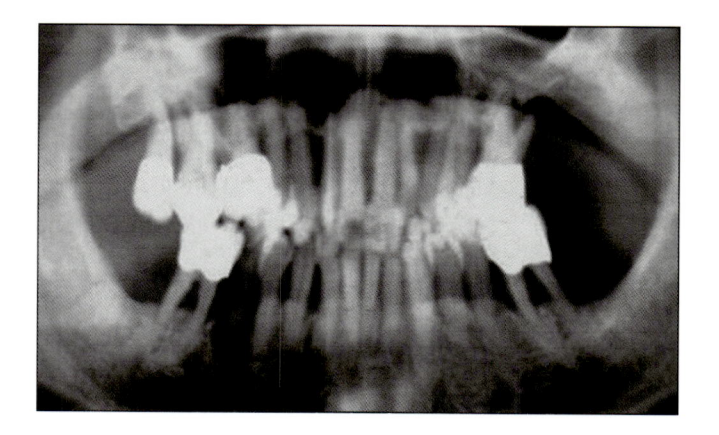

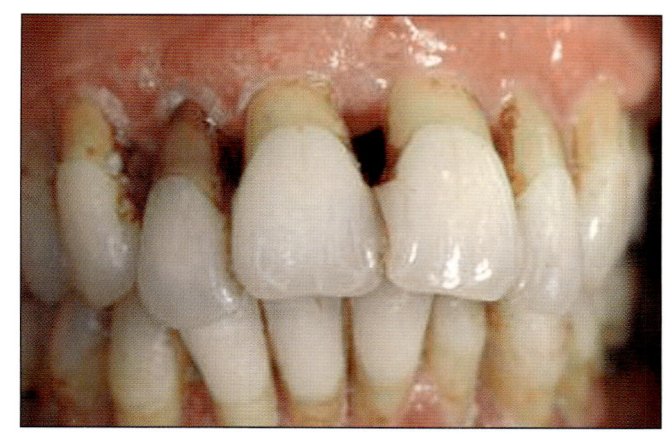

Fig 13-1b Frontal view of the patient before treatment.

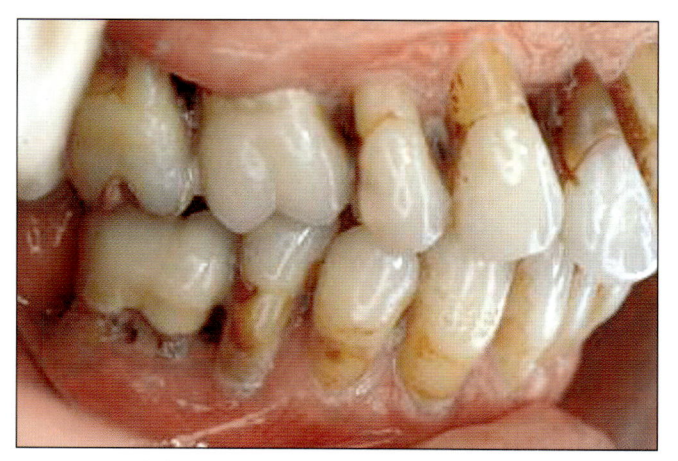

Fig 13-1c Right lateral view.

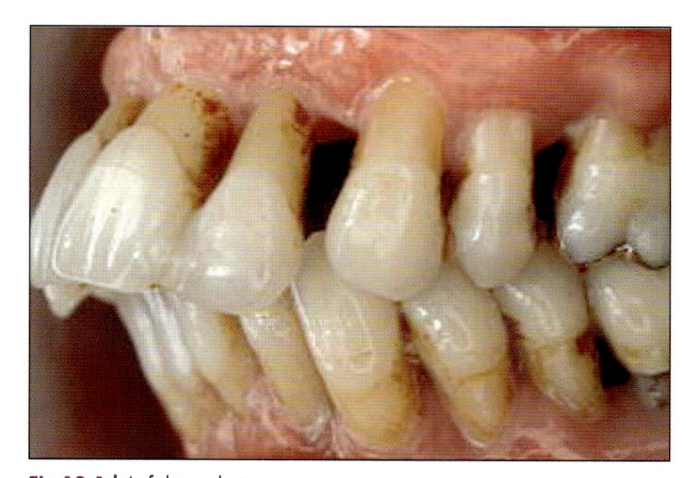

Fig 13-1d Left lateral view.

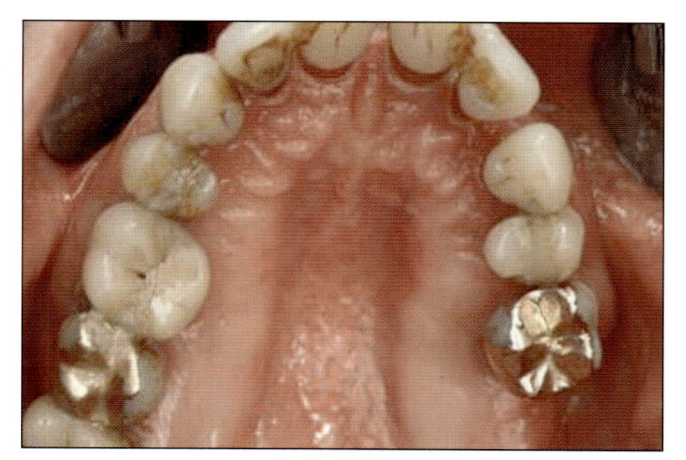

Fig 13-1e Maxillary occlusal view.

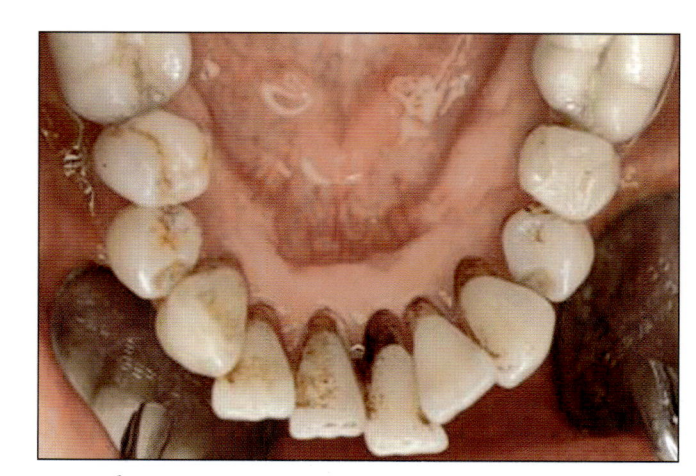

Fig 13-1f Mandibular occlusal view.

Fig 13-1g Radiographic examination showing advanced periodontal destruction and insufficient bone volume in the anterior maxilla.

## Case Reports

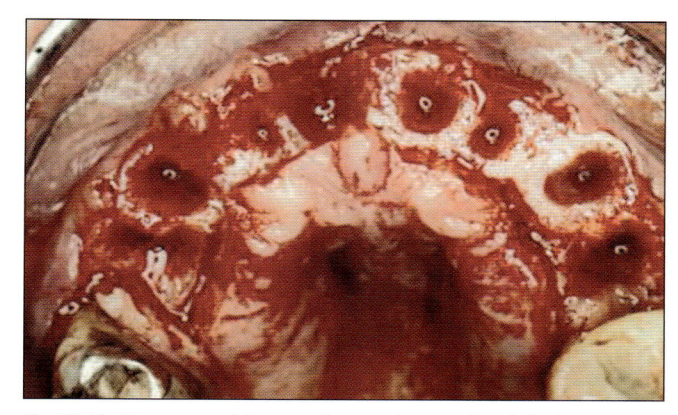

Fig 13-1h Extraction of the maxillary teeth immediately before implant placement.

Fig 13-1i Alveolar sockets in the mandible immediately before implant placement.

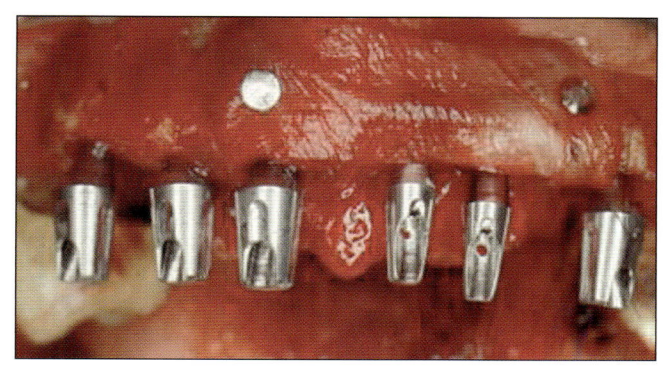

Fig 13-1j Implant placement in fresh extraction sockets with abutment connection. The buccal dehiscences were augmented with autogenous bone and covered with collagen membranes.

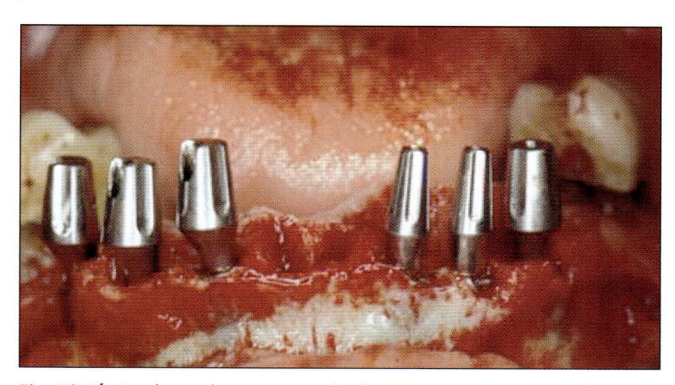

Fig 13-1k Implant placement and abutment connection in the mandible for immediate loading.

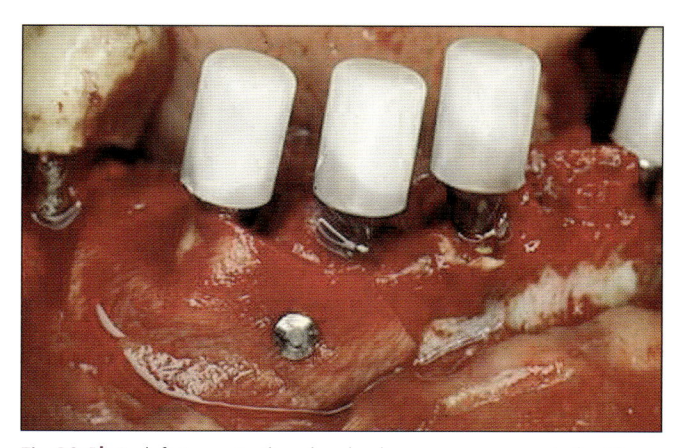

Fig 13-1l A deficiency in the alveolar bone was augmented with autogenous bone and covered with a collagen membrane in order to regenerate bone on the distal site of the implant in the first premolar site.

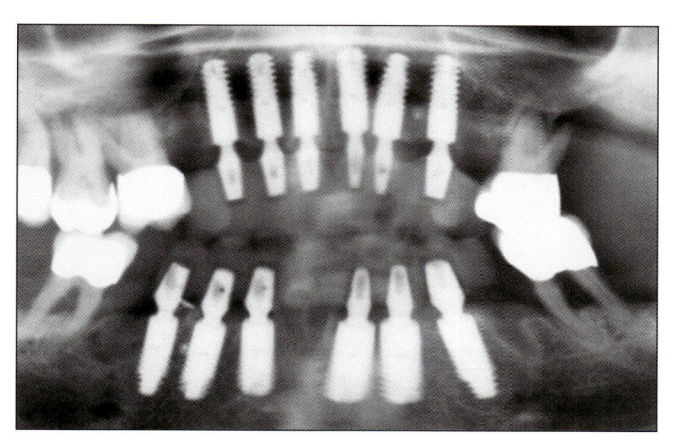

Fig 13-1m Postoperative situation 3 months after loading.

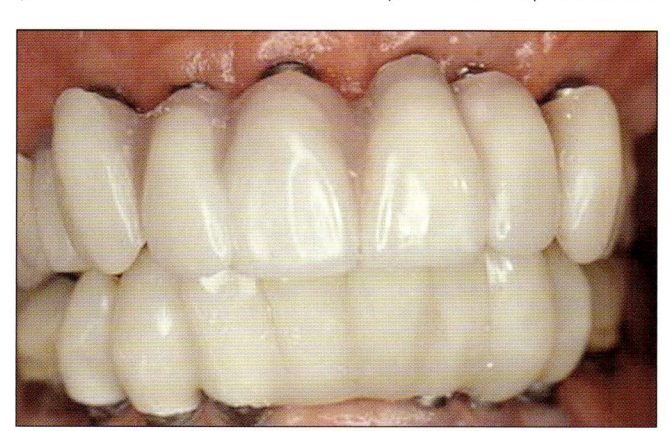

Fig 13-1n New provisional restorations in place 3 months after loading.

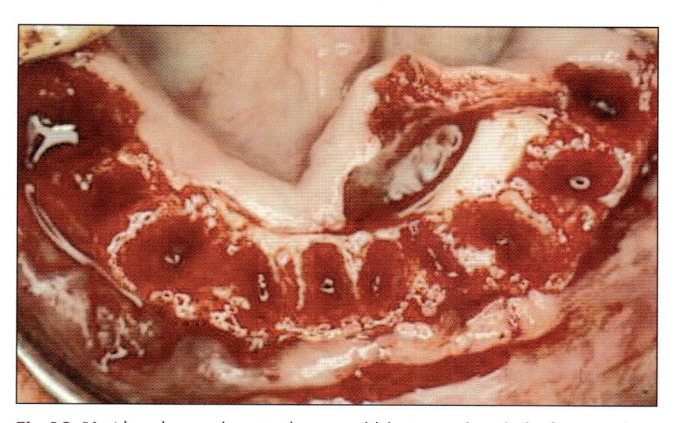

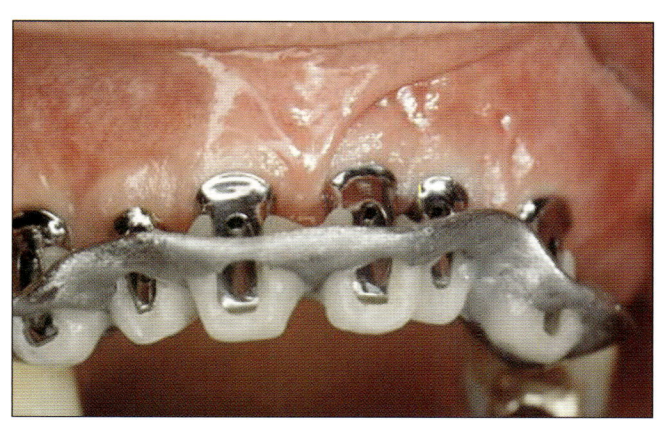

Fig 13-1o Abutments in place using a rigid jig.

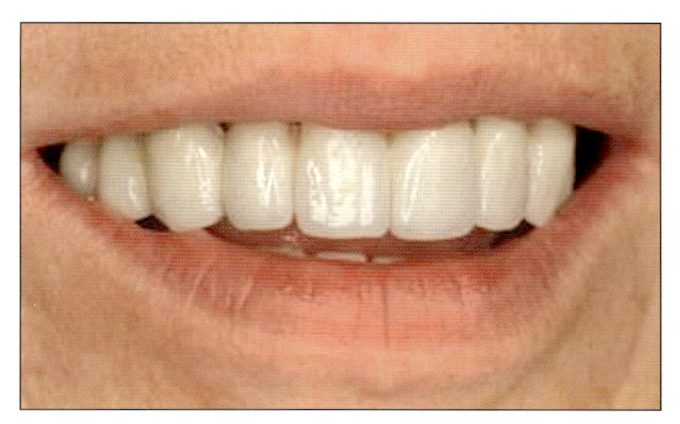

**Fig 13-1p** Smile line of the patient 2 years after loading. The patient was very satisfied with the final outcome.

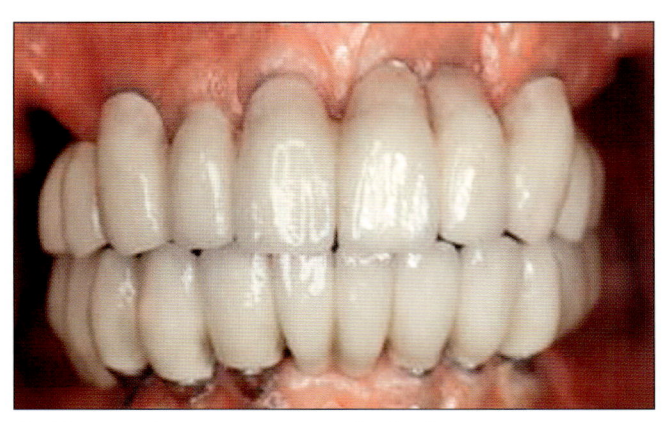

**Fig 13-1q** Final restoration 2 years after loading.

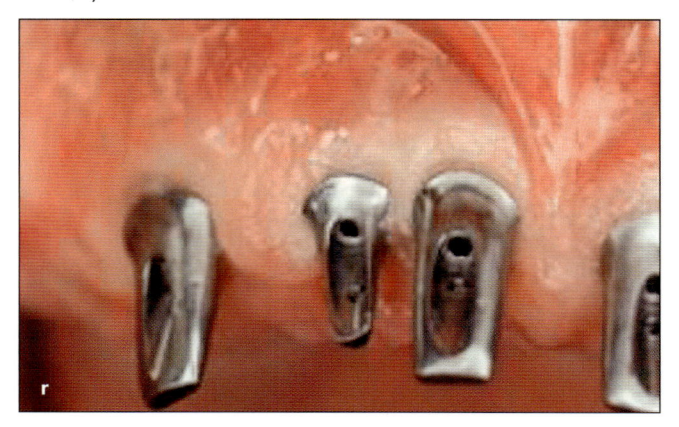

**Figs 13-1r and 13-1s** Peri-implant soft tissue condition in the right *(r)* and left *(s)* sides of the maxilla 2 years after loading.

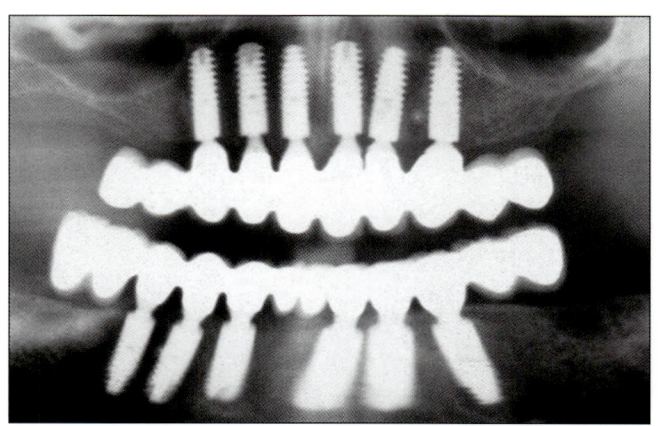

**Fig 13-1t** Panoramic radiograph 2 years after immediate loading presenting the bone gain over the implant platform.

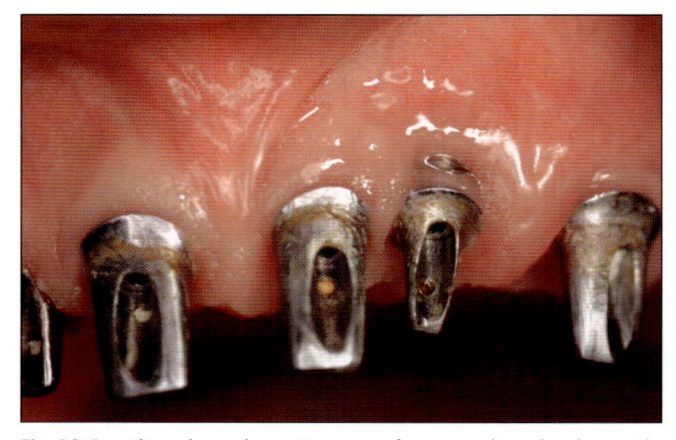

**Fig 13-1u** Clinical condition 3 years after immediate loading. Observe the buccal dehiscence at the maxillary left lateral incisor.

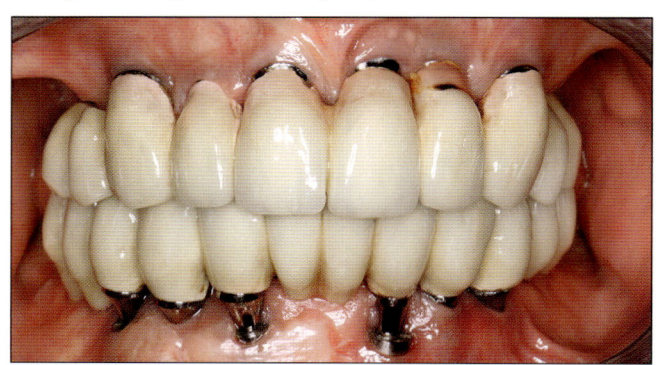

**Fig 13-1v** Clinical appearance at 11-year follow-up.

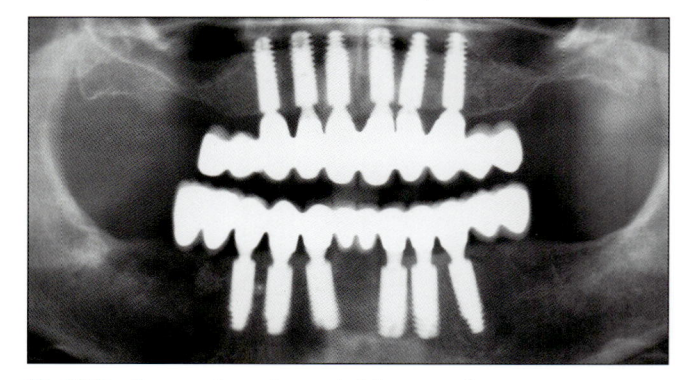

**Fig 13-1w** Panoramic radiograph 11 years after treatment presenting more bone in the mandible, where the abutments were never removed. Bone stability in the interproximal areas is due to the platform switching and the subcrestal implant placement. (Dental technician: M. Biaesch, Frankfurt, Germany.)

## Case Reports

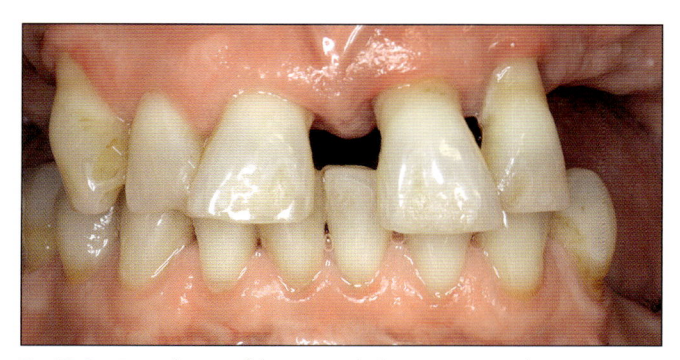

**Fig 13-2a** Frontal view of the patient before treatment. The patient complained of the diastema between her maxillary central incisors.

**Fig 13-2b** Lateral window preparation and sinus elevation procedure on the right side.

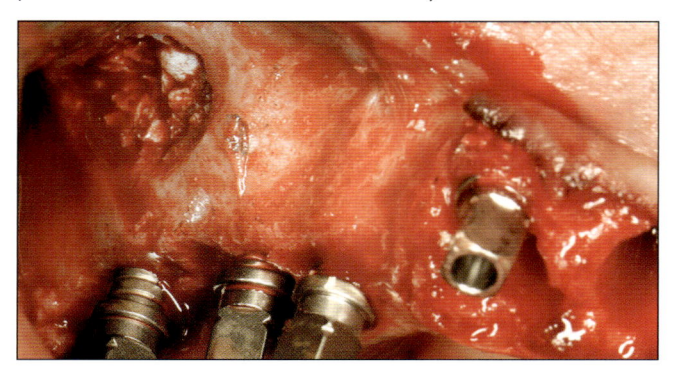

**Fig 13-2c** Augmentation with a composite graft of autogenous bone and bone mineral (cancellous form). Implants placed on the right side.

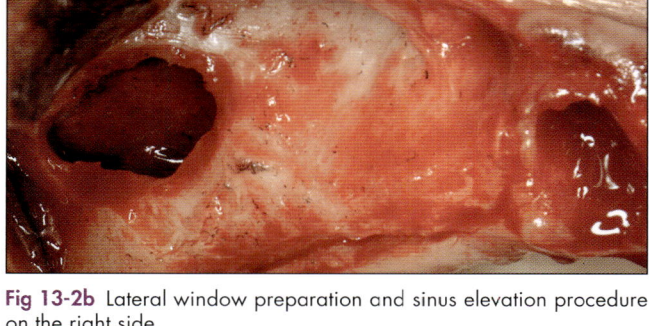

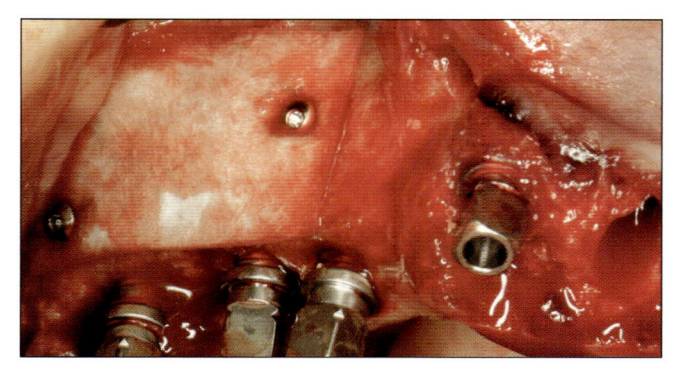

**Fig 13-2d** Coverage of the right-side lateral window with a collagen membrane.

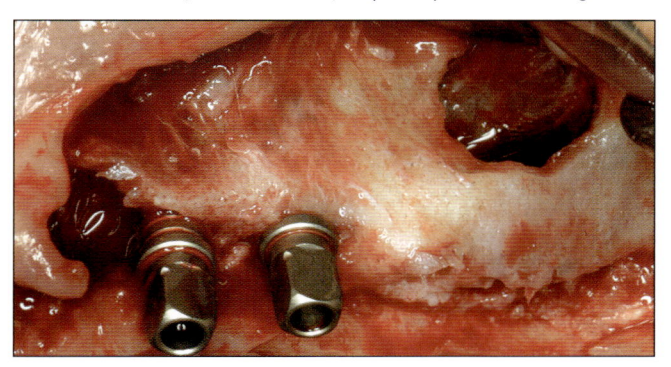

**Fig 13-2e** Lateral window preparation and sinus elevation procedure on the left side.

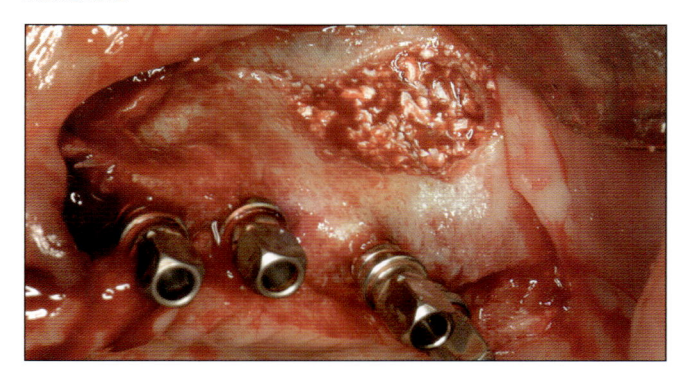

**Fig 13-2f** Augmentation with composite graft of autogenous bone and bone mineral (cancellous form). Implants placed on left side.

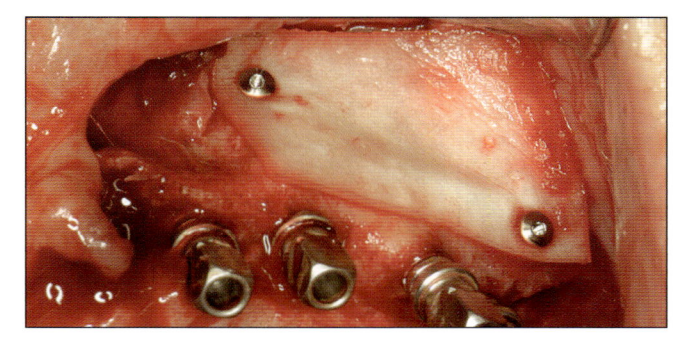

**Fig 13-2g** Coverage of the left-side lateral window with a collagen membrane.

## Case 2: Immediately loaded implants in the maxilla in conjunction with sinus elevation

A woman presented with a chief complaint of a diastema between her maxillary central incisors (Fig 13-2a). The periodontal condition was very poor except for the maxillary right canine. The treatment plan involved extracting all maxillary teeth, performing simultaneous sinus elevation (bilaterally), and placing implants and abutments for immediate loading.

The grafting procedures used Bio-Oss cancellous and autogenous bone from the tuberosity as well as collagen membranes to cover the lateral sinus windows (Figs 13-2b to 13-2g).

151

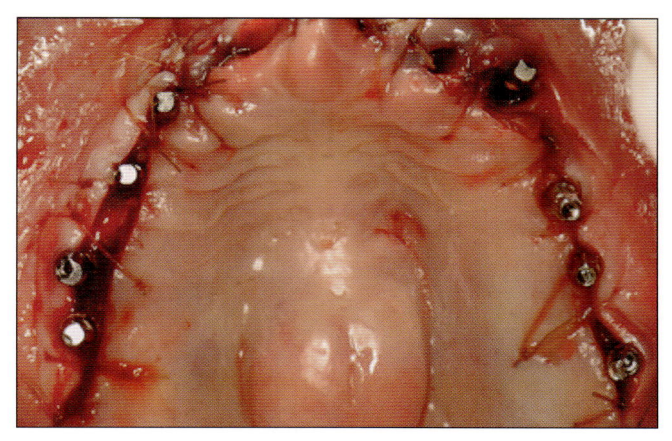

**Fig 13-2h** Abutment connection for immediate loading.

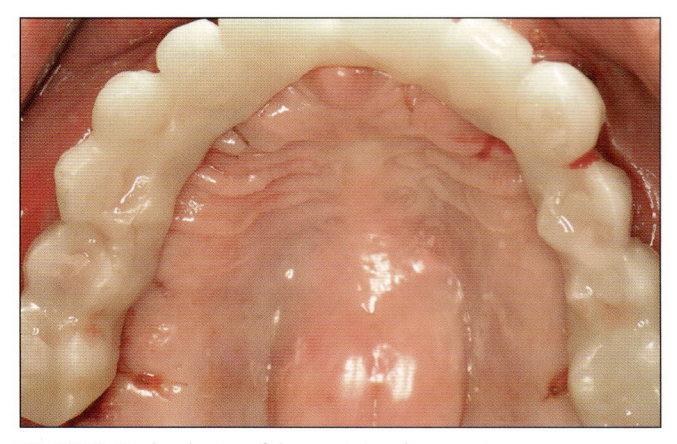

**Fig 13-2i** Occlusal view of the provisional restoration.

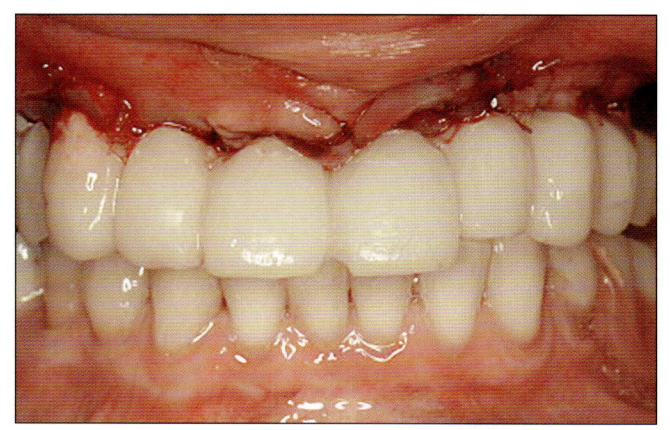

**Fig 13-2j** Frontal view of the provisional restoration. There is no longer a diastema between the central incisors.

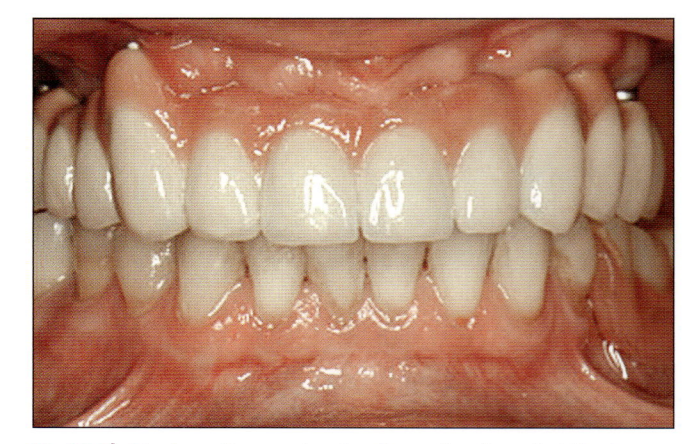

**Fig 13-2k** Final maxillary restoration 9 months after rehabilitation.

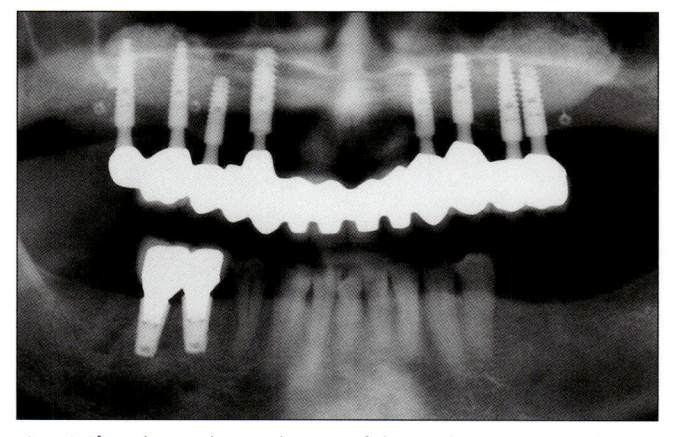

**Fig 13-2l** Radiographic evaluation of the implants 5 years after immediate loading.

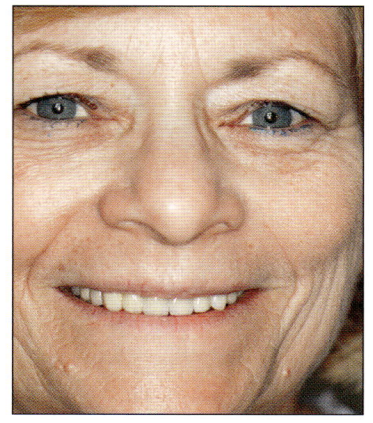

**Fig 13-2m** Frontal view of the patient and her smile line 5 years after rehabilitation of the maxilla. (Surgery and restoration by G. E. Romanos and A. Basha, New York, NY.)

Final abutments were placed with the final torque and were never removed (Fig 13-2h). The provisional prosthesis was fabricated using the OST protocol, which did not replicate the diastema between the central incisors. The patient was very satisfied with the esthetic result immediately after surgery (Figs 13-2i and 13-2j).

The implants were evaluated for stability and peri-implant complications over 9 months. The final prosthesis was fabricated using an abutment-level impression without abutment removal (Fig 13-2k). The patient was still very happy with the final result at the 5-year follow-up (Figs 13-2l and 13-2m).

Case Reports

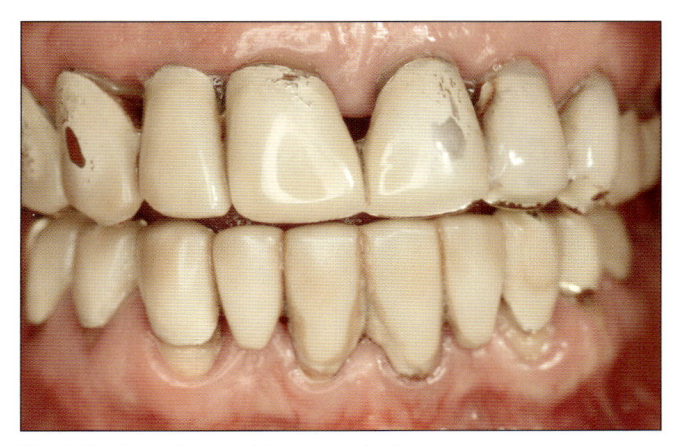

Fig 13-3a Frontal view of the patient before treatment.

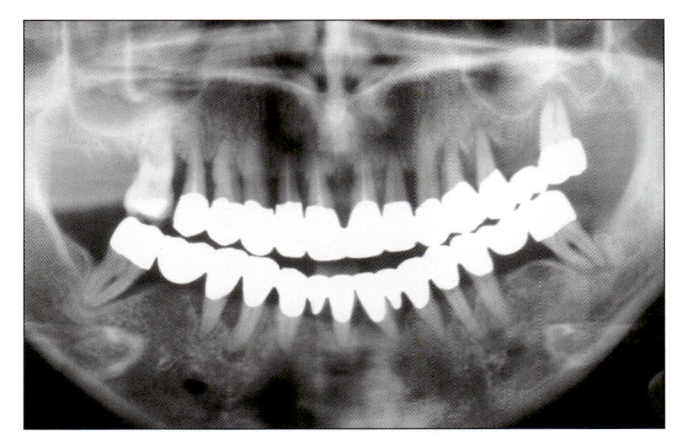

Fig 13-3b Panoramic radiograph presenting the hopeless dentition.

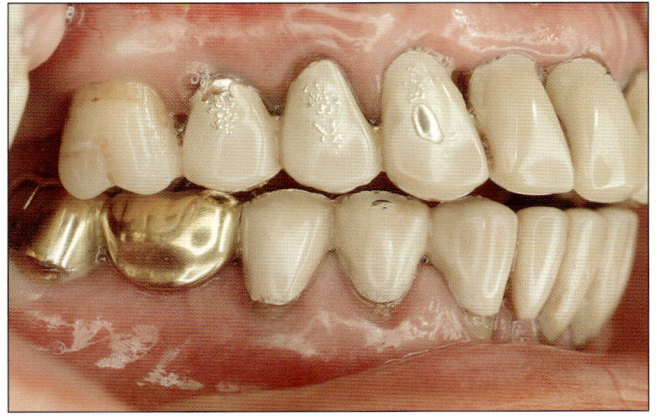

Fig 13-3c Right lateral view.

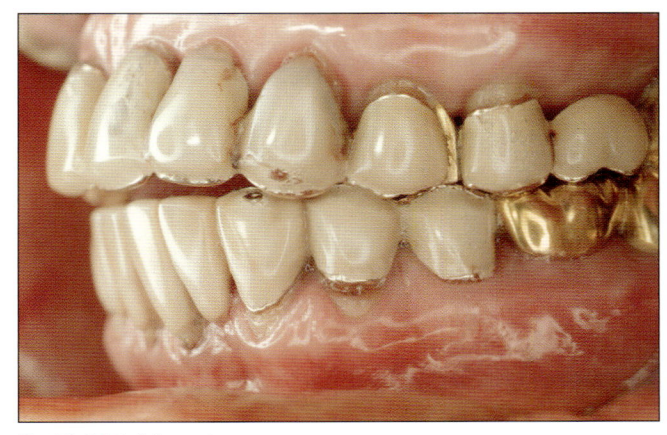

Fig 13-3d Left lateral view.

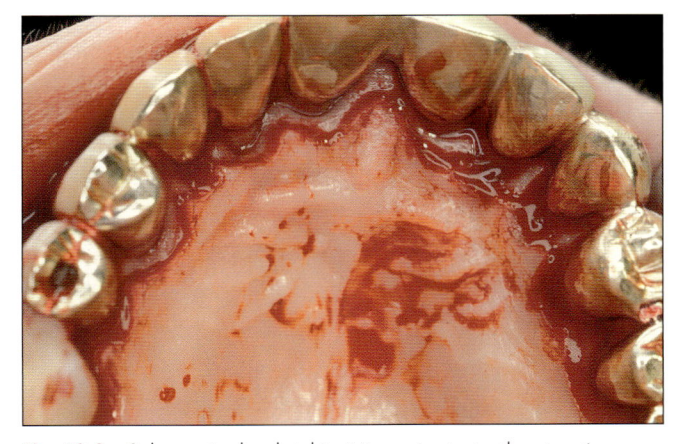

Fig. 13-3e Submarginal palatal incision prior to tooth extraction.

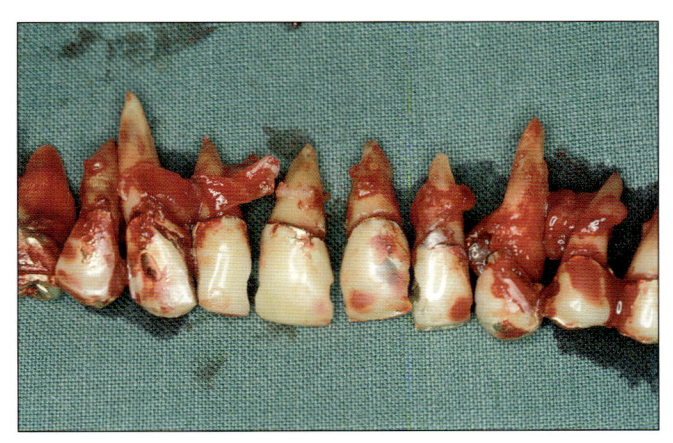

Fig 13-3f Extracted maxillary teeth.

## Case 3: Advanced immediate loading in the maxilla and mandible

This similar case documents an immediate loading protocol for a woman who presented with generalized severe periodontal disease and a hopeless dentition (Figs 13-3a to 13-3d).

The teeth were extracted after a combination of a split- and then full-thickness periodontal flap (buccally and palatally with a submarginal incision) to remove the entire inflamed pocket epithelium (Figs 13-3e and 13-3f). The implants were placed in the maxilla and mandible, and the sockets were filled with autogenous bone from the residual ridges (Figs 13-3g to 13-3j). Abutments were placed for immediate loading with OST provisional restorations (Fig 13-3k). The postoperative panoramic radiograph showed the implant positioning (Fig 13-3l). The delivery of the final prosthesis was performed 3 to 4 months after implant placement. The patient was very

## 13 Immediate Loading of Implants Placed in Fresh Extraction Sockets

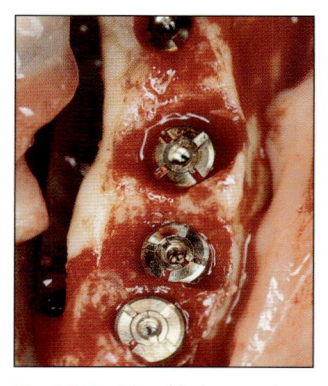

**Fig 13-3g** Mandibular implants placed in fresh extraction sockets.

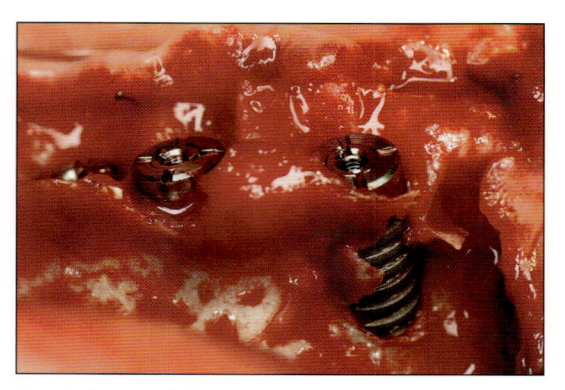

**Fig 13-3h** Bone dehiscences prior to augmentation.

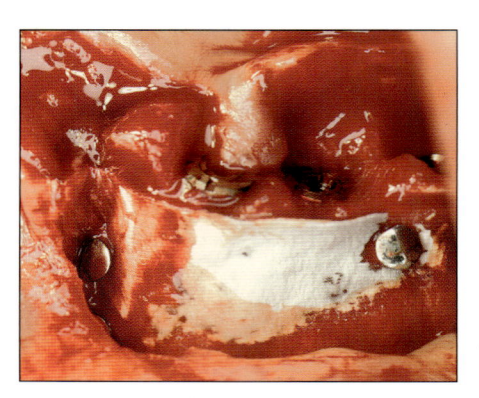

**Fig 13-3i** Sockets filled with particulate and autogenous bone graft and covered with a collagen membrane.

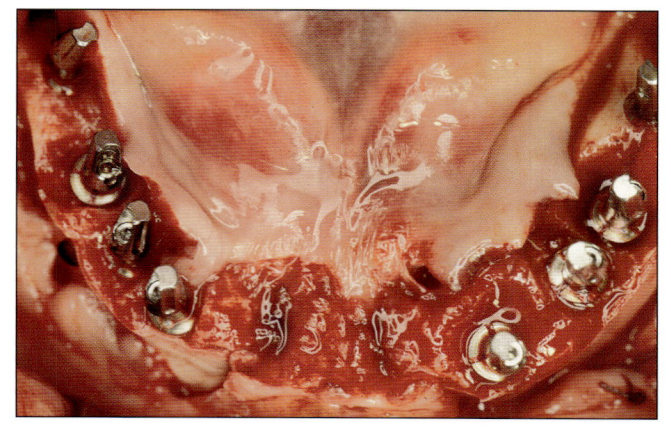

**Fig 13-3j** Abutment connection in the mandible for immediate loading.

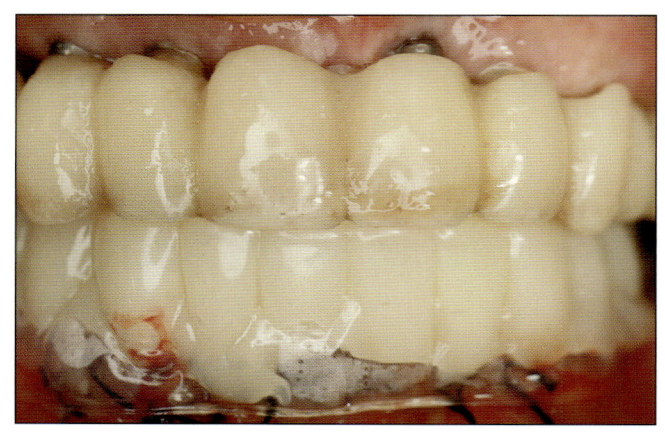

**Fig 13-3k** Full-mouth provisional restorations made using the OST protocol.

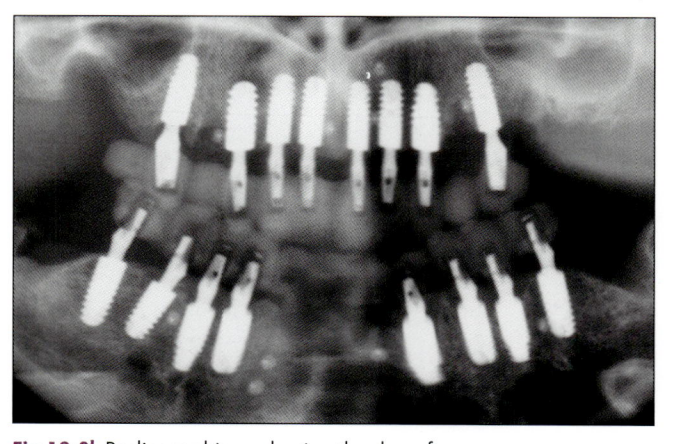

**Fig 13-3l** Radiographic evaluation the day after surgery.

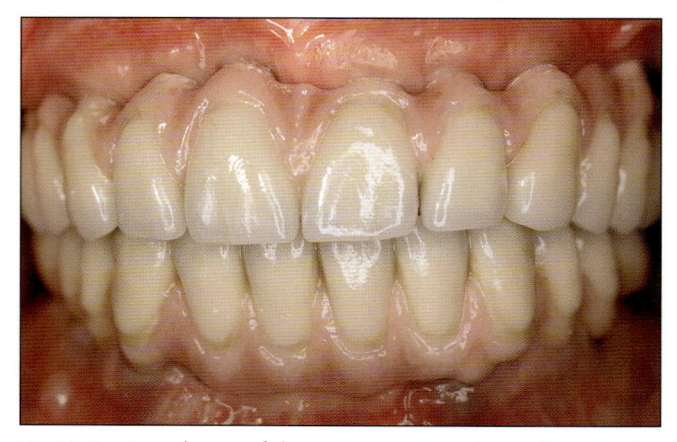

**Fig 13-3m** Frontal view of the restoration in occlusion 2 years after immediate loading.

satisfied with the clinical outcome. The abutments were removed, and new customized abutments were delivered with subgingival shoulders to improve esthetics.

After 2 years of loading, the patient was very happy with the excellent result (Figs 13-3m to 13-3p). Crestal bone stability was verified according to the radiographic evaluation (Fig 13-3q). Within the first 5 years of loading, some soft tissue dehiscence was observed, and free gingival grafts were placed to stabilize it. The implants were stable over the 8 years of observation, and no further changes in the soft tissues were observed clinically and radiographically at the final follow-up visit (Figs 13-3r to 13-3u).

## Case Reports

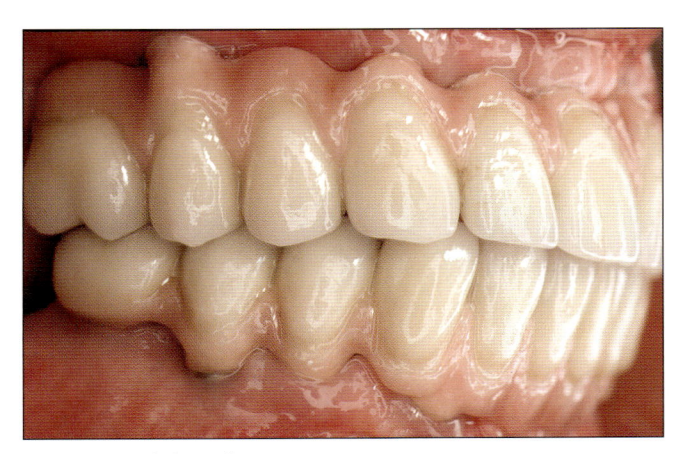

**Fig 13-3n** Right lateral view.

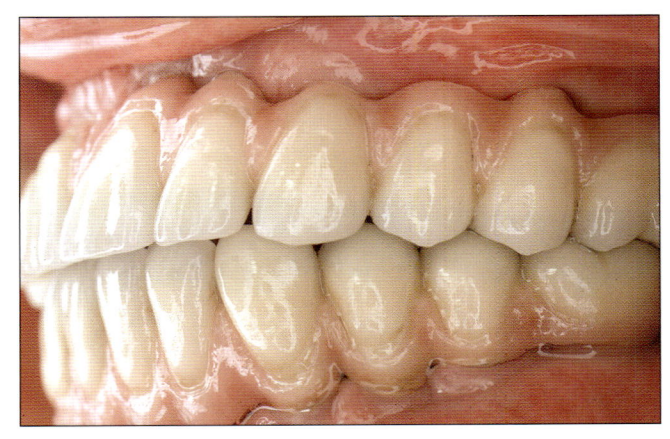

**Fig 13-3o** Left lateral view.

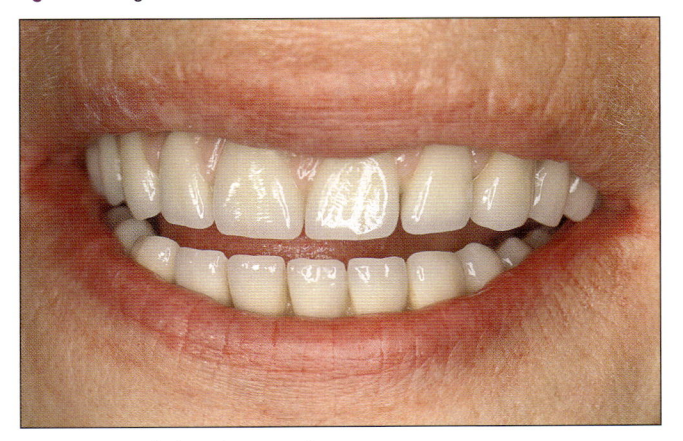

**Fig 13-3p** Smile line 2 years after treatment.

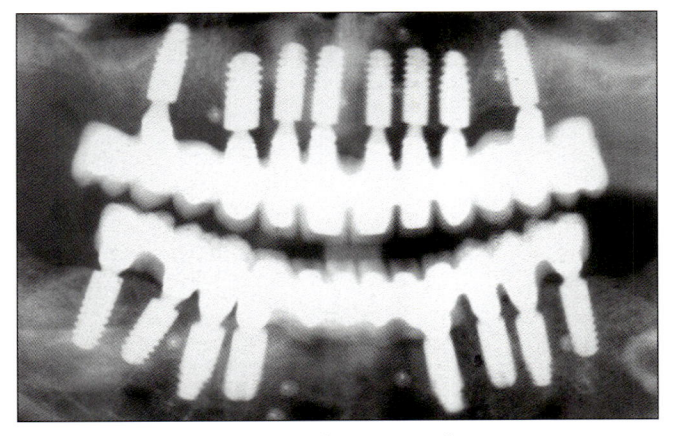

**Fig 13-3q** Panoramic radiograph 2 years after surgery presenting crestal bone stability.

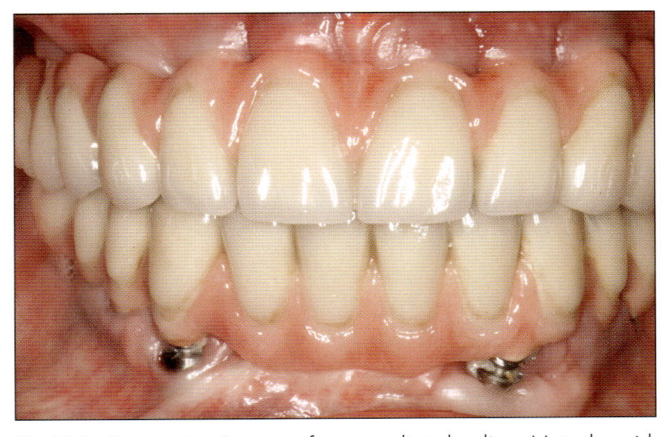

**Fig 13-3r** Restoration 8 years after immediate loading. Note the midfacial recessions in some areas due to buccal bone resorption.

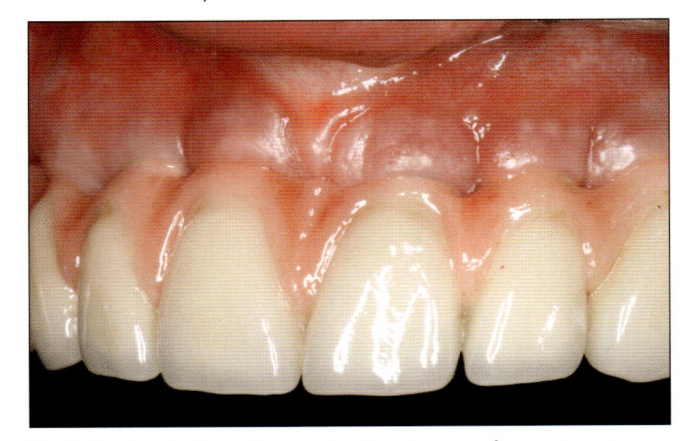

**Fig 13-3s** Detail of maxillary restoration 8 years after treatment.

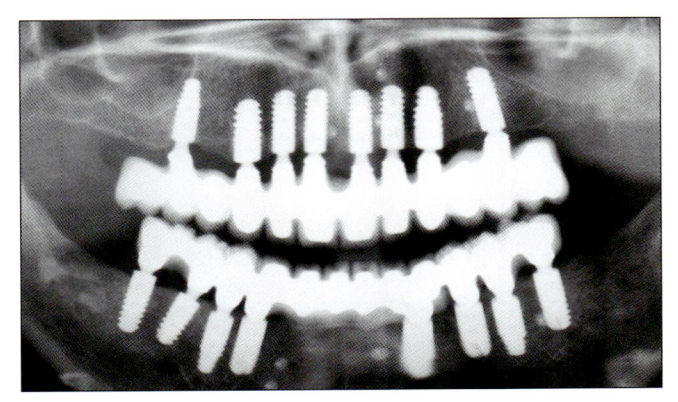

**Fig 13-3t** Panoramic radiograph 8 years after immediate loading. There is no interproximal bone loss.

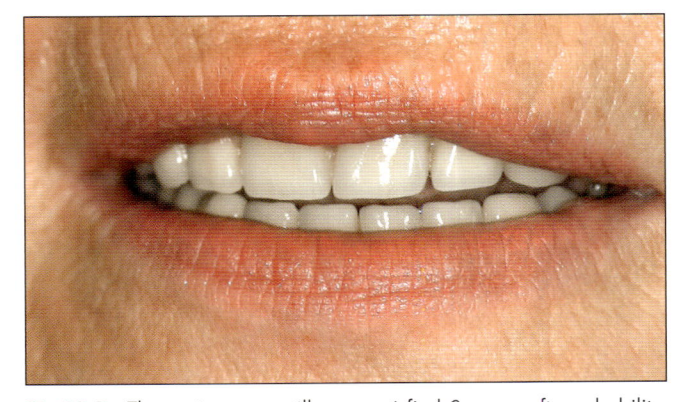

**Fig 13-3u** The patient was still very satisfied 8 years after rehabilitation. (Dental technician: M. Funk, Reichelsheim, Germany.)

## 13 — Immediate Loading of Implants Placed in Fresh Extraction Sockets

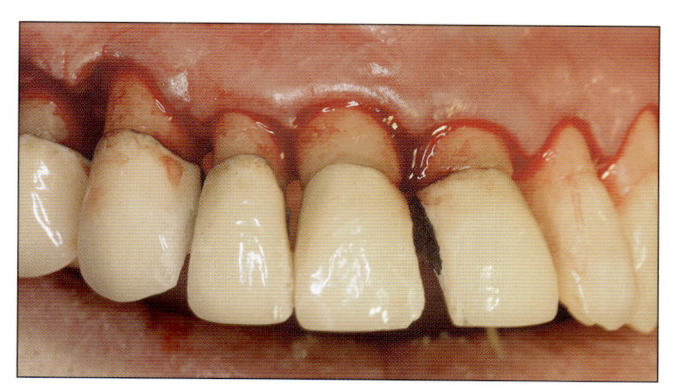

**Fig 13-4a** Intrasulcular incision prior to tooth extraction with the goal of removing the inflamed pocket epithelium.

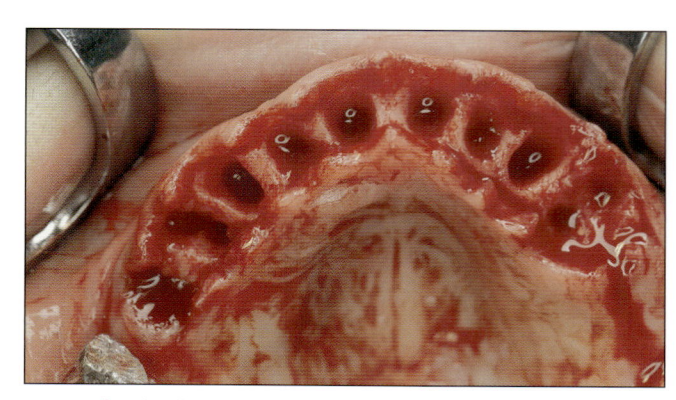

**Fig 13-4b** Alveolar sockets after tooth extraction and debridement. Note the thick bony walls and the horizontal bone loss. The flap was not elevated excessively due to the sufficient buccal wall thickness.

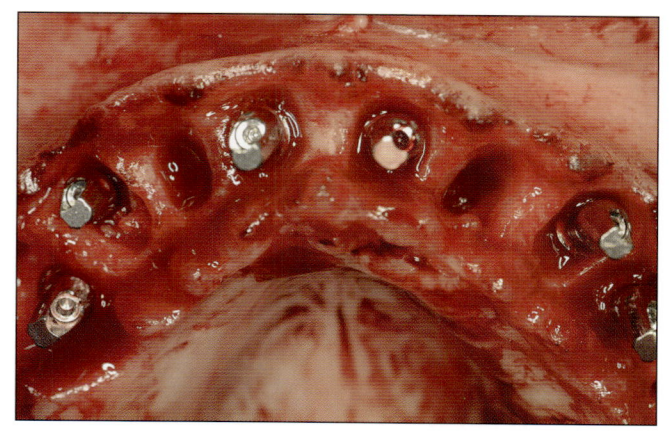

**Fig 13-4c** Subcrestal implant placement without the use of any grafting materials. Abutments were connected for immediate loading.

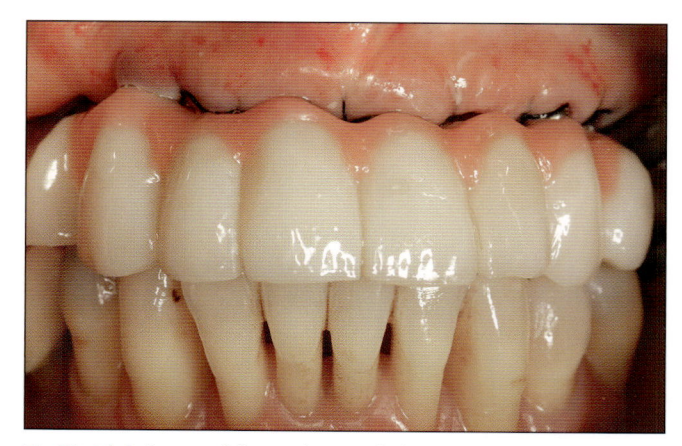

**Fig 13-4d** Splinting of the implants with the provisional restoration for immediate loading.

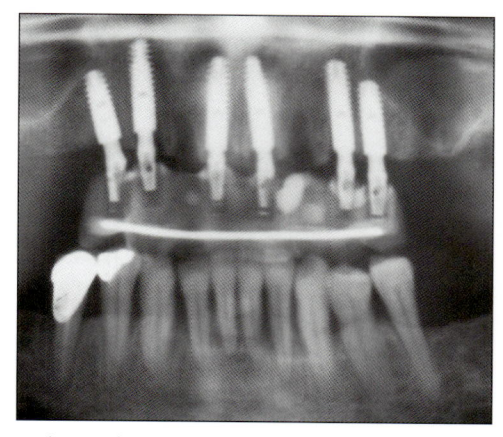

**Fig 13-4e** Radiographic evaluation with the splinted provisional restoration in place.

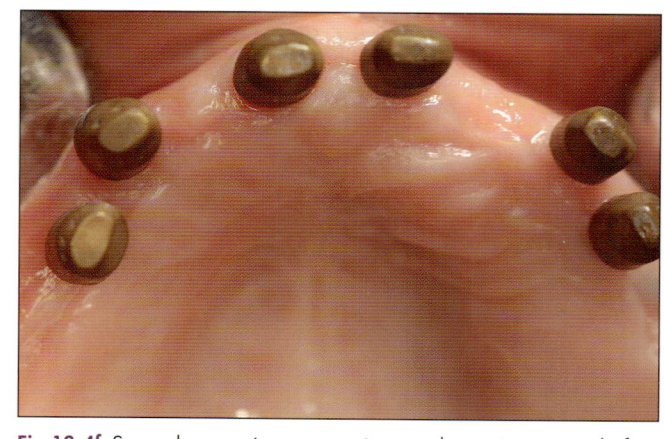

**Fig 13-4f** Secondary copings over primary telescopic copings before intraoral cementation of the final restoration.

## Case 4: Maxillary rehabilitation with immediate loading and a removable restoration

This case presents the treatment of a patient with mobile teeth due to periodontal disease with severe attachment loss. The maxillary teeth were extracted and the sockets were cleaned from granulation tissues (Figs 13-4a and 13-4b). Implants were placed in the sockets subcrestally, and the abutments were connected with the final torque (Fig 13-4c). The implants were splinted together with a provisional restoration (Figs 13-4d and 13-4e). After a period of 3 to 4 months of healing, the final impressions were taken without removing the abutments, and primary telescopes were fabricated (Fig 13-4f). Secondary copings were connected with a metal-reinforced, implant-retained prosthesis. The crest of bone was evaluated every year, and after 8 years of immediate loading, the bone levels presented a stable result (Figs 13-4g). The patient was satisfied with the final clinical outcome (Fig 13-4h).

Case Reports

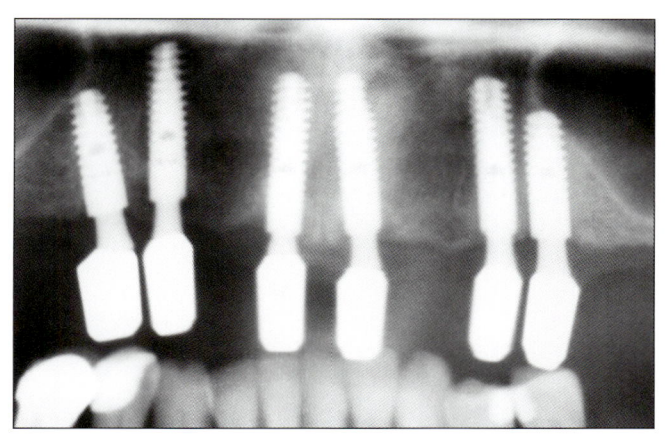

**Fig 13-4g** Radiographic evaluation of the bone levels at the 8-year follow-up.

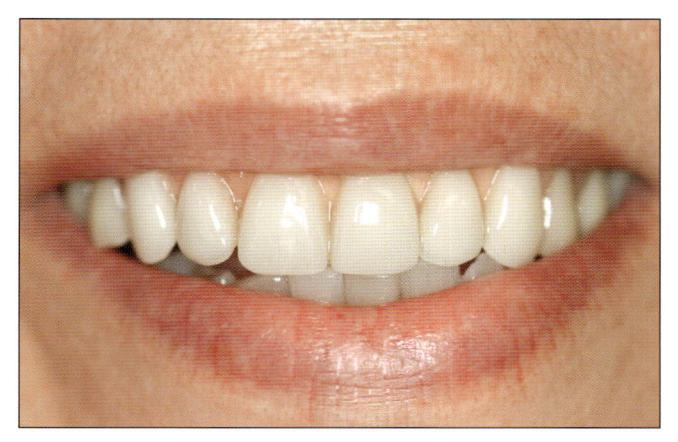

**Fig 13-4h** View of prosthesis after 8 years of loading.

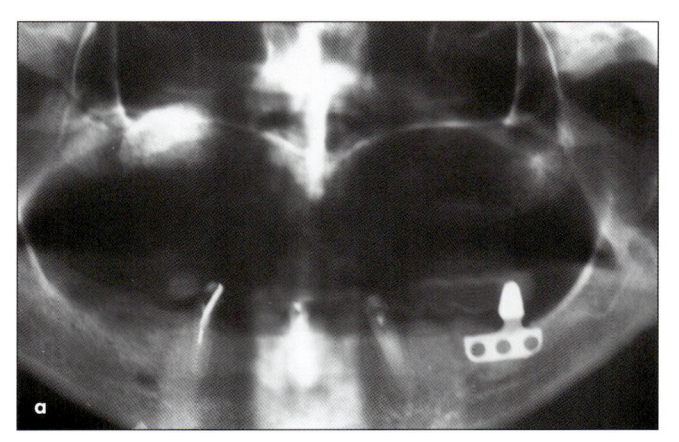

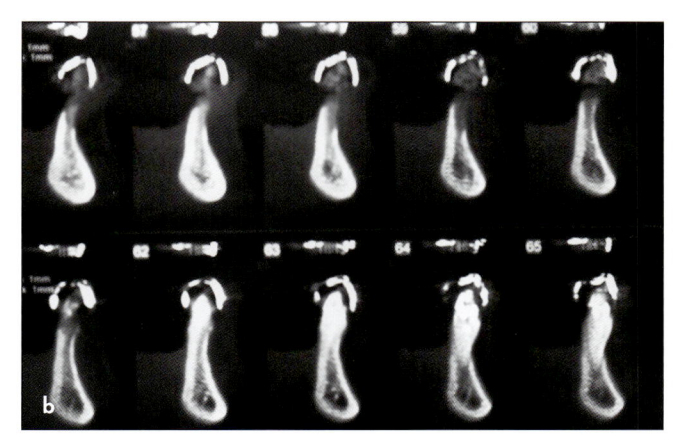

**Figs 13-5a and 13-5b** Radiographic evaluation demonstrating an extremely atrophic mandible.

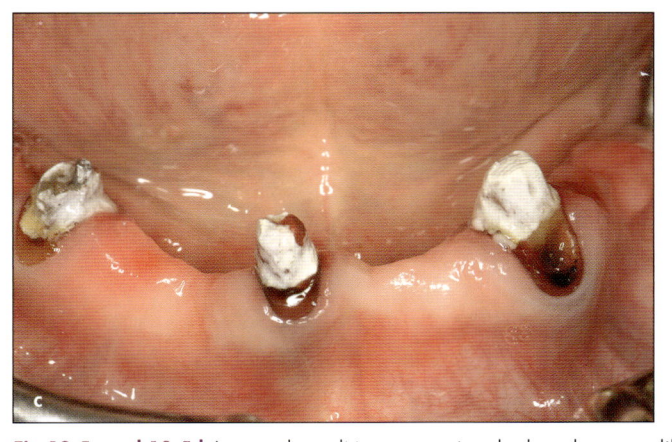

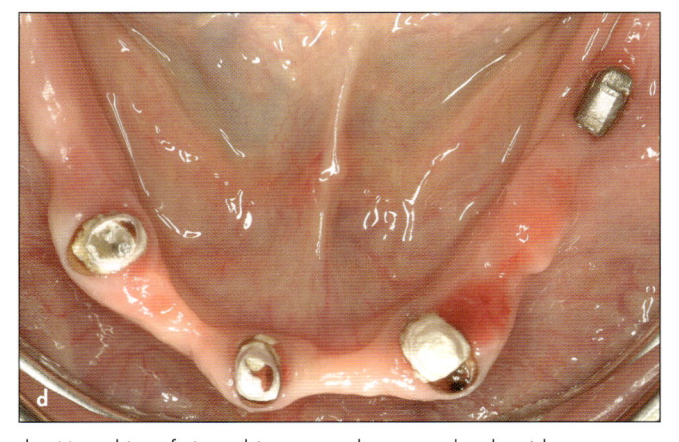

**Fig 13-5c and 13-5d** Intraoral condition presenting the hopeless mandibular dentition, thin soft tissue biotype, and narrow alveolar ridge.

## Case 5: Management of an extreme atrophic mandible with immediate loading in conjunction with grafting

The following case demonstrates the use of an advanced treatment protocol on a woman with a low smile line, thin soft tissue biotype, and extremely narrow mandibular alveolar ridge (Figs 13-5a to 13-5-d). The remaining mandibular teeth were deemed hopeless, and the narrow anterior alveolar ridge was treated with bone spreading (Figs 13-5e to 13-5-g). In other areas of the mandible, treatment included bilateral augmentation (buccal and lingual) to increase the ridge width for simultaneous implant placement and immediate loading. Implants were

157

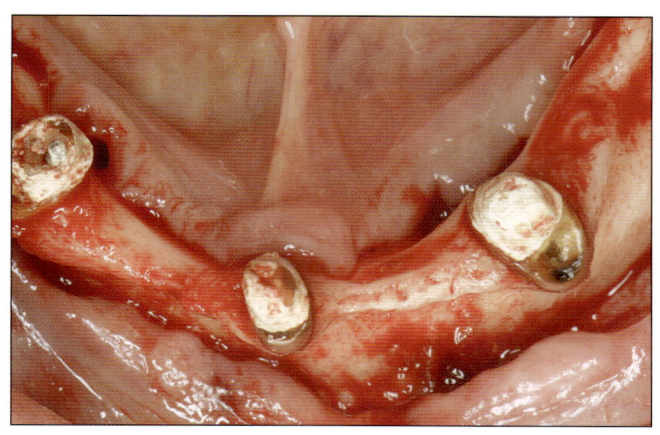

**Fig 13-5e** Flap elevation and preparation of the narrow alveolar ridge presenting undercuts.

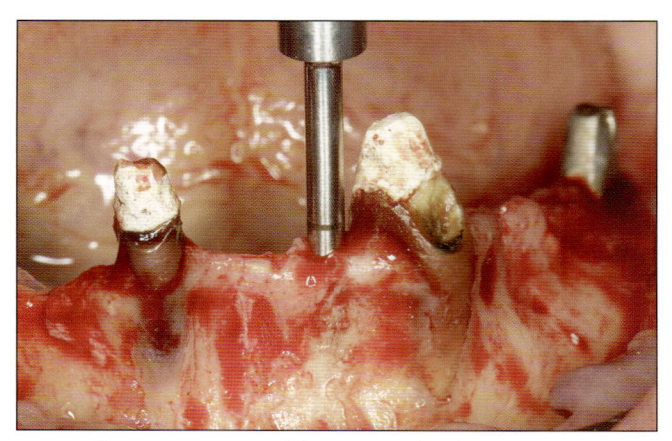

**Fig 13-5f** Bone spreading of the narrow alveolar ridge using Stoma osteotomes.

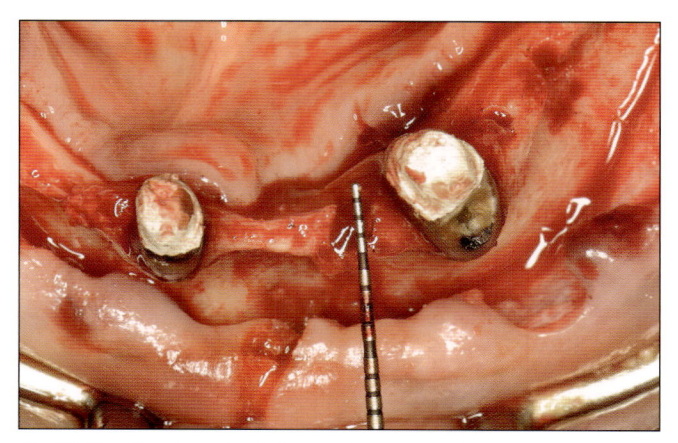

**Fig 13-5g** Alveolar ridge following bone spreading.

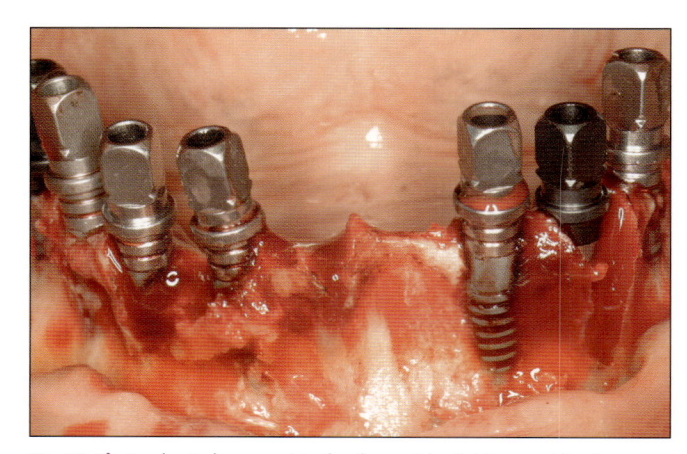

**Fig 13-5h** Implant placement in the the residual ridge and fresh extraction sockets with high primary stability.

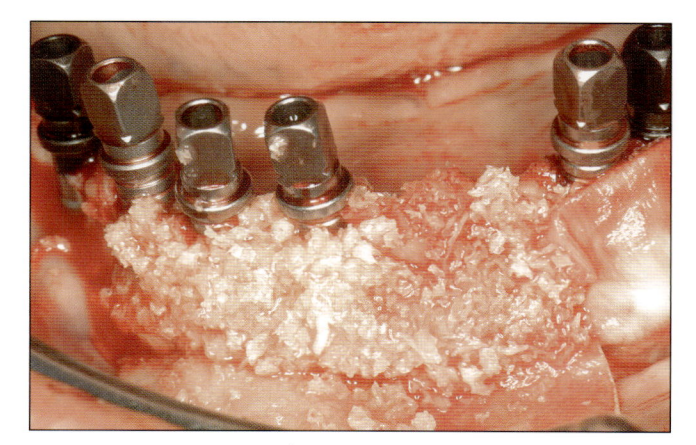

**Fig 13-5i** Augmentation with autogenous bone and human allograft (Puros) in a sandwich technique to increase the bone volume.

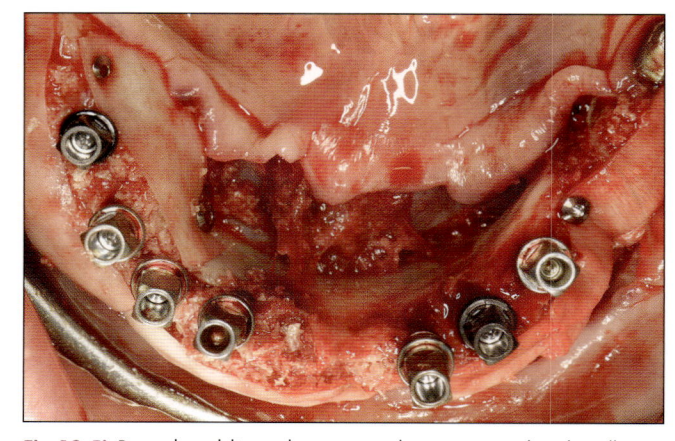

**Fig 13-5j** Buccal and lingual augmented sites covered with collagen membranes (Biomend Extend).

placed into the residual ridge and, after the remaining mandibular dentition was extracted, also in the fresh extraction sockets (Fig 13-5h). The exposed implant surfaces were covered with autogenous, particulated bone and a second layer of human allograft in a cancellous form (Puros, Zimmer) (Fig 13-5i). The augmented sites were finally covered with collagen membranes (Biomend Extend, Zimmer), which were fixed in place via titanium tacks (Fig 13-5j). All implants achieved primary stability and were connected with their abutments for im-

Case Reports

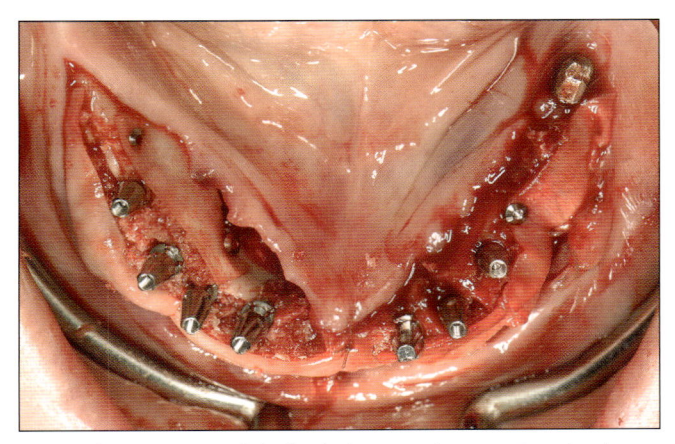

Fig 13-5k Connection of the final abutments for immediate loading.

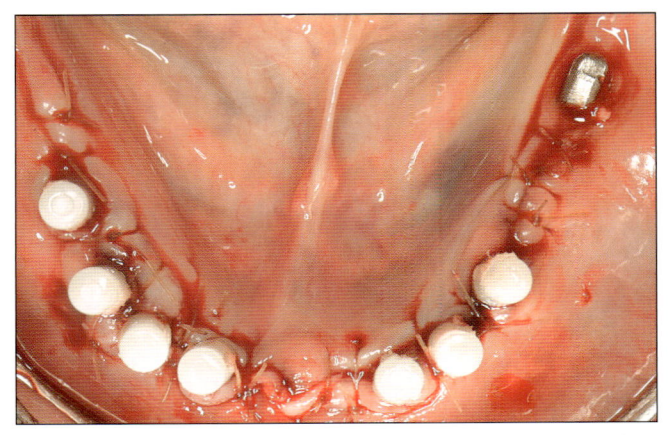

Fig 13-5l Mandibular flap sutured in preparation for provisionalization. Note the significant increase in the width of the ridge.

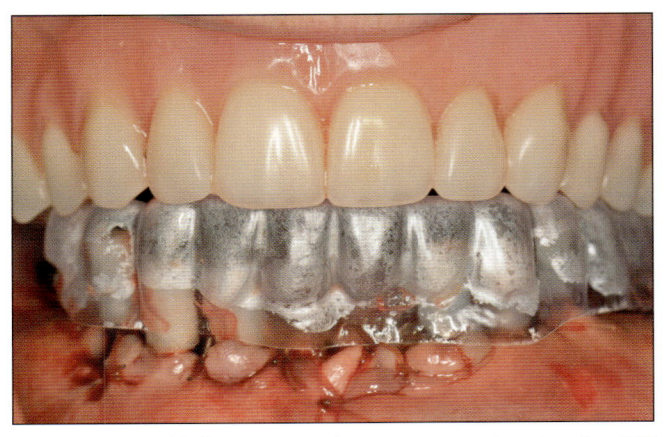

Fig 13-5m Mandibular provisional restoration made using the OST protocol.

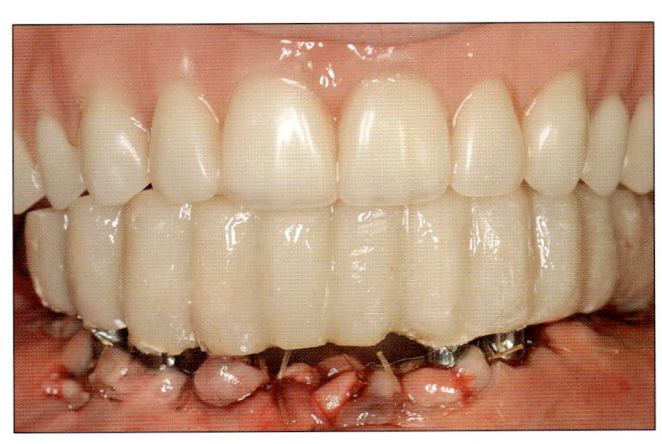

Fig 13-5n Provisional mandibular restoration in place.

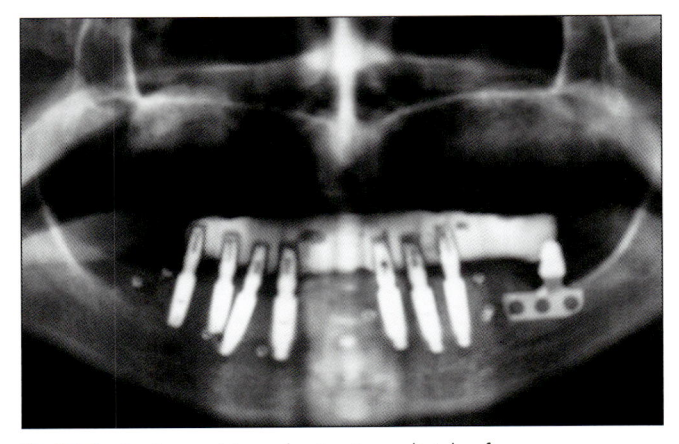

Fig 13-5o Radiographic evaluation immediately after surgery.

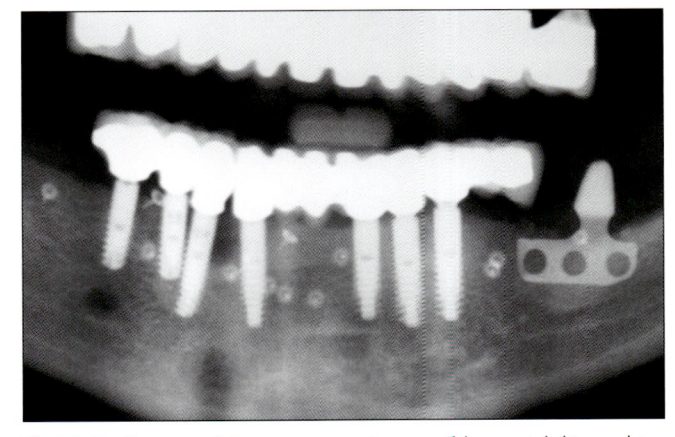

Fig 13-5p Five-year follow-up presenting good bone stability and implant success. (Restoration by H. C. Luu, New York, NY.)

mediate loading using a provisional resin bridge (Figs 13-5k to 13-5o). The implants were covered by bone during the augmentation and evaluated every 6 months after delivery of the final prosthesis. The final restoration was fabricated after impression without removal of the abutments. The 5-year follow-up visit showed stability of the crest of bone (Fig 13-5p), and the patient was satisfied with the final clinical outcome.

# 13 | Immediate Loading of Implants Placed in Fresh Extraction Sockets

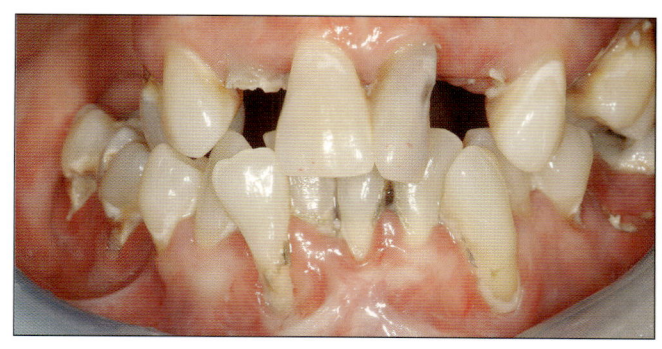

**Fig 13-6a** Pretreatment view showing generalized caries, tooth loss, tooth malposition, attachment loss, and inflammation.

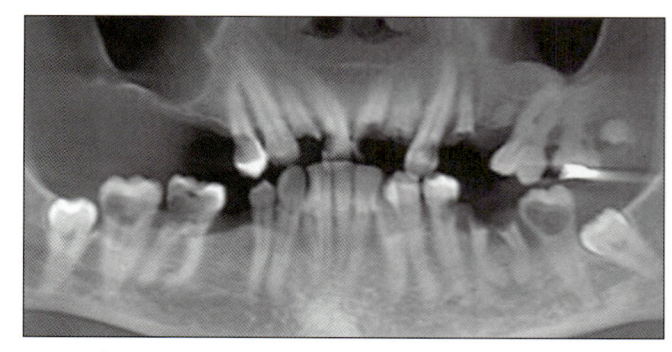

**Fig 13-6b** Panoramic radiograph (taken from CBCT) illustrating generalized caries, moderate periodontal bone loss, opacified maxillary sinuses, and partially erupted mandibular third molars.

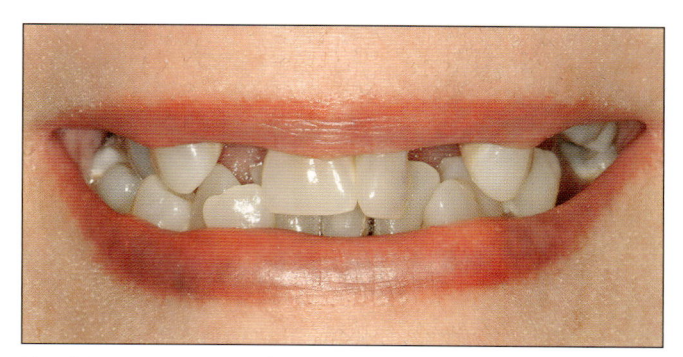

**Fig 13-6c** Pretreatment smile esthetics.

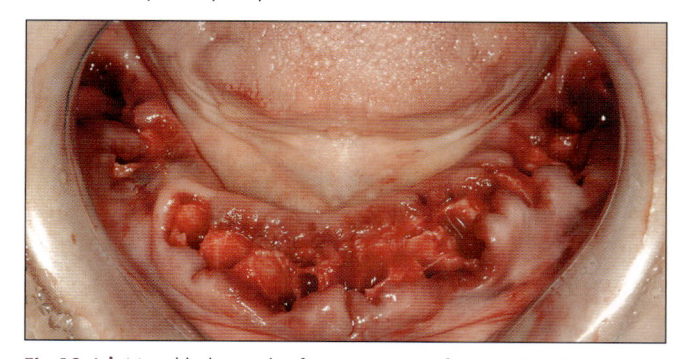

**Fig 13-6d** Mandibular arch after extraction of erupted teeth.

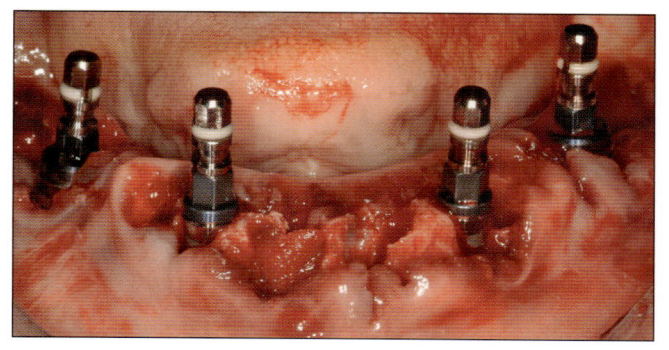

**Fig 13-6e** Mandibular implants placed in positions of the first molars and canines in relative parallel alignment.

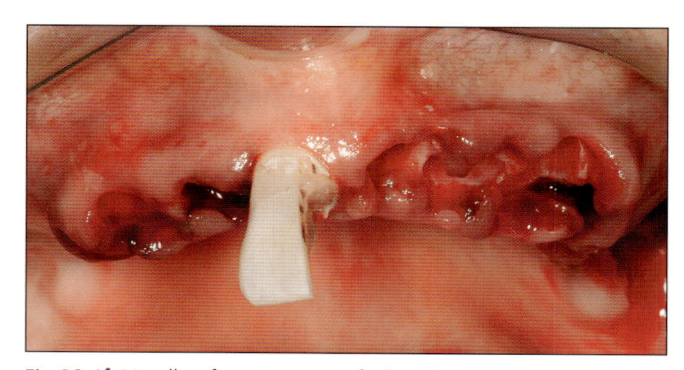

**Fig 13-6f** Maxilla after extraction of all teeth except the right central incisor, which was reduced to simulate the anticipated new midline.

## Case 6: Multiple caries and immediate loading

A 46-year-old woman presented with poor dental hygiene, a high susceptibility for caries, and a history of drinking soda. She had generalized moderate periodontal bone loss, generalized recession, and lack of keratinized tissue and soft tissue. She experienced depression, social withdrawal, and poor self-image related to her dental condition and appearance (Figs 13-6a to 13-6c).

When she had sought dental care previously, she was scolded for allowing her dentition to deteriorate, for not having better oral hygiene, and for her poor dietary habits. Previous treatment options had not met her desire to maintain a fixed dentition, reduce treatment time to a reasonable number of scheduled appointments, and ensure a positive long-term prognosis. After discussing treatment options, she opted for simultaneous extraction, implant placement, and immediate loading. Diagnostic evaluation included casts, cone beam computed tomography (CBCT), and photos. A diagnostic wax-up opening her bite approximately 2 mm in the incisors was completed to visualize the anticipated tooth positioning and alignment.

In a single surgical procedure beginning in the mandible, all teeth were extracted except the impacted third molars (Fig 13-6d). Straumann regular neck (RN) and wide neck (WN) SLActive-surface, tissue-level implants were placed parallel in the first molar and canine sockets (Fig 13-6e). Solid abutments were torqued to 35 Ncm. Matching impression copings were attached, and flap closure was done with interrupted chromic gut sutures. A closed-tray impression was taken with polyvinyl siloxane (PVS) impression material for impression coping pickup.

In the maxilla, all teeth were extracted except the right central incisor (Fig 13-6f). To facilitate shifting the midline approximately 3 mm to the patient's right, the mesial 3 mm of the tooth was removed with a bur. Straumann

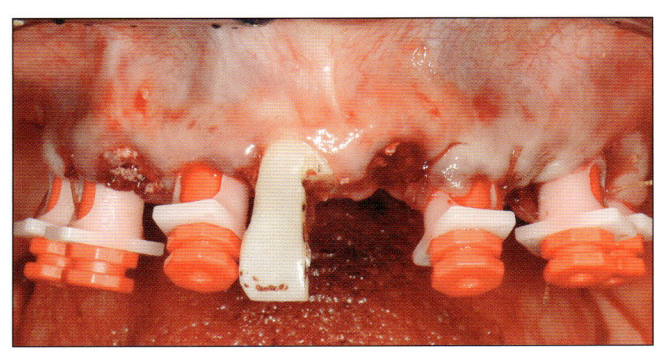

**Fig 13-6g** Implants in the lateral incisor and first and second premolar positions with implant-level impression copings.

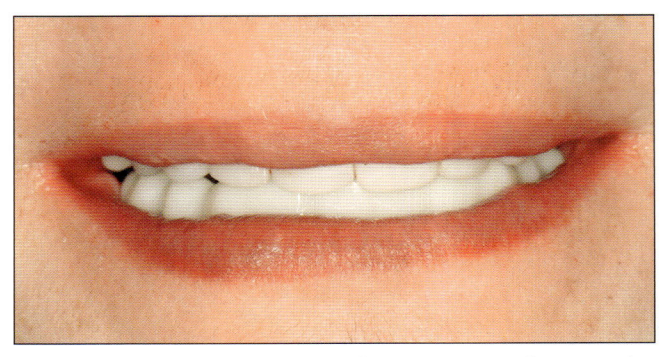

**Fig 13-6h** Smile esthetics immediately postsurgery with "overnight" self-cure composite provisional restorations retained by friction and no cement.

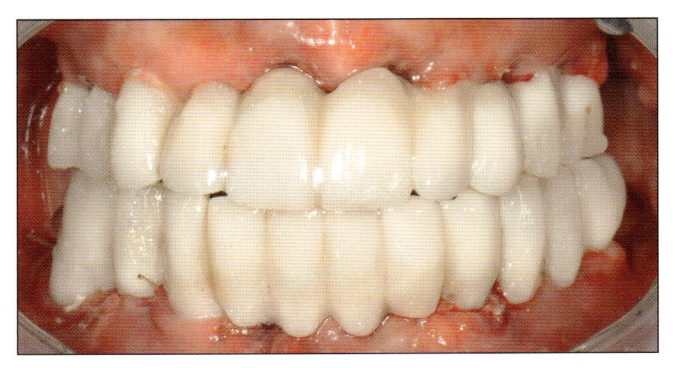

**Fig 13-6i** Laboratory processed, metal-reinforced provisional restorations adjusted, polished, and cemented 1 day following surgery.

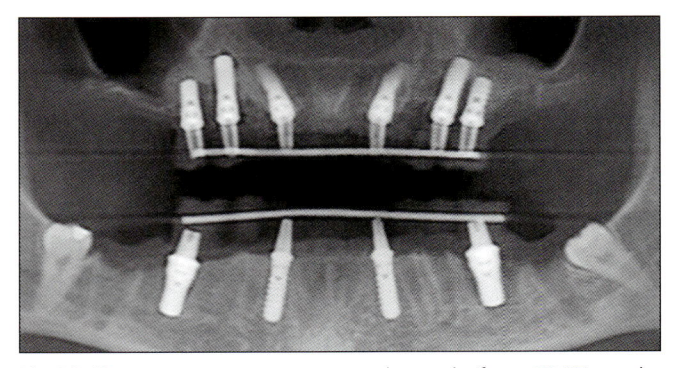

**Fig 13-6j** Postoperative panoramic radiograph (from CBCT) on the day of provisional insertion.

RN SLActive-surface, tissue-level implants were placed axially along the palatal aspects of the sockets of the lateral incisors and first and second premolars, without consideration for parallelism (Fig 13-6g). Straumann synOcta closed-tray impression copings were attached, flaps were closed (see Fig 13-6g), and a PVS impression was taken. Three- and 4.5-mm healing abutments were attached to the maxillary implants.

Prefabricated clear acrylic occlusal registration devices were seated over the abutments to verify vertical dimension, tooth position, and fit. Bite registration material was syringed into the registrations and placed in the mouth while the patient was guided into centric relation at the correct vertical dimension. Once the bite registration was set, additional material was syringed onto the occlusal surface to index the registrations to each other. Following the occlusal registration, the right maxillary central incisor was extracted.

All impressions, analogs, occlusal registrations, healing abutments, Straumann synOcta 15- and 20-degree angled abutments (for the maxilla), and the diagnostic wax-up were sent to the dental laboratory for fabrication of metal-reinforced acrylic provisional restorations. "Overnight" provisional restorations were created using the OST (Fig 13-6h).

The day following surgery, the OST composite provisionals were gently removed, and the mandibular provisional restoration was inserted and checked. The maxillary healing abutments were removed, and angled synOcta abutments were transferred from the maxillary cast into the patient's mouth in accordance with the orientation selected by the technician during fabrication. Once the abutments were seated, the maxillary provisional restoration was checked. Occlusal adjustment established even contact in centric occlusion and shallow anterior group function guidance in protrusive and lateral movements. The provisionals were polished and cemented using sparing amounts of polycarboxylate cement (Figs 13-6i and 13-6j). The patient was counseled to avoid tough, sticky, or crunchy foods for 4 to 6 weeks. She was thrilled with the immediate esthetic improvement.

The patient returned 3 months later for final restoration. All implants healed with evidence of clinical success, although the mandibular canine implants showed approximately 1 mm of recession on the facial surfaces (Fig 13-6k). Prosthetic procedures began in anticipation of computer-aided design/computer-assisted manufactured (CAD/CAM), one-piece nonprecious frames for metal-ceramic cemented restorations. The mandibular restoration was retained on the existing abutments and the maxilla received CAD/CAM–milled angled abutments (Fig 13-6l). New impressions were taken along with occlusal registration, and verification jigs were tried in to confirm the accuracy of the casts. Final restorations used pink ceramic to simulate interproximal gingiva and improve esthetics. Following occlusal adjustments, the final restorations were cemented with polycarboxylate (Figs 13-6m to 13-6q).

Gingival augmentation of the mandibular canine implants was recommended but not yet accepted by the patient. Overall, the patient was extremely satisfied with the final results including esthetics, comfort, and function. More importantly, the patient's personality was transformed with a renewed positive attitude, increased self-confidence, and radiant appearance.

## 13 Immediate Loading of Implants Placed in Fresh Extraction Sockets

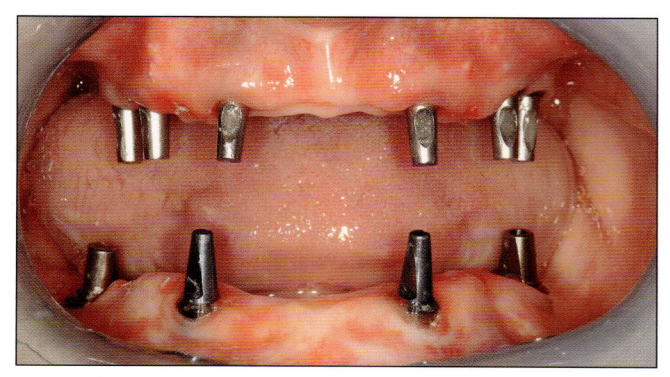

**Fig 13-6k** Provisional restorations removed after 3 months. Note the angled abutments in the maxilla and solid abutments in the mandible. Recession is visible on the mandibular canine implants.

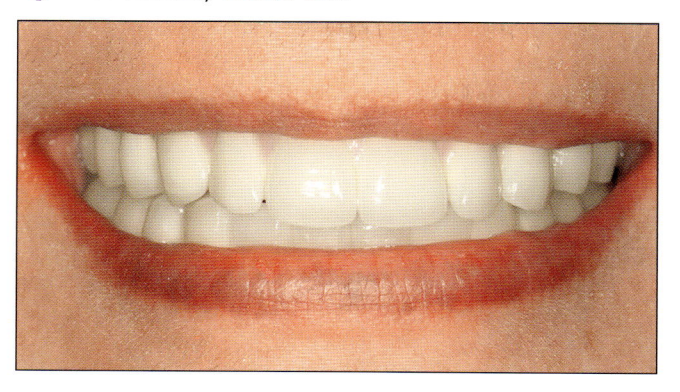

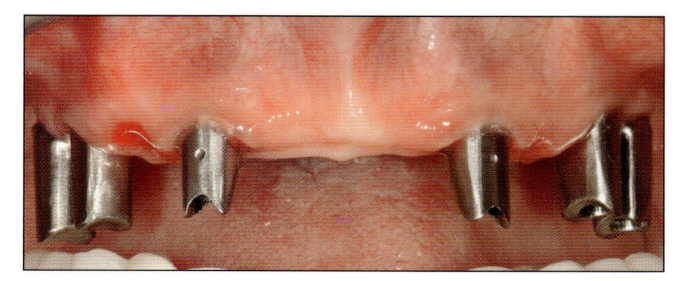

**Fig 13-6l** Maxillary milled custom abutments positioned for verification jig.

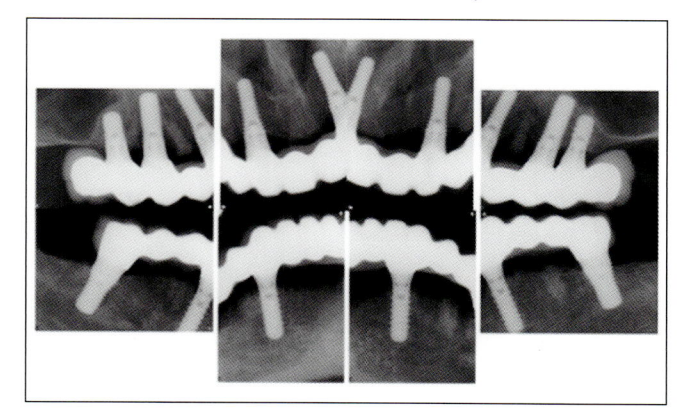

**Fig 13-6m** Follow-up periapical radiographs show normal peri-implant bone levels as well as resolution of radiopaque maxillary sinuses. Inorganic bovine bone in many extraction sockets simulates root tips.

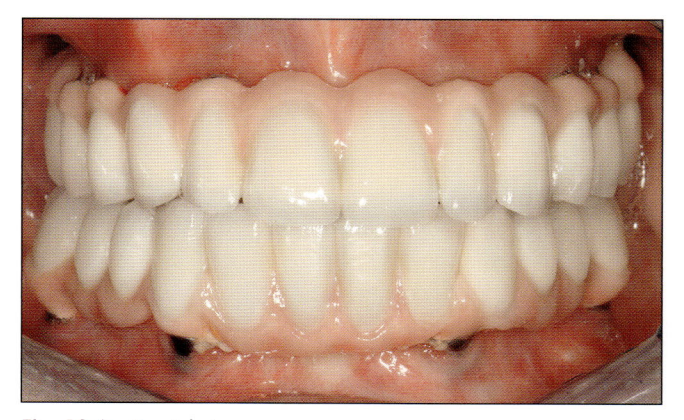

**Figs 13-6n** Frontal view.

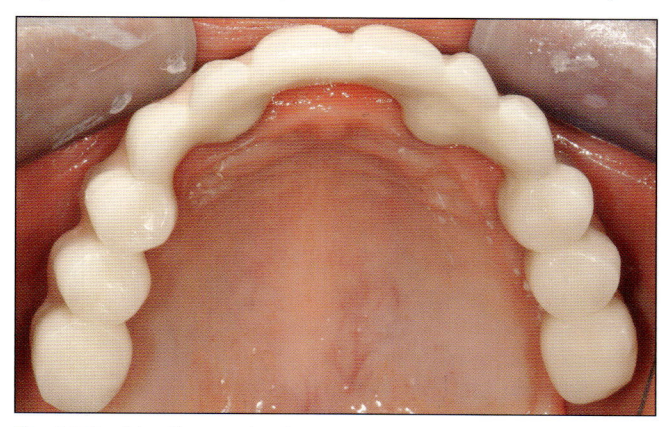

**Figs 13-6o** Maxillary occlusal view.

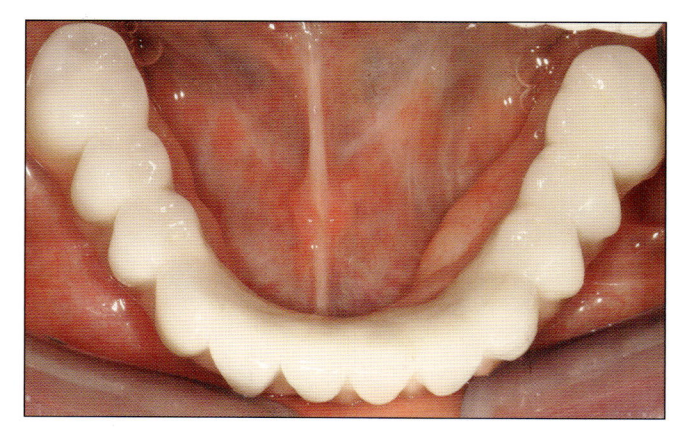

**Figs 13-6p** Mandibular occlusal view.

**Figs 13-6q** Final CAD/CAM–milled metal-ceramic restorations illustrating excellent esthetics, function, and patient satisfaction. (Surgery and prosthodontics by J. Ganeles, Boca Raton, FL.)

Case Reports

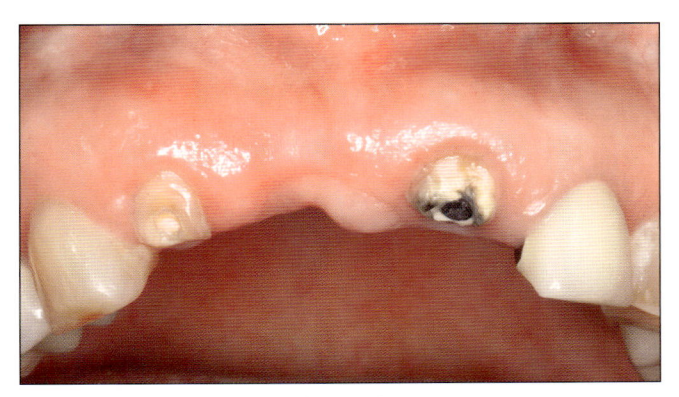

Fig 13-7a Clinical situation before tooth extraction.

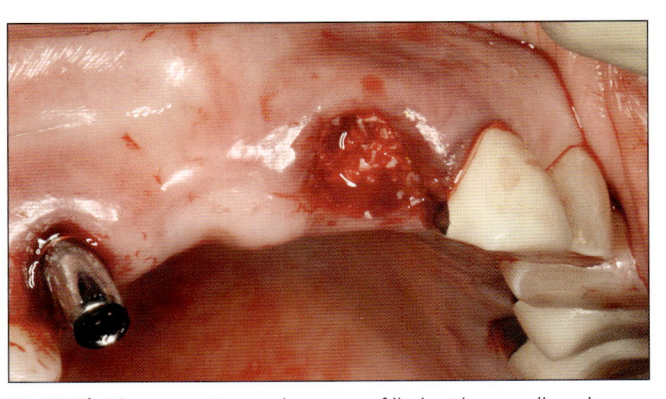

Fig 13-7b The extraction sockets were filled with cancellous human allograft (Straumann) immediately before implant placement.

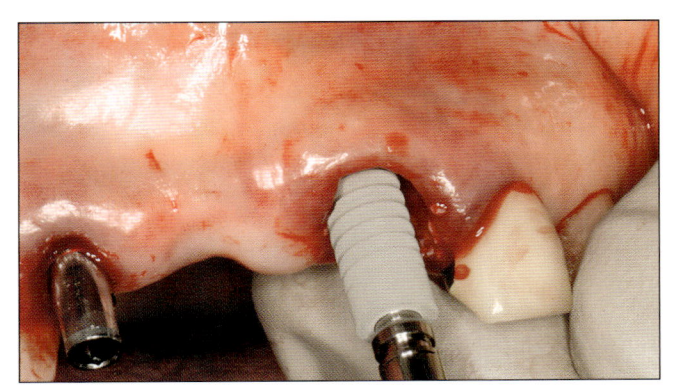

Fig 13-7c Implants with a progressive thread design were placed to condense the grafting material during insertion.

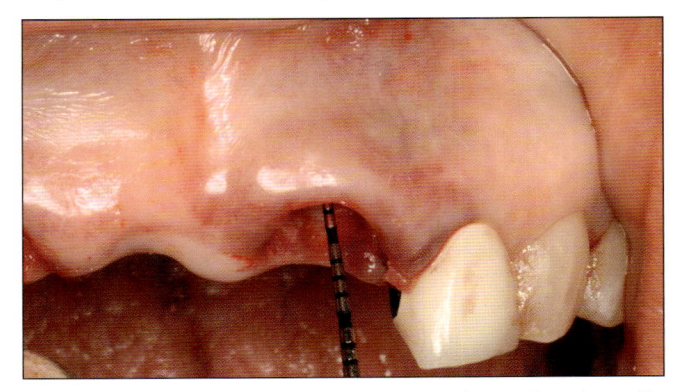

Fig 13-7d Subcrestal implant placement 1 mm deeper than the midfacial aspect of the buccal bone (3 mm from the gingival margin).

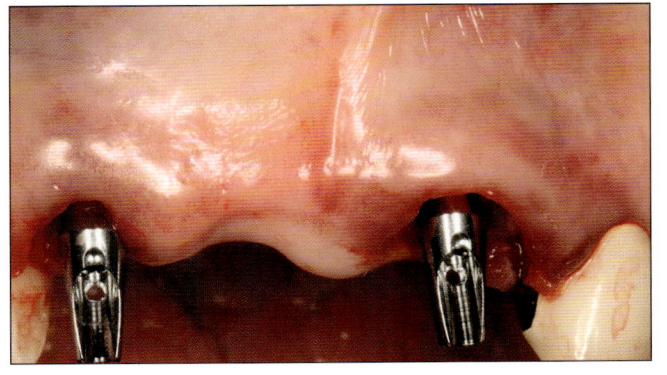

Fig 13-7e Abutment connection for immediate functional loading.

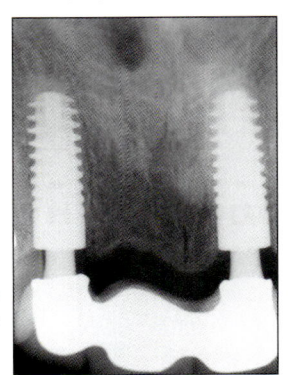

Fig 13-7f After 1 year of loading, the radiographic evaluation presents excellent crestal bone. (Restoration by G. E. Romanos and J. Lim, Rochester, NY).

## Case 7: Immediate loading in a partially edentulous patient

A patient presented with a poor prognosis for her maxillary anterior dentition (Fig 13-7a). The maxillary left central incisor and right lateral incisor were deemed hopeless and were extracted. Osteotomies were prepared in the fresh extraction sockets according to a surgical template, and after the drilling was completed, the sockets were filled with human allograft material to increase the primary stability of implants after implant placement (Fig 13-7b).

Two Ankylos C/X implants (Dentsply Friadent) were placed 1 mm subcrestally from the midfacial aspect of the buccal bone and were splinted together with a provisional 3-unit partial denture after final abutment connection (Figs 13-7c to 13-7e). The Ankylos C/X implants have a progressive thread design for high primary stability. One year after loading, the implants were stable and the crestal bone presented excellent healing without resorption (Fig 13-7f). Bone stability over the implant platform resulted from the use of platform switching and the lack of abutment removal over the entire observation period.

163

# 13 Immediate Loading of Implants Placed in Fresh Extraction Sockets

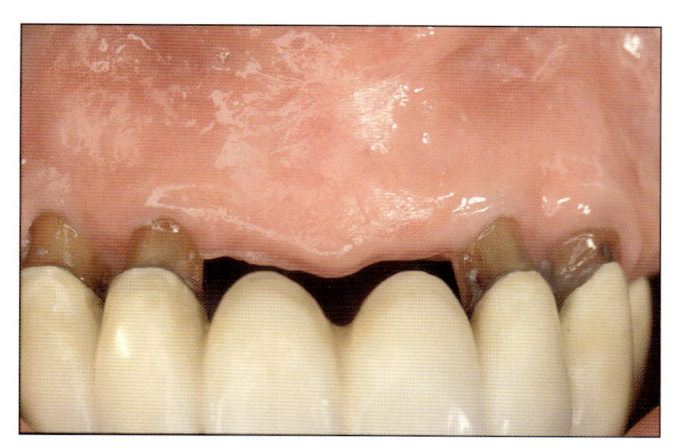

**Fig 13-8a** Clinical situation before implant therapy.

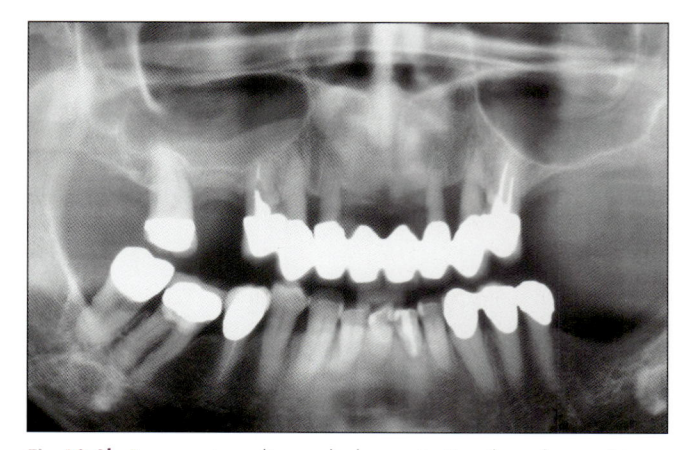

**Fig 13-8b** Panoramic radiograph demonstrating the advanced bone loss in the maxilla.

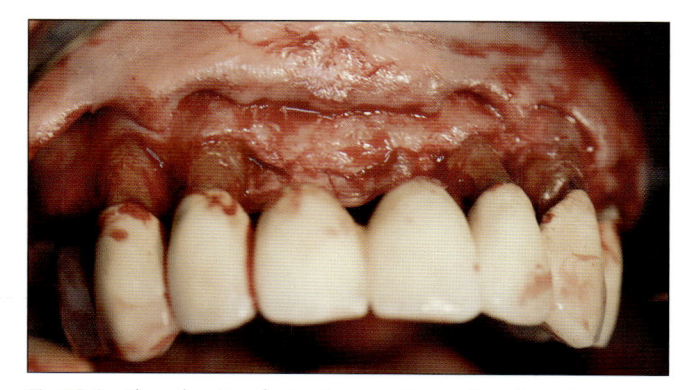

**Fig 13-8c** Flap elevation for tooth extraction and implant placement.

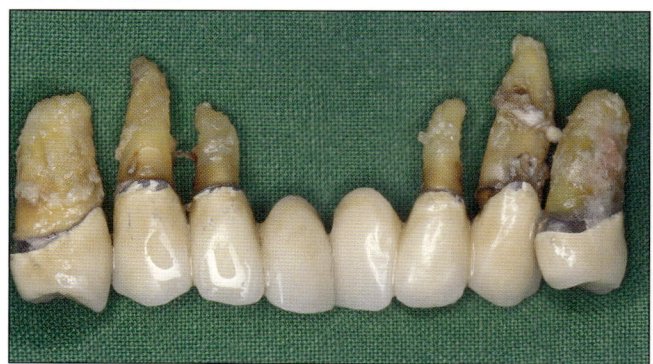

**Fig 13-8d** Extracted hopeless teeth.

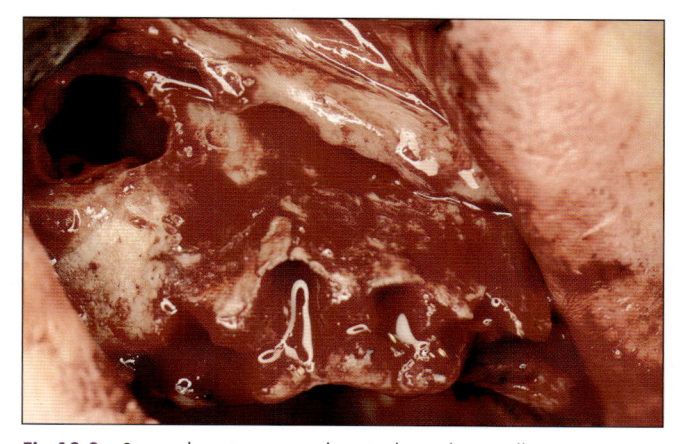

**Fig 13-8e** Sinus elevation procedure in the right maxilla.

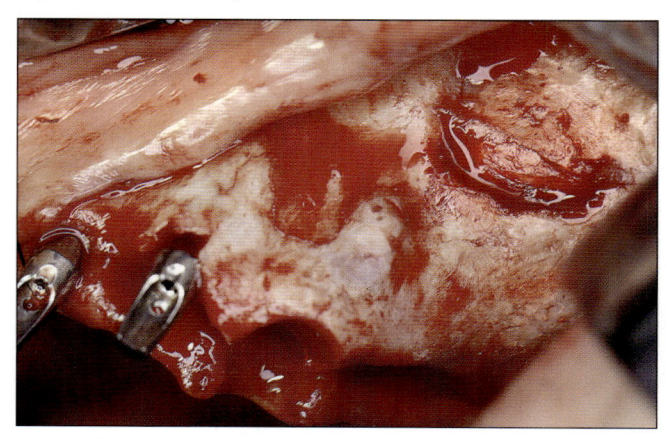

**Fig 13-8f** Simultaneous sinus augmentation and implant placement in the grafted sinus prepared for immediate loading.

## Case 8: Advanced protocol in the maxilla with simultaneous grafting and immediate loading

This case illustrates the implant therapy of a woman with advanced attachment loss of the residual maxillary teeth. For esthetic and phonetic reasons, she had used a gingival mask (Fig 13-8a). Radiographic examination revealed that the maxillary teeth had short roots and an unfavorable prognosis (Fig 13-8b). The patient was informed about the possibility of extracting the maxillary teeth and immediately placing implants in conjunction with bilateral sinus elevation. She agreed to the treatment plan. The teeth were extracted atraumatically without advanced flap elevation in the anterior esthetic zone, where the alveolar ridge was very thin (Figs 13-8c and 13-8d).

Bilateral sinus elevation was performed, and bone grafting material was placed prior to implant placement (Figs 13-8e and 13-8f). The donor site for the grafting material was corticocancellous bone blocks from the anterior mandible, which were particulated with a bone mill. Six implants with a progressive thread design were placed in the fresh extraction sockets and the residual ridge according to a prosthetic guide. Bio-Gide (Geistlich) collagen membranes were used to cover the lateral windows. The final abutments were inserted using final torque (15 Ncm), and provisional caps were placed prior to flap closure (Fig 13-8g). The provisional restoration was made using Protemp (Espe) resin material in the Omnivac template in accordance with the

# Case Reports

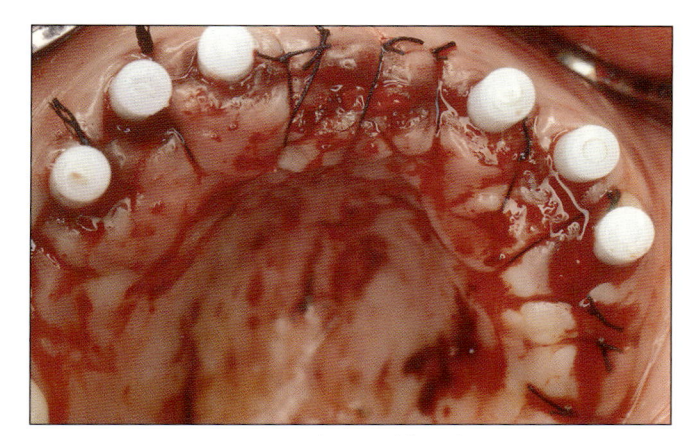

**Fig 13-8g** Temporary caps in place and flap closure.

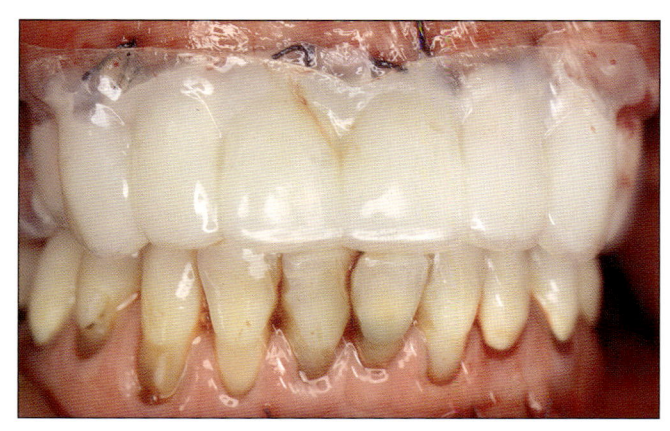

**Fig 13-8h** Provisional restoration fabricated with the OST protocol.

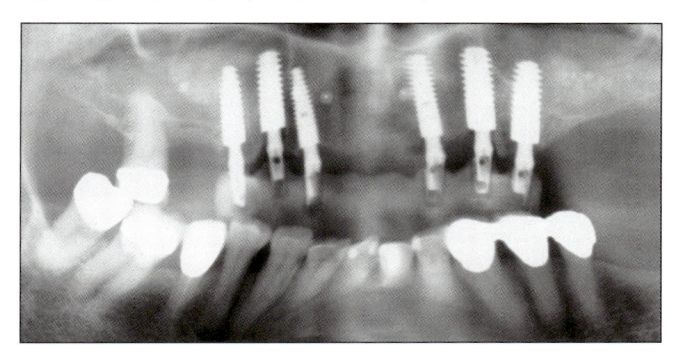

**Fig 13-8i** Postoperative radiograph.

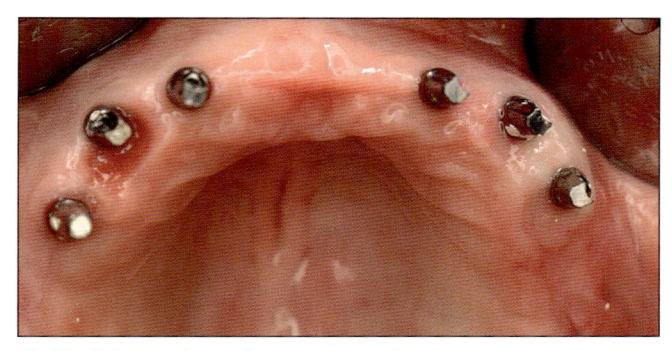

**Fig 13-8j** Peri-implant soft tissues 3 months after surgery.

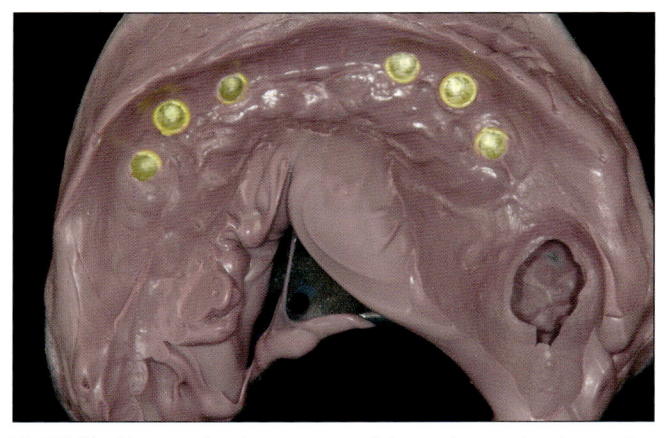

**Fig 13-8k** Abutment-level impression of the implants using impression caps and without removal of the abutments.

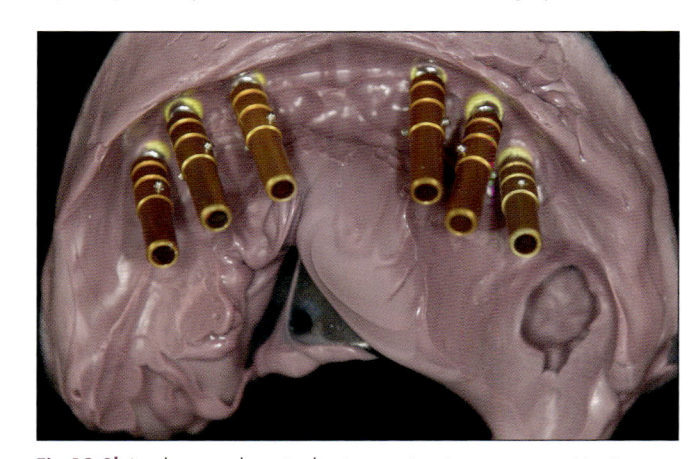

**Fig 13-8l** Implant analogs in the impression in correct positioning.

OST protocol (Fig 13-8h). The panoramic radiograph after surgery presents the placement of the implants and the grafting procedures (Fig 13-8i).

Postoperative healing was uneventful. The patient followed the recommended soft/liquid diet for the first 3 months after surgery, and the provisional restoration was cemented in place without removal for the entire healing period. After 3 months, the prosthesis was removed and the implant stability was evaluated (Fig 13-8j).

An impression using impression caps over the implant abutments was taken, so as not to remove the abutments, and a master cast was made using abutment analogs (Figs 13-8k and 13-8l). Primary telescopic galvano copings were fabricated in a high-quality dental laboratory, and the secondary copings were made later (Fig 13-8m). The final framework for the prosthesis was made on the master cast and evaluated for passive fit intraorally (Figs 13-8n and 13-8o). The secondary telescopic copings were fixed intraorally with Nimetic Cem (Espe), and a new impression was made to pick up the soft tissue shape. A couple of weeks later, the primary galvano copings were placed for permanent cementation (Fig 13-8p). The final removable prosthesis represented the perioprosthetic considerations for good implant maintenance and optimal patient comfort (Figs 13-8q and 13-8r). The patient was very happy with the esthetic and phonetic result. The patient was evaluated every 6 months for the first 2 years and then annually. The final result 8 years after implant placement and immediate loading showed excellent implant stability, soft tissue health, and patient satisfaction (Figs 13-8s and 13-8t).

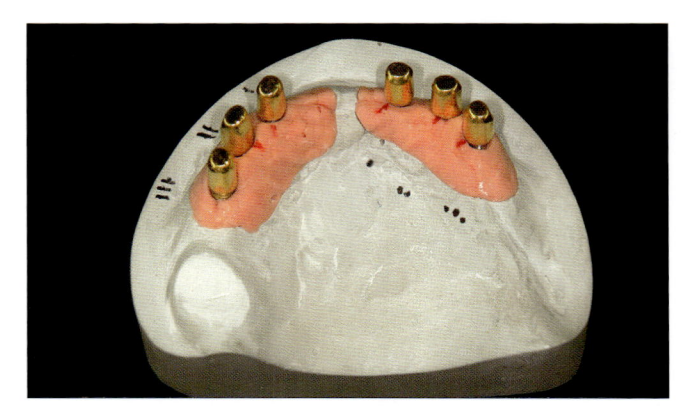

## 13 Immediate Loading of Implants Placed in Fresh Extraction Sockets

**Fig 13-8m** Master cast with primary galvano copings in place.

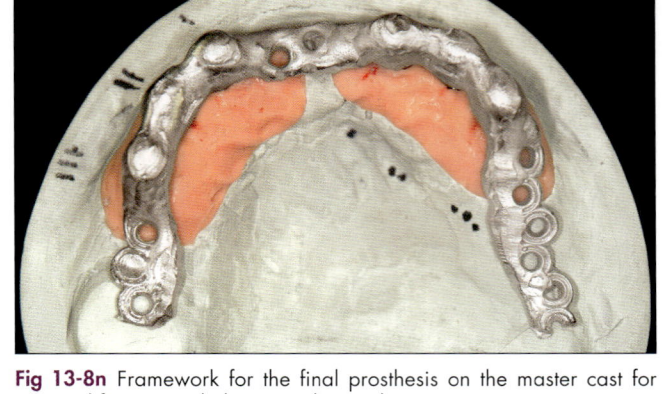

**Fig 13-8n** Framework for the final prosthesis on the master cast for intraoral fixation with the secondary galvano copings.

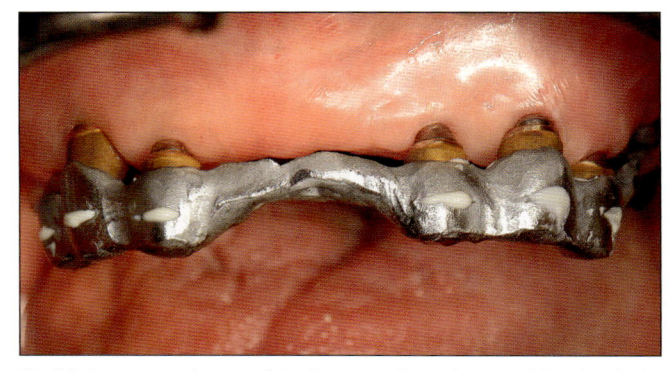

**Fig 13-8o** Intraoral view of the framework in place and fixed with the secondary copings.

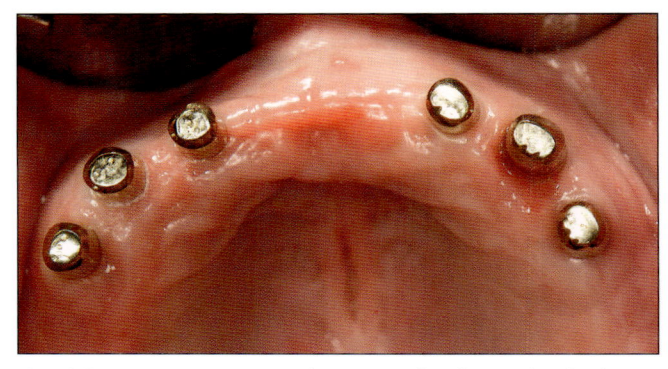

**Fig 13-8p** Primary copings in place 3 months after implant healing.

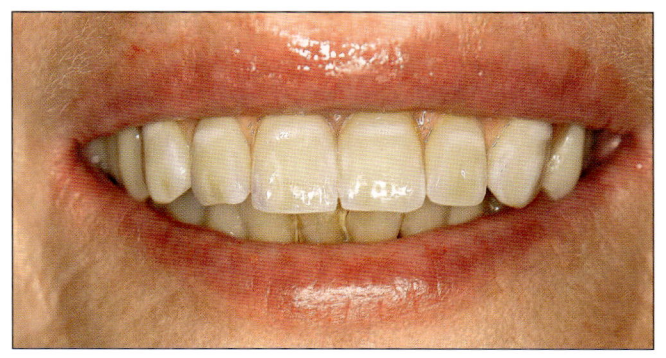

**Fig 13-8q** Final restoration in place.

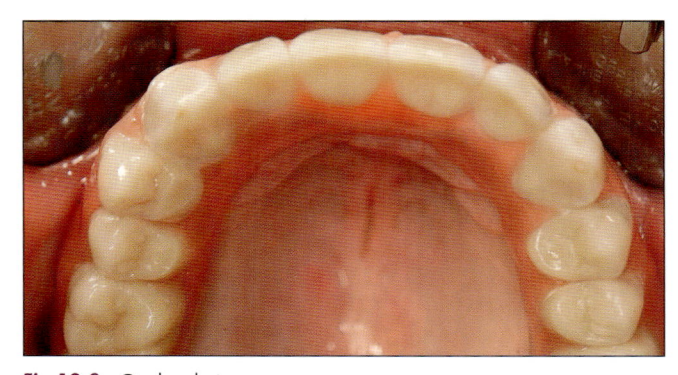

**Fig 13-8r** Occlusal view.

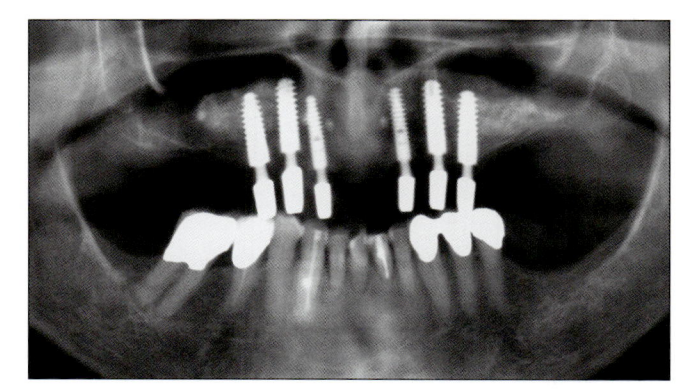

**Fig 13-8s** Radiographic evaluation after 8 years of loading presenting excellent condition of the implants.

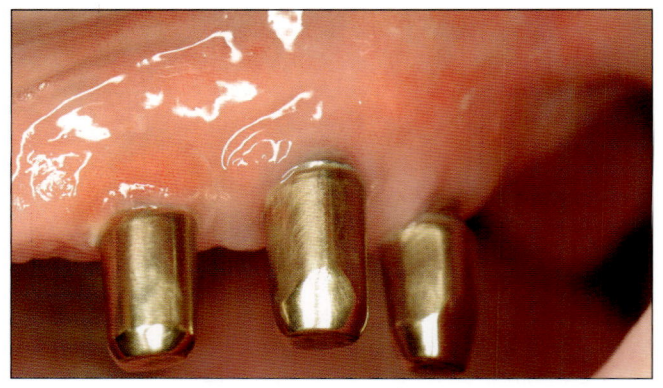

**Fig 13-8t** Healthy peri-implant soft tissues after 8 years of loading. (Dental technician: J. Lee, Frankfurt, Germany.)

Case Reports

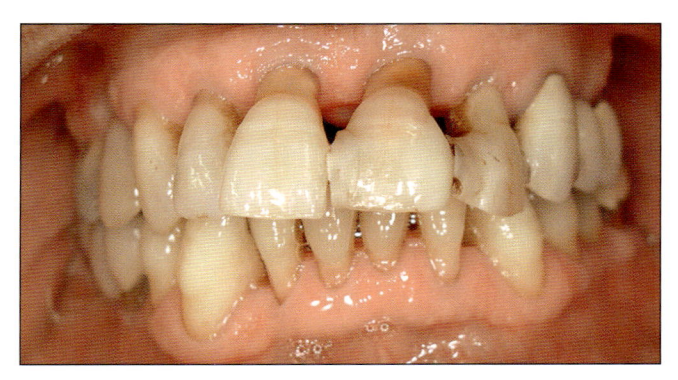

**Fig 13-9a** Anterior view of the initial situation.

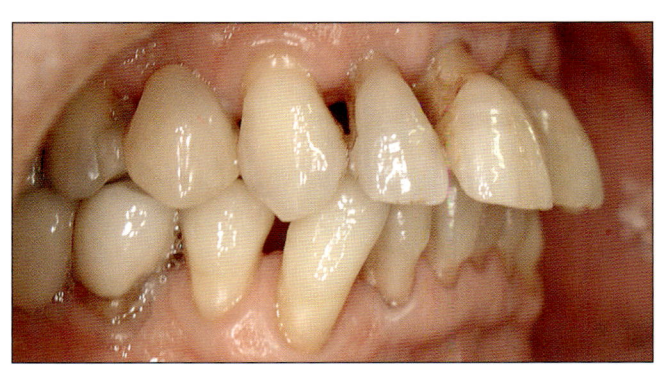

**Fig 13-9b** Lateral view of the initial situation.

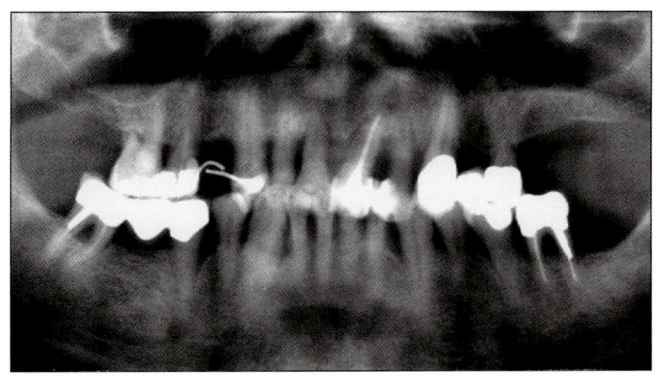

**Fig 13-9c** Panoramic radiograph of the initial situation.

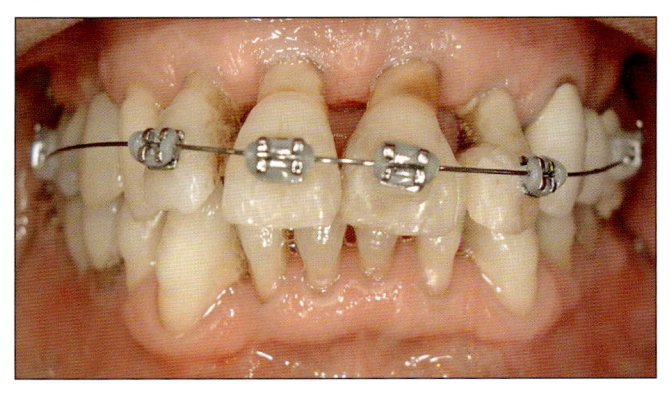

**Fig 13-9d** Anterior view of first phase of orthodontic treatment.

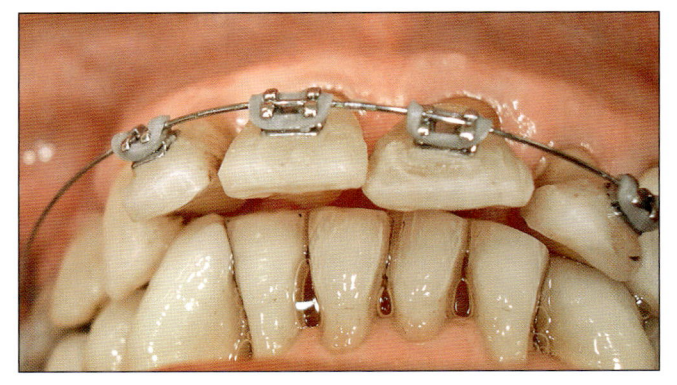

**Fig 13-9e** Inferior view showing the misalignment of the anterior teeth at the beginning of orthodontic treatment.

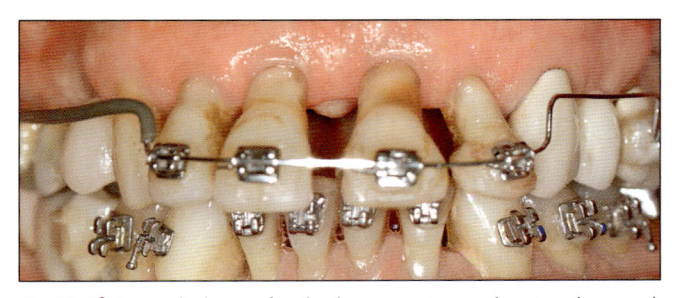

**Fig 13-9f** Second phase of orthodontic treatment showing the maxillary incisors after 1 month of orthodontic extrusion. Buccal displacement of the four anterior teeth has achieved the objective of repositioning the gingival contour.

## Case 9: Esthetic maxillary restoration involving orthodontic extrusion, soft tissue contouring, and immediate loading

A man presented with hopeless maxillary central and lateral incisors (Figs 13-9a to 13-9c). The patient opted for esthetic restoration of the anterior maxilla with four adjacent implants with immediate restoration. An integrated clinical approach was taken with transdisciplinary treatment planning, starting with orthodontic treatment of the maxillary incisors (Figs 13-9d and 13-9e). The goal was to restore the gingival esthetics before placing implants for immediate restoration. As in all advanced restorative cases, time and patience are essential for obtaining an excellent outcome. The first orthodontic phase took about 8 months in order to obtain the intended extrusion of the maxillary anterior teeth, as well as the soft tissue and alveolar ridge changes in both width and length[38–42] (Fig 13-9f). In order to diminish the pronounced interdental spaces created in the anterior maxilla by orthodontic extrusion (because of conical root anatomy), provisional composite restorations were completed (Figs 13-9g).

After the completion of orthodontic treatment, the surgical and prosthetic phases were planned with attention to tooth anatomy, number of implants, restorative scheme (eg, splinted restoration or individual crowns, presence of pontics and/or cantilever or individual fixtures), establishment of primary stability, and immediate loading (Figs 13-9h and 13-9i). Based on the width and length of the alveolar ridge, it was decided to place one implant for each tooth in the fresh extraction sockets (Figs 13-9j and 13-9k).

It is important to know the advantages and limitations of an implant system prior to the surgery. In Fig 13-9l,

167

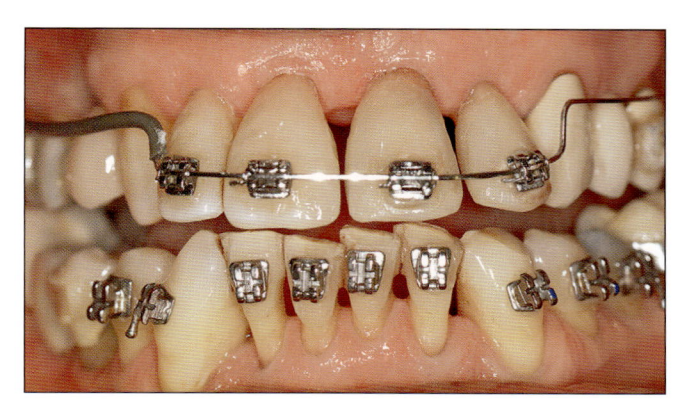

**Fig 13-9g** Provisional composite restorations in the anterior maxilla close the pronounced interdental spaces resulting from the orthodontic extrusion.

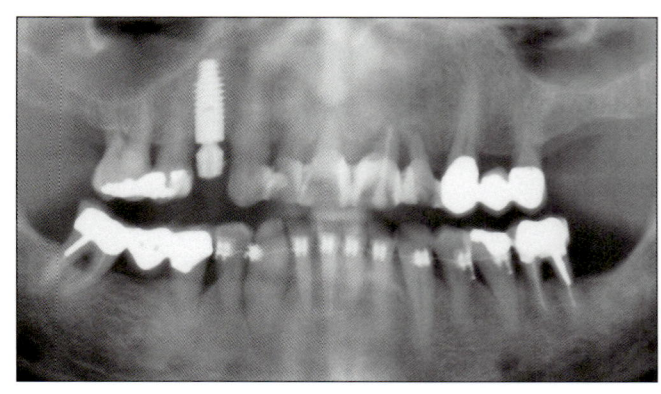

**Fig 13-9h** Radiographic evaluation showing bone levels after orthodontic extrusion.

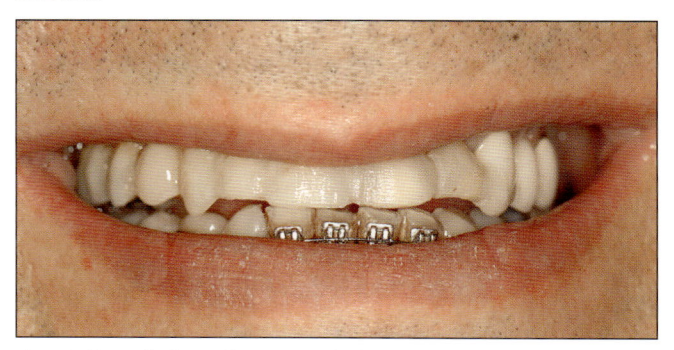

**Fig 13-9i** Smile line after removal of the orthodontic appliance just prior to surgery.

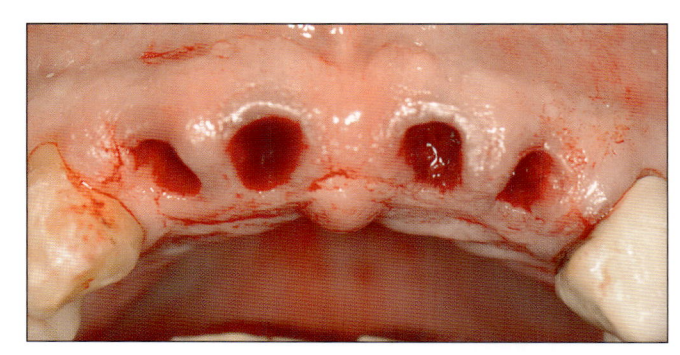

**Fig 13-9j** Occlusal view of anterior maxillary ridge after extraction of the incisors.

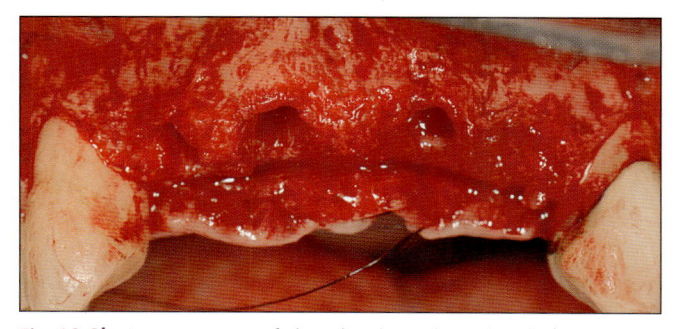

**Fig 13-9k** Anterior view of the alveolar ridge after flap elevation. Note the length of the ridge, especially in interproximal regions.

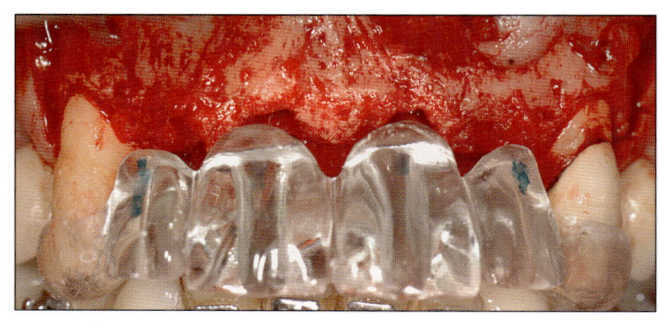

**Fig 13-9l** Prepared prosthetic guide in position. Note the length of the cervical contour of the anterior teeth and the contour of the alveolar ridge. Because of the implant system being used, it was necessary to maintain adequate space for the transgingival portion of the implants.

the gingival margin of the surgical template shows a small amount of vertical space added to accommodate the transgingival portion of the tissue-level Straumann implants. For this particular situation, it was necessary to create vertical space through sculpting the scallop contour of the alveolar ridge in keeping with the gingival margin highlighted by the prosthetic template for the planned restoration.[43] This clinical procedure provides the necessary amount of vertical space for correct implant placement in the mesiodistal, buccopalatal, and coronoapical dimensions.

For the central incisors, two Straumann RN implants were placed with a 4.1-mm diameter and 12-mm length, and for the lateral incisors, two Straumann narrow neck (NN) implants were placed with a 3.3-mm diameter and 12-mm length (Fig 13-9m). In accordance with the treatment plan, immediate restorations were possible because of the excellent primary stability.

Two 7.0-mm solid abutments were connected to the RN implants in the central incisor sites, and conventional abutments were connected to the NN implants in the lateral incisor sites (Fig 13-9n). After abutment placement, splinted provisional crowns were relined, polished, and cemented in place (Figs 13-9o and 13-9p).

After 6 months, final impressions were taken for fabrication of the final restorations. Eight months after loading, individual crowns were cemented in place that followed the soft tissue contours obtained over the previous months (Figs 13-9q to 13-9t). After 4 years of loading, clinical examination showed a successful restoration with healthy tissues, and computed tomography (CT) scans demonstrated the clear presence of a buccal plate as well as a crestal bone that maintained the clinical soft tissue contour over 4 years (Figs 13-9u to 13-9y).

Case Reports

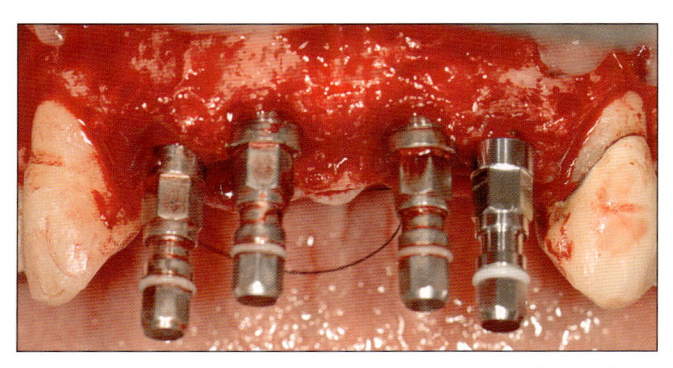

**Fig 13-9m** Four anterior implants positioned according to the prosthetic-surgical planning.

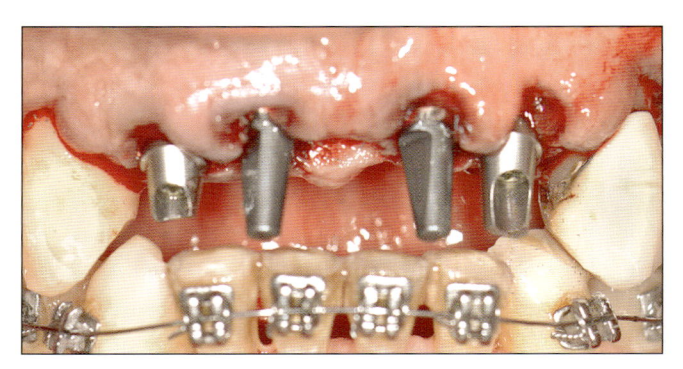

**Fig 13-9n** Prosthetic abutments connected prior to provisional relining.

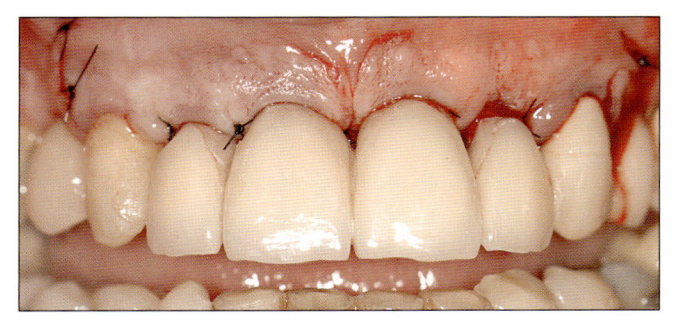

**Fig 13-9o** Cemented provisional restorations.

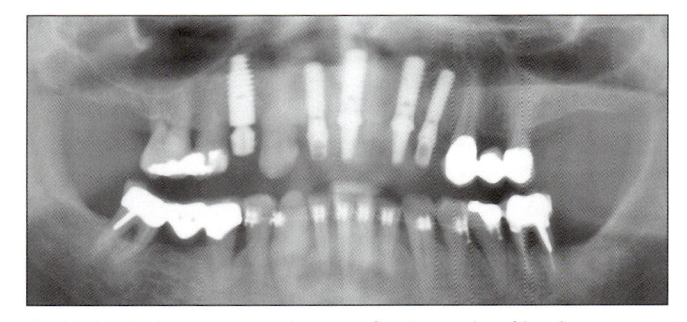

**Fig 13-9p** Radiographic evaluation after 3 months of loading.

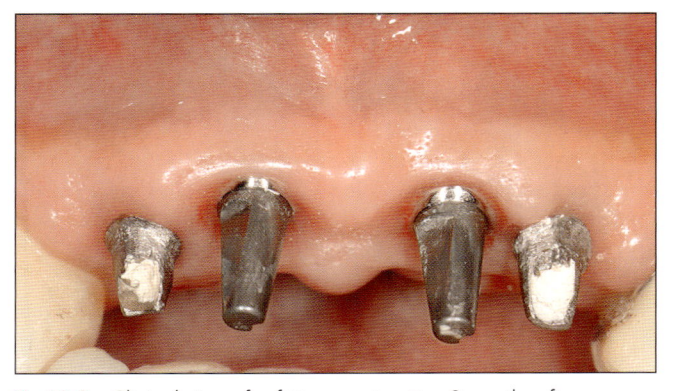

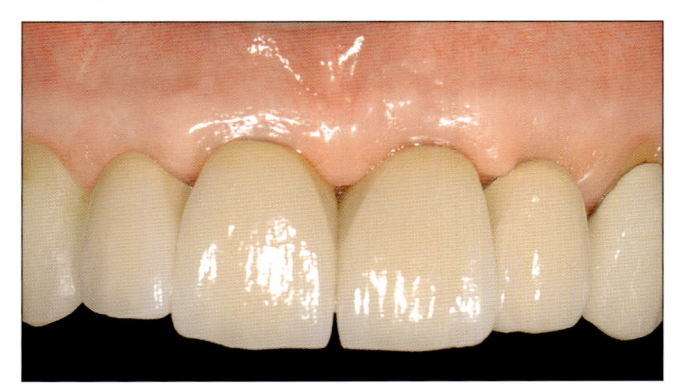

**Fig 13-9q** Clinical view of soft tissue maturation 8 months after surgery.

**Fig 13-9r** Anterior view of individual maxillary incisor crowns cemented in place.

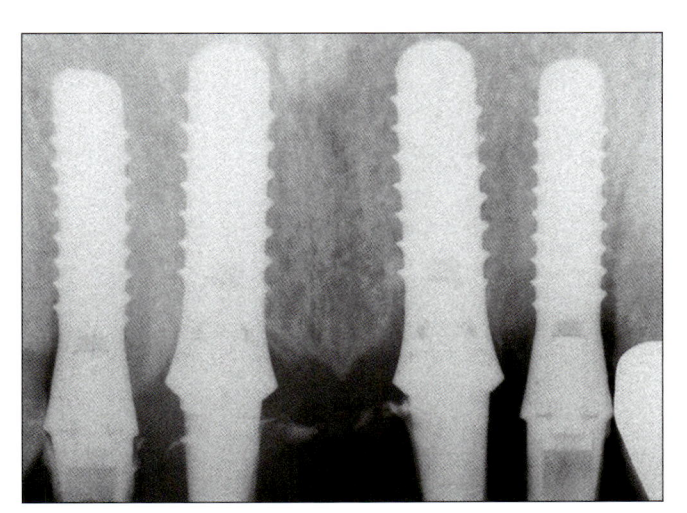

**Fig 13-9s** Radiographic evaluation after 8 months of loading.

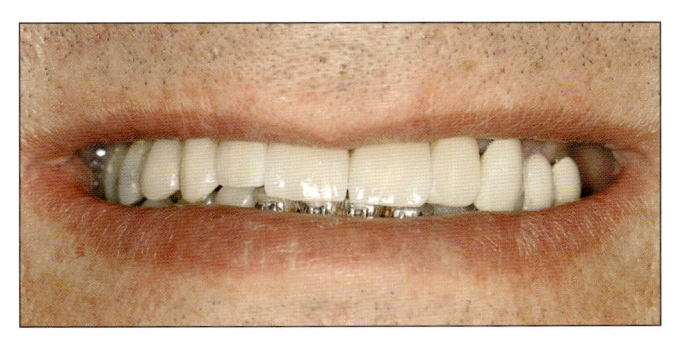

**Fig 13-9t** Anterior view of the patient's smile with the final crowns in place.

# 13 | Immediate Loading of Implants Placed in Fresh Extraction Sockets

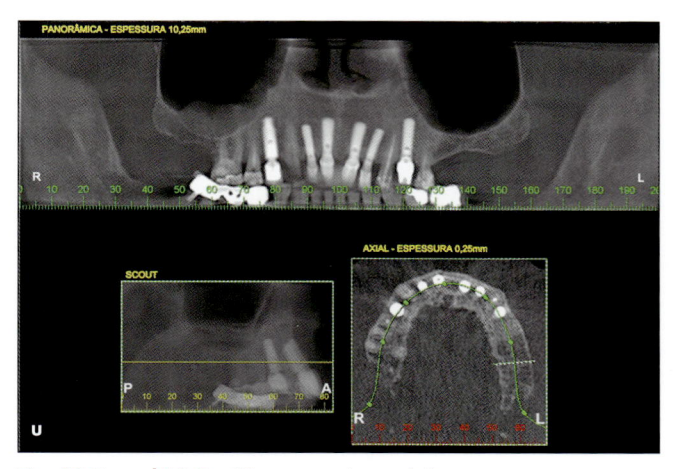

**Figs 13-9u and 13-9v** CT scans at 4-year follow-up.

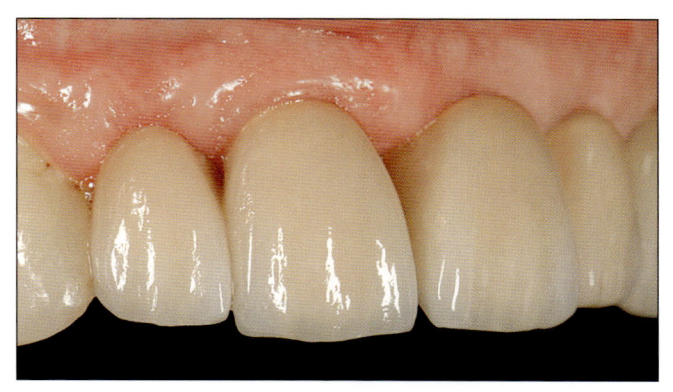

**Fig 13-9w** Right lateral view of final crowns 4 years after loading.

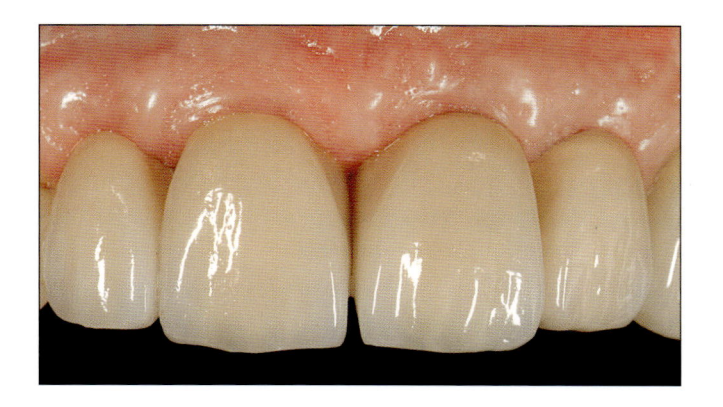

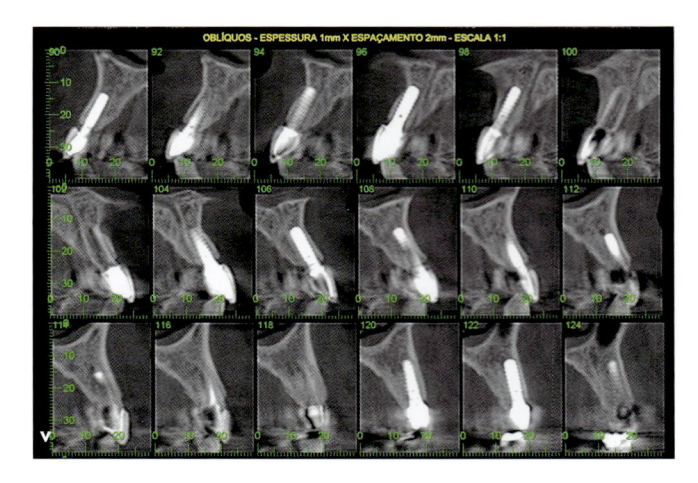

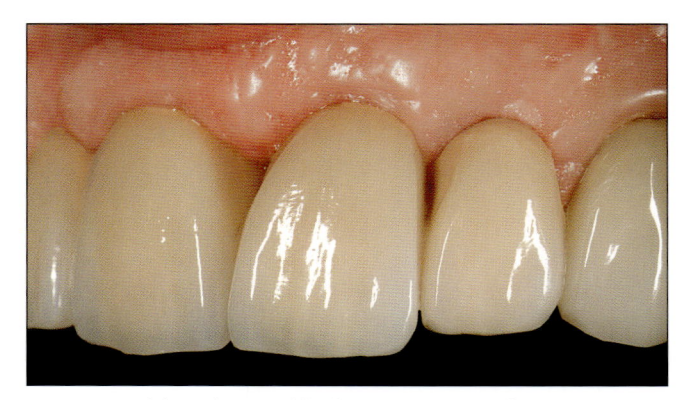

**Fig 13-9x** Left lateral view of final crowns 4 years after loading.

**Fig 13-9y** Anterior view of final crowns 4 years after loading. (Orthodontics, surgery, and prosthodontics by C. A. Arita and C. C. Arita.)

## Conclusion

- Integrated treatment planning in implant dentistry is the key to successful restorative treatment, especially in the esthetic region.
- Immediate loading strongly depends on following correct restorative treatment planning, in addition to the essential factors of primary stability and control of micromovements.
- Knowledge of the implant system—its advantages and limitations—is paramount to the success of every restorative treatment outcome.

## References

1. Steinhardt G. Pathologisch-anatomische Untersuchungen zur Heilung von Zahnextraktionswunden und ihrer Komplikation beim Menschen. Paradentium 1932;4:122–128.
2. Claflin RS. Healing of disturbed and undisturbed extraction wounds. J Am Dent Assoc 1936;23:945–959.
3. Euler H. Die Heilung von Extraktionswunden. Eine tierexperimentelle Studie. Dtsch Monatsschr Zahnheilk 1923;41:685–700.
4. Mangos JF. The healing of extractions wounds. NZ Dent J 1941;37:4–23.

5. Amler MH, Johnson PL, Salman I. Histological and histochemical investigation of human alveolar socket healing in undisturbed extraction wounds. J Am Dent Assoc 1960;61:32–44.
6. Amler MH. The time sequence of tissue regeneration in human extraction wounds. Oral Surg 1969;27:309–318.
7. Amler MH. The age factor in human extraction wound healing. J Oral Surg 1977;35:193–197.
8. Carlsson GE, Thilander H, Hedegard B. Histologic changes in the upper alveolar process after extractions with or without insertion of an immediate full denture. Acta Odontol Scand 1967;25:21–43.
9. Trombelli L, Farina R, Marzola A, Bozzi L, Liljenberg B, Lindhe J. Modeling and remodeling of human extraction sockets. J Clin Periodontol 2008;35:630–639.
10. Araujo M, Lindhe J. The edentulous alveolar ridge. In: Lindhe J, Lang NP, Karring T (eds). Clinical Periodontology and Implant Dentistry, ed 5. Oxford: Blackwell Munksgaard, 2008.
11. Cardaropoli G, Araújo M, Lindhe J. Dynamics of bone tissue formation in tooth extraction sites. An experimental study in dogs. J Clin Periodontol 2003;30:809–818.
12. Cardaropoli G, Araújo M, Hayacibara R, Sukekava F, Lindhe J. Healing of extraction sockets and surgically produced—augmented and non-augmented—defects in the alveolar ridge. An experimental study in the dog. J Clin Periodontol 2005;32:435–440.
13. Araújo M, Linder E, Wennström J, Lindhe J. The influence of BioOss collagen on healing of an extraction socket: An experimental study in the dog. Int J Periodontics Restorative Dent 2008;28:123–135.
15. Lekovic V, Carmargo P, Klokkevold P, et al. Preservation of alveolar bone in extraction sockets using bioabsorbable membranes. J Periodontol 1998;69:1044–1049.
14. Lekovic V, Kenney E, Weinlaender M, et al. A bone regenerative approach to alveolar ridge maintenance following tooth extractions. Report of 10 cases. J Periodontol 1997;68:563–570.
16. Artzi Z, Nemcowski C. The application of deproteinized bovine bone mineral for ridge augmentation prior to implantation. Clinical and histologic observations in a case report. J Periodontol 1998;69:1062–1067.
17. Becker W, Clokic C, Sennerby L, Urist MR, Becker BE. Histologic findings after implantation and evaluation of different grafting materials and titanium microscrews into extraction sockets: Case reports. J Periodontol 1998;69:414–421.
18. Carmagnola D, Adriaens P, Berglundh T. Healing of human extraction sockets filled with Bio-Oss. Clin Oral Implants Res 2003;14:137–143.
19. Iasella J, Greenwell H, Miller R, Hill M, Drisko C, Bohra A, Scheetz J. Ridge preservation with freeze-dried bone allograft and a collagen membrane compared to extraction alone for implant site development: A clinical and histologic study in humans. J Periodontol 2003;74:990–999.
20. Nevins M, Camelo M, De Paoli S, et al. A study of the fate of the buccal wall of extraction sockets of teeth with prominent roots. Int J Periodontics Restorative Dent 2006;26:19–29.
21. Molly L, Vandromme H, Quirynen M, Schepers E, Adams JL, van Steenberghe D. Bone extraction following implantation of bone biomaterials into extraction sites. J Periodontol 2008;79:1108–1115.
22. Araújo MG, Lindhe J. Ridge alterations following tooth extraction with and without flap elevation: An experimental study in the dog. Clin Oral Implants Res 2009;20:545–549.
23. Fickl S, Schneider D, Zuhr O, et al. Dimensional changes of the ridge contour after socket preservation and buccal overbuilding: An animal study. J Clin Periodontol 2009;36:442–448.
24. Schulte W, Kleineikenscheidt H, Lindner K, Schareyka R. The Tübingen immediate implant in clinical studies [in German]. Dtsch Zahnarztl Z 1978;33:348–359.
25. Covani U, Cornelini R, Barone A. Bucco-lingual bone remodeling around implants placed into immediate extraction sockets: A case series. J Periodontol 2003;74:268–273.
26. Covani U, Cornelini R, Barone A. Vertical crestal bone changes around implants placed into fresh extraction sockets. J Periodontol 2007;78:810–815.
27. Crespi R, Cappare P, Gherlone E. Fresh-socket implants placed in periapical infected sites in humans. J Periodontol 2010;81:378–383.
28. Crespi R, Cappare P, Gherlone E, Romanos GE. Immediate versus delayed loading of dental implants placed in fresh extraction sockets in the maxillary esthetic zone: A clinical comparative study. Int J Oral Maxillofac Implants 2008;23:753–758.
29. Crespi R, Cappare P, Gherlone E. Radiographic evaluation of marginal bone levels around platform-switched and non-platform-switched implants used in an immediate loading protocol. Int J Oral Maxillofac Implants 2009;24:920–926.
30. Canullo L, Rasperini G. Preservation of peri-implant soft and hard tisues using platform switching of implants placed in immediate extraction sockets: A proof-of-concept study with 12- to 36-month follow-up. Int J Oral Maxillofac Implants 2007;22:995–1000.
31. Canullo L, Fedele GR, Iannello G, Jepsen S. Platform switching and marginal bone-level alterations: The results of a randomized-controlled trial. Clin Oral Implants Res 2010;21:115–121.
32. Grunder U. Immediate functional loading of immediate implants in edentulous arches: Two-year results. Int J Periodontics Restorative Dent 2001;21:545–551.
33. Romanos GE. Surgical and prosthetic concepts for predictable immediate loading of oral implants. J Calif Dent Assoc 2004;32:991–1001.
34. Romanos GE. Present status of immediate loading of oral implants. J Oral Implantol 2004;30:189–197.
35. Guida L, Iezzi G, Annunziata M, et al. Immediate placement and loading of dental implants: A human histologic case report. J Periodontol 2008;79:575–581.
36. Small PN, Tarnow DP. Gingival recession around implants: A 1-year longitudinal prospective study. Int J Oral Maxillofac Implants 2000;15:527–532.
37. Shin SW, Bryant SR, Zarb GA. A retrospective study on the treatment outcome of wide-bodied implants. Int J Prosthodont 2004;17:52–58.
38. Salama H, Salama M. The role of orthodontic extrusive remodeling in the enhancement of soft and hard tissue profiles prior to implant placement: A systematic approach to the management of extraction site defects. Int J Periodontics Restorative Dent 1993;13:313–333.
39. Salama M, Salama H, Garber DA. Options and implant site enhancement: The utilization of orthodontic extrusion. Pract Proced Aesthet Dent 2002;14:125–130.
40. Chambrone L, Chambrone LA. Forced orthodontic eruption of fractured teeth before implant placement: Case report. J Can Dent Assoc 2005;71:257–261.
41. Korayem M, Flores-Mir C, Nassar U, Olfert K. Implant site development by orthodontic extrusion—A systematic review. Angle Orthod 2008;78:752–760.
42. Arita CA. Estética em implantes: O "momento mágico" do dente restaurando a estética rosa. Rev Dental Press Periodontia Implantol 2008;2(3):68–76.
43. Buser D, Martin WC, Belser UC. Achieving optimal esthetic results. In: Buser D, Belser U, Wismeijer D (eds). ITI Treatment Guide. Vol 1: Implant Therapy in the Esthetic Zone—Single-Tooth Replacements. Berlin: Quintessence, 2007:26–37.

# Management of Immediate Loading Complications

## 14

In every treatment concept, there are complications to be considered, and it is important for every clinician to know how to manage them. This chapter discusses ways to avoid and manage complications related to immediate loading. Keep in mind the exact definition of *immediate loading* (functional or occlusal) and *immediate provisionalization*: the provisional restoration is placed and occlusal contacts are engaged immediately after implant placement.

Good primary stability is the main factor for success.[1-6] Primary stability will decrease during the first 3 to 4 weeks due to the resorptive processes at the interface; however, as bone remodeling occurs, this implant stability will increase (secondary or biologic stability), especially when implants are placed with functional loading.[7] Immediate loading is a therapeutic concept that can provide long-term success. Different types of restorations in various clinical indications (single-tooth, partial denture, and full-arch restorations) can be successful using implants placed in the residual bone or fresh extraction sockets under immediate loading conditions (see chapters 6 to 8 and 13).

From the scientific standpoint, there is clinical as well as histologic evidence that the immediate loading concept provides high success rates similar to conventional loading protocols,[8-12] even in patients with compromised bone metabolism[12,13] (see chapter 10). When some requirements are considered, such treatment protocols can be used with different implant designs in varying bone qualities as well as simultaneously with grafting techniques (see chapters 9 and 11).

There are factors, such as the tongue and lip musculature and parafunctional habits, that may affect the implant interface during the initial stages of healing. However, the main complications in the immediate loading concept are related to surgical and prosthetic complications.

## Surgical Complications

Surgical complications are classified as intra- and postoperative complications.

### Intraoperative complications

#### Drilling in poor-quality bone

The main intraoperative surgical complication is drilling in areas of poor bone quality, which may decrease the primary implant stability and compromise the outcome. The selection of tapered implant systems and the characteristics of the thread design (see chapter 4) can increase implant stability in poor-quality bone. In addition to the implant design, an extremely important factor is the advanced surgical experience of the surgeon. Undersizing the osteotomy and avoiding the use of final drills recommended by the manufacturer can lead to better primary stability. The osteotomy (drilling) technique is very sensitive and should be performed with attention and care. Instead of drills, special osteotomes (condensers) may be used to condense the bone in order to increase the bone-implant contacts and provide better implant stability.

#### Overtorquing an implant

Overtorque of an implant may increase the pressure at the bone, leading to crestal bone necrosis and defect formation and inhibiting osseous replacement during the normal healing period.[14] Bone fracture may also result from the overtorque of an implant, especially when advanced resorption of the ridge is present (Fig 14-1).

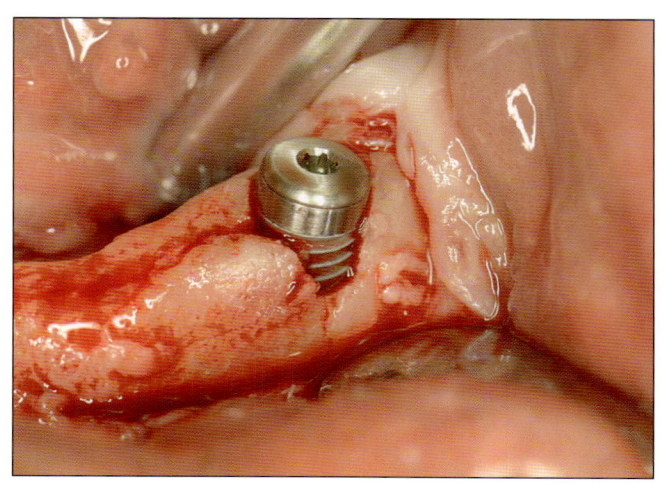

**Fig 14-1** In an attempt to obtain better primary stability for immediate loading, an implant with a larger diameter was placed and overtorqued, resulting in an alveolar ridge fracture.

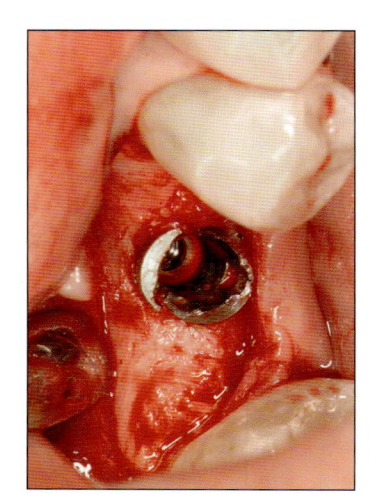

**Fig 14-2** Implant fracture due to overtorquing for immediate loading.

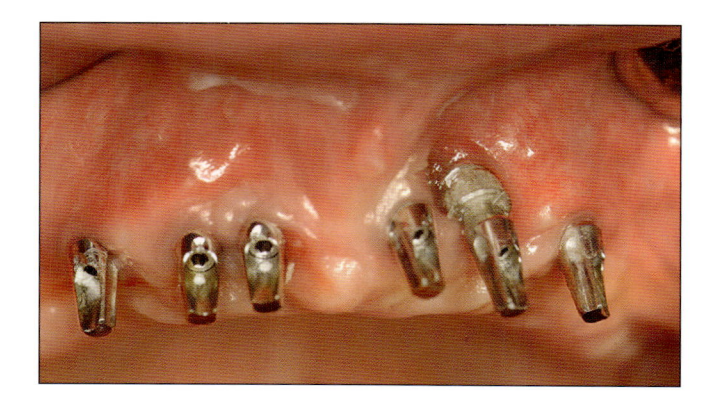

**Fig 14-3** Resorption of the buccal plate due to excessively buccal implant placement.

Excessive torque of an implant in order to increase primary stability could be responsible for fracture of the mounting instrument, damage to the implant-abutment connection, or fracture of the implant (Fig 14-2). This significant clinical problem may occur in dense bone when an overtorque of the implant is used in an improper osteotomy; if necessary, the implant will have to be removed using trephines or other techniques (eg, piezosurgery, lasers), resulting in loss of the surrounding bone and compromising the site for future implant placement. In some cases, a wider implant can be placed simultaneously.

In order to avoid these surgical complications, the author strongly recommends having experience with the specific implant system used and performing the osteotomy in a gentle and careful manner. Before excessive torque is applied to the implant, a step-back technique with implant removal and deeper preparation and tapping of the osteotomy should be considered as an alternative technique. In addition, self-tapping implants decrease bone compression during implant placement.

## Buccal implant placement

Implant placement at an excessively buccal angulation or position leads to significant intraoperative and long-term postoperative complications. Placing an implant with a buccal angulation increases the risks of buccal dehiscences, which necessitate guided bone regeneration treatment. Also, placement of an implant too buccally will lead to buccal plate perforations or a decrease in the buccal plate thickness, resulting in long-term implant failure or compromised esthetics (Fig 14-3). Comprehensive three-dimensional preoperative planning as well as the use of the prosthetic guide is recommended to decrease the risk of excessively buccal positioning.

## Implants placed in fresh extraction sockets with immediate loading

An implant placement at the level of the bone crest immediately after tooth extraction may lead to bone resorption and implant thread exposure at the early or late stages of healing. This is a significant complication when implants are placed in the esthetic zone. Bone resorption is also greater in cases with advanced augmentative procedures in conjunction with immediate loading concepts. An alternative plan with extraction, socket (ridge) preservation, and a conventional loading protocol should always be considered. Deeper implant placement and final abutment connection (ie, without subsequent removal) have been recommended; using

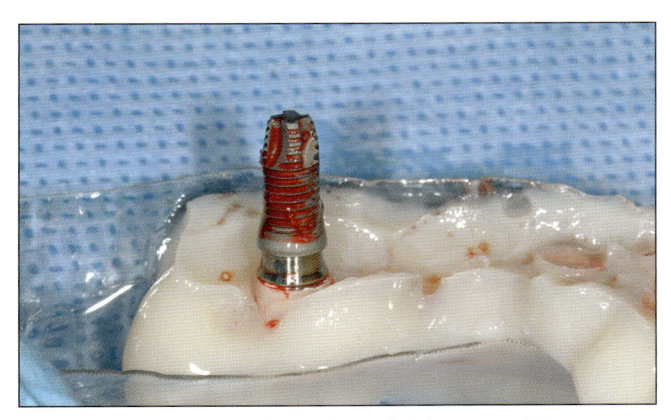

**Fig 14-4** Implant removal during chairside fabrication of the provisional restoration immediately after implant placement in very poor-quality bone in the posterior mandible.

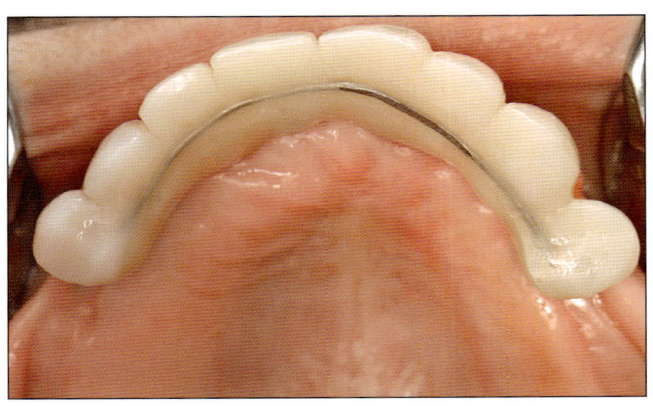

**Fig 14-5** Metal (wire) reinforcement of a provisional restoration 3 weeks after immediate implant placement and immediate loading to control implant micromovements.

implant systems with platform switching is also advised. In such cases, the final impression should be performed at the abutment level and not at the implant level.[15–17]

## Immediate postoperative complications

Mobility or removal of insufficiently stable implants may occur when impressions are taken the day of the surgery. The excessive tensile forces at the implant-abutment interface during impression removal (especially in the maxilla and when implant placement is performed simultaneously with augmentation) may result in implant mobility, dislocation, or failure. Therefore, the author strongly recommends not taking impressions the day of the surgery in compromised clinical cases. Special care also should be used during provisional removal on the day of surgery when implants were placed in very poor-quality bone (Fig 14-4). The restorative dentist who takes the impressions must be very well informed about the surgical technique used and the bone quality; otherwise, the surgeon has responsibility for the implant stability and the final impression should be completed after healing.

# Prosthetic Complications

Sufficient implant immobilization through splinting of adjacent implants is mandatory for implant success. The provisional restoration has to be fabricated using stable materials to avoid fractures in the healing stage. In full-arch immediate loading cases, the design of the provisional restoration must manage direct occlusal forces as well as successful splinting of the implants and control of micromovements. Provisional restorations should be rigid and strong and remain well attached to the implant abutments throughout the healing process. In cases of excessive loading or long-term provisionalization, metal reinforcement of the provisional restoration is important (Fig 14-5). Some clinicians recommend screw-retained immediate restorations and others cement-retained restorations.[18–20] Both types of provisional restorations have advantages and disadvantages, and the clinician should know exactly what the expected limitations are in order to avoid complications with immediate loading. The occlusal contacts should be symmetric, and only slight (or no) contacts should be maintained in the lateral mandibular movements. The cusp tips should be rounded to avoid sharp edges that lead to parafunctional contacts during function.

If a provisional restoration loosens from the supporting implants too early during the healing process or if the implant support and restoration are inadequately engineered, implant failure may occur. For that reason, the author recommends a strict follow-up schedule as well as immobilization of the provisional restoration using resin-based cementation materials (eg, ImplaCem [Equinox], Retrieve [Parkell]).

However, the removal of the provisional prosthesis has to be performed with care in order to avoid excessive forces at the implant-abutment interface and subsequent implant failure. In case of implant mobility during the healing period, it is important to know the exact cause of the mobility. If the implant is mobile and radiographic findings confirm progressive peri-implant bone loss with suppuration (ie, peri-implantitis), implant loss is to be expected. In the experience of the author, only one case in 15 years of experience presented this kind of bone loss within the healing period due to insufficient plaque control and compliance of the patient. If the implant-abutment connection becomes loose, the abutment should be tightened with the final prosthetic torque. Additional immobilization of the implant with the adjacent implants for a further 4 to 6 weeks, as well as a soft diet protocol, is mandatory in order to prevent implant failure.

The soft or liquid diet has been recommended by many clinicians,[20–22] especially during the initial healing stages, because it reduces the compressive and tensile forces at the implant-abutment interface. Higher failure rates with immediately loaded implants have been documented in patients with a history of bruxism.[23,24] In case of continuous fractures of the provisional restoration during the healing stage, the patient's diet protocol should be evaluated and the possibility of bruxism considered. In such cases, a more rigid provisional restoration using metal reinforcement is always recommended (see Fig 14-5).

# Conclusion

There is evidence in the scientific literature that immediate loading of dental implants can be used successfully in the long term and for various clinical indications. The basis for long-term success is an understanding of the biology, the wound-healing mechanisms, the process of osseointegration, and how to achieve and maintain implant stability. The implant design, implant surface chemistry, bone metabolic activity, patient health status, and applied forces dictate the timing and success of the healing process.

Although the literature shows immediately loaded implants to be as predictable as conventionally loaded implants, readers should be aware that the majority of the authors are highly skilled clinicians with experience in implant surgery and implant prosthodontics working under controlled clinical conditions with careful case selection. The risks for complications and failures using immediate loading are increased because the surgical and restorative treatments take place within the same visit. Therefore, excellent and precise treatment planning, use of an implant system with high primary stability, and treatment by clinicians experienced in advanced surgical and restorative techniques are the main requirements for reducing the risk for failures and achieving long-term success. Patient compliance is an absolute requirement for further control of biomechanical risks, resulting in prevention and elimination of complications with these complex treatment protocols.

# References

1. Szmukler-Moncler S, Piattelli A, Favero GA, Dubruille JH. Considerations preliminary to the application of early and immediate loading protocols in dental implantology. Clin Oral Implants Res 2000;11:12–15.
2. Cameron H, Pilliar RM, MacNab I. The effect of movement on the bonding of porous metal to bone. J Bio Mater Res 1973;7:301–311.
3. Schatzker J, Horne JG, Sumner-Smith G. The effect of movement on the holding power of screws in bone. Clin Orthodont Relat Res 1975;111:257–262.
4. Soballe K, Hansen ES, Brockstedt-Rasmussen H, Bunger C. Tissue ingrowth into titanium and hydroxyapatite-coated implants during stable and unstable mechanical conditions. J Orthop Res 1992;10:285–299.
5. Szmukler-Moncler S, Salama H, Reingewirtz Y, Dubruille JH. Timing of loading and effect of micromotion on bone dental implant interface: Review of experimental literature. J Biomed Mater Res 1998;43:192–203.
6. Brunski JB, Moccia AF, Pollock SR, Korostoff E, Trachtenberg DI. The influence of functional use of endosseous dental implants on the tissue implant interface: 1. Histological aspects. J Dent Res 1979;58:1953–1963.
7. Raghavendra S, Wood MC, Taylor TD. Early wound healing around endosseous implants: A review of the literature. Int J Oral Maxillofac Implants 2005;20:425–431.
8. Del Fabbro M, Testori T, Francetti L, Taschieri S, Weinstein R. Systematic review of survival rates for immediately loaded dental implants. Int J Periodontics Restorative Dent 2006;26:249–263.
9. Romanos GE. Bone quality and the immediate loading of implants. Critical aspects based on literature, research and clinical experience. Implant Dent 2009;18:203–209.
10. Romanos GE, Froum S, Hery C, Cho SC, Tarnow DP. Survival rate of immediately vs. delayed loaded implants: Analysis of the current literature. J Oral Implantol 2010;36:315–324.
11. Romanos GE, Testori T, Degidi D, Piattelli A. Histologic and histomorphometric findings from retrieved, immediately occlusally loaded implants in humans. J Periodontol 2005;76:1823–1832.
12. Romanos GE, Nentwig GH. Immediate loading using cross-arch fixed restorations in heavy smokers: Nine consecutive case reports for edentulous arches. Int J Oral Maxillofac Implants 2008;23:513–519.
13. Romanos GE, Johansson C. Immediate loading with complete implant-supported restorations in an edentulous heavy smoker: Histologic and histomorphometric analyses. Int J Oral Maxillofac Implants 2005;20:282–290.
14. Bashutski JD, D'Silva NJ, Wang HL. Implant compression necrosis: Current understanding and case report. J Periodontol 2009;80:700–704.
15. Romanos GE. Treatment of advanced periodontal destruction with immediately loaded implants and simultaneous bone augmentation. A case report. J Periodontol 2003;74:255–261.
16. Romanos GE. Present status of immediate loading of oral implants. J Oral Implantol 2004;30:189–197.
17. Romanos GE. Surgical and prosthetic concepts for predictable immediate loading of oral implants. J Calif Dent Assoc 2004;32:991–1001.
18. Tarnow DP, Emtiaz S, Classi A. Immediate loading of threaded implants at stage 1 surgery in edentulous arches: Ten consecutive case reports with 1- to 5-year data. Int J Oral Maxillofac Implants 1997;12:319–324.
19. Ganeles J, Rosenberg MM, Holt RL, Reichman LH. Immediate loading of implants with fixed restorations in the completely edentulous mandible: Report of 27 patients from a private practice. Int J Oral Maxillofac Implants 2001;16:418–426.
20. Romanos GE, Nentwig GH. Immediate functional loading in the maxilla using implants with platform switching: Five-year results. Int J Oral Maxillofac Implants 2009;24:1106–1112.
21. Degidi M, Piattelli A. Immediate functional and non-functional loading of dental implants: A 2- to 60-month follow-up study of 646 titanium implants. J Periodontol 2003;74:225–241.
22. Aparicio C, Ouazzani W, Aparicio A, et al. Immediate/early loading of zygomatic implants: Clinical experiences after 2 to 5 years of follow-up. Clin Implant Dent Relat Res 2010;12(suppl):e77–e82.
23. Balshi TJ, Wolfinger GJ. Immediate loading of Brånemark implants in edentulous mandibles: A preliminary report. Implant Dent 1997;6:83–88.
24. Glauser R, Rée A, Lundgren AK, Gottlow J, Hämmerle CH, Schärer P. Immediate loading of Brånemark implants applied in various jawbone regions: A prospective, 1-year clinical study. Clin Implant Dent Relat Res 2001;3:204–213.

# Index

Page numbers followed by "f" indicate figures; those followed by "t" indicate tables; those followed by "b" indicate boxes

## A
Abutments
  ceramic, 135, 135f
  connection of, 81f, 142f
  provisional, 70f
  telescopic, 61, 61f–62f
Acid-etched implant surface, 31f, 31–32
Advanced immediate loading, in maxilla, 73f–75f, 73–75
Advanced lateral and vertical augmentation
  in mandible, 92–96, 93f–96f
  in maxilla, 96, 97f–99f
Alveolar ridge
  augmentation of, 99, 101, 101f–105f
  deficiency of, 97f
  expansion of, 80f
  tapered implants in, 143
Angiogenesis, 3
Animal studies
  bone response, 43–44, 45f
  peri-implant soft tissue response, 46–48
Anterior mandible
  implant-supported bar-retained overdentures in, 55–56, 56f
  telescopic-retained overdentures in, 56, 57b, 57f–60f, 58
Appositional growth, 6
Atrophic mandible, 75f–77f, 75–76, 157f–159f, 157–159

## B
Bar-retained overdentures, implant-supported, 55–56, 56f
Bar-retained restorations, 12, 13f, 20
Bioceramic coating, 33–35, 35f
Biologic width, 47
Biomaterials, 28
Biomechanics, 19
Blood clot stabilization, 131
Bone
  anatomy of, 1
  formation of, 4
  healing of, 4–6, 5f, 8, 17
  loading effects on, 4
  microvasculature of, 2–3
  physiology of, 3–4
  remodeling of, 1–2, 19
  strain on, 3f, 3–4
Bone augmentation
  alveolar, 99, 101f
  single-tooth implants after, 137, 137f–139f, 140f–141f, 140–141
Bone grafting
  in heavy smoker, 114, 114b
  in mandible, 63–68, 64f–68f
  in maxilla, 69f–72f, 69–72
  single-implant placement after, 143, 143f
Bone quality
  description of, 7
  immediate loading affected by, 18, 18f
  poor, drilling in, 173
Bone response
  animal studies of, 43–44, 45f
  human studies of, 48–49, 49f
Bone-implant contact, 6–8, 11, 41t
Bone-implant interface
  bone density at, 11
  histomorphometric analysis of, 43
  micromovement at, 40–41
Brånemark implants, 17
Buccal implant placement, 174, 174f

## C
Calcium phosphate discrete crystalline deposition, 34, 35f
Capillaries, 2–3
Caries, 160f–161f, 160–161
Cement line, 6
Cement-retained provisional restorations, 175
Ceramic abutment, 135, 135f
Clot formation, 6, 7f
Complications
  buccal implant placement, 174, 174f
  drilling in poor-quality bone, 173
  implants placed in fresh extraction sockets, 174–175
  intraoperative, 173–175, 174f
  overtorquing of implant, 173–174, 174f
  postoperative, 175
  prosthetic, 175–176
Cone beam computed tomography, 98f
Connective tissue contact, 47–48
Contact osteogenesis, 8
Cortical bone, 1–2
Corticocancellous block
  maxilla augmentation using, 97f
  maxilla loading after horizontal augmentation with, 89–92, 90f–92f
Cross-arch implant-supported prosthesis, 124, 125f–128f, 127
Cylindric implants, 40f

## D
Delayed loading
  animal studies of, 44
  histologic analysis of, 44
Diet protocol, 78, 175
1,25-Dihydroxyvitamin $D_3$, 2
Dynamic osteogenesis, 5f, 5–6

## E
Early loading, 11, 41
Edentulous arches, 77–78
Edentulous patients. *See also* Partial edentulism.
  implant-supported bar-retained overdentures in, 55–56, 56f
  mandible, 112f
  maxilla, 112f
Extraction sockets
  fresh, implant placement in
    advanced protocol for, 147, 148f–150f, 153f–154f, 153–154
    case reports, 147–169, 148f–170f
    complications of, 174–175
    maxilla, 151f–157f, 151–156
    multiple caries, 160f–161f, 160–161
    studies of, 146–147
  healing of, 145–146
  remodeling of, 146

# Index

**F**
Fibrin clot, 6, 7f
Fixed restorations, 14–15

**G**
Grafted bone, maxilla loading after horizontal augmentation with, 89–92, 90f–92f. *See also* Bone grafting.
Grit blasting, 31f, 31–33, 35
Growth factors, 2
Guided bone regeneration, 93

**H**
Haversian systems, 44
Healing, of bone, 4–6, 5f, 8, 17
Hemiosteonal remodeling, 1
HIV-positive patients, 115, 116f–118f, 119t
Hong Kong Bridge Protocol, 15
Horizontal augmentation with corticocancellous block, maxilla loading after, 89–92, 90f–92f

**I**
Immediate loading
 definition of, 11–12
 functional, 11
 methods of, 11
 nonfunctional, 11
 rationale for, 12
 survival rates, 12–13
Immediate provisionalization, 12
Immediately loaded implants
 bone formation around, 44, 45f
 bone response to. *See* Bone response.
 description of, 17
 histologic findings, 44, 49f
 peri-implant soft tissue response of, 46
 survival rate of, 131
Implant(s)
 buccal placement of, 174, 174f
 cylindric, 7
 healing of, 17
 immediate, 17
 narrow-diameter, 7
 nontapered, 49–51, 50f
 overtorquing of, 173–174, 174f
 in partially edentulous patients, 16
 removal of, 101
 scalloped, 132
 screw-type, 12, 39, 41, 50
 single-tooth. *See* Single-tooth implants.
 tapered. *See* Tapered implants.
 threaded. *See* Threaded implants.
 titanium-free, 7
Implant design
 healing affected by, 7
 immediate loading affected by, 17
Implant retrieval analysis, 30
Implant stability
 definition of, 12
 primary, 6–8, 13, 39–40, 78, 173
 secondary, 39
Implant surface
 acid-etched, 31f, 31–32
 bioceramic coating, 33–35, 35f
 biocompatibility testing of, 28–29
 bone metabolism affected by, 43
 calcium phosphate discrete crystalline deposition, 34, 35f
 clinical evaluation of, 29–30
 definition of, 27
 grit blasting of, 31f, 31–33, 35
 illustration of, 7f
 immediate loading affected by, 17–18
 machined, 31f
 modifications of, 30–35
 nanotechnology application to, 34–35
 osseointegration affected by, 27
 plasma-sprayed hydroxyapatite, 30, 33–34
 rough, 7, 30–31
 saline-blasted, large-gritty, acid-etched, 32
 testing of, 28–30
 titanium plasma-sprayed surface, 13, 17, 20, 30, 31f
 topographic modifications of, 30–33
 treatments for changing, 27
Implant-abutment connection, 20
Intraoperative complications, 173–175, 174f
Ion beam–assisted deposition, 34

**J**
Junctional epithelium, 47–48

**L**
Lacunocanalicular system, 4
Lamellar bone, 4, 5f, 44
Lateral and vertical augmentation, advanced
 in mandible, 92–96, 93f–96f
 in maxilla, 96, 97f–99f

**M**
Mandible. *See also* Anterior mandible; Posterior mandible.
 after advanced lateral and vertical augmentation in, 92–96, 93f–96f
 atrophic, 75f–77f, 75–76, 157f–159f, 157–159
 bone quality in, 18
 edentulous, 112f
 of heavy smoker, 108–110, 110f–114f
 peri-implant soft tissue in, 113f
 posterior, 82, 83f–87f
Maxilla
 advanced lateral and vertical augmentation in, 96, 97f–99f
 bone grafting in, 69f–72f, 69–72
 bone quality in, 18
 edentulous, 112f
 of heavy smoker, 108–109
 immediate loading in
  advanced, 73f–75f, 73–75, 164–165
  with cross-arch implant-supported prosthesis and bilateral sinus elevation, 124, 125f–128f, 127
  fresh extraction sockets, 151f–157f, 151–156
  after horizontal augmentation with corticocancellous block, 89–92, 90f–92f
  sinus elevation performed simultaneously with, 129, 129f–130f, 151f–152f, 151–152, 164f–166f, 164–165
 orthodontic extrusion in, 167f–170f, 167–168
 peri-implant soft tissue in, 113f
 posterior, 79–81, 80f–81f
Maxillary left lateral incisor, 134, 134f
Mechanostat theory, 3–4
Metal-ceramic restorations, 67
Midcrestal incision, 77

**N**
Nanoindentation, 29
Nanotechnology, 34–35, 35f
Narrow-diameter implants, 7
Nontapered implants, 49–51, 50f

**O**
Occlusal contacts, 132
Omnivac shell technique, 91f–92f, 91–92, 115

One-stage protocol, 46
Osseointegration
 animal studies of, 43–44
 definition of, 1
 factors that affect, 29, 43
 implant surface effects on, 27
 mechanisms of, 4
Osteoblasts, 2, 4
Osteoclasts, 2, 4
Osteoconduction, 6, 7f
Osteocytes, 2, 4
Osteogenesis, 5f
Osteotomy, 6
Overdentures, 12–14, 13f
 implant-supported bar, 55–56, 56f
 telescopic-retained, 56, 57b, 57f–60f, 58
Overtorquing, of implant, 173–174, 174f

# P
Partial dentures, 16
Partial edentulism
 immediate loading in, 163, 163f
 implant placement in, 16
 telescopic abutments in, 61, 61f–62f
Peri-implant soft tissues
 in maxilla, 113f
 response of, 46–48, 86f
Periodontal disease, 107, 153
Plasma-sprayed hydroxyapatite, 30, 33–34
Platelet-derived growth factor, 6
Platform switching, 56, 135, 135f, 143
Posterior implants, 15
Posterior mandible
 advanced augmentation in, 99, 100f–101f
 immediate loading in, 82, 83f–87f, 99, 100f–101f
 resorption in, 93f
 single-tooth implants in, 133, 133f
Posterior maxilla, 79–81, 80f–81f
Primary implant stability, 6–8, 13, 39–40, 78, 173
Progressive bone loading, 11–12
Prostacyclin, 2
Prostaglandin $E_2$, 2
Prosthetic complications, 175–176
Provisional abutments, 70f
Provisional restorations
 cement-retained, 175
 fixed, 20, 78
 metal reinforcement of, 175, 175f
 screw-retained, 175

# R
Remodeling of bone, 1–2, 19
Removable restoration, 156, 156f–157f
Resonance frequency analysis, 40
Rough-surface implants, 27, 30–31

# S
Saline-blasted, large-gritty, acid-etched implant surface, 32
Scalloped implants, 132
Screw-retained provisional restorations, 175
Screw-type implants
 case reports of, 50
 description of, 12, 39, 41
Secondary implant stability, 39
Self-tapping implants, 40
Single-tooth implants
 in adolescent patient, 142, 142f
 in augmented bone, 137, 137f–139f
 case reports of, 133f–144f, 133–144
 clinical results of, 131, 132t
 customized ceramic abutment and platform switching, 135, 135f
 description of, 16, 131
 hard and soft tissue augmentation with, 140f–141f, 140–141
 maxillary left lateral incisor, 134, 134f
 in posterior mandible, 133, 133f
 tapered implants, 136, 136f–137f
Sinus elevation, simultaneous
 autograft for, 122, 123f–124f
 case reports of, 122–129, 123f–130f
 cross-arch implant-supported prosthesis and, 124, 125f–128f, 127
 lateral window preparation for, 122f
 in maxilla, 124, 125f–130f, 127, 129, 151, 151f–152f, 164f–165f, 164–165
 radiographs of, 122f
 technique for, 121
Smokers/smoking
 bone grafting in, 114, 114b
 clinical study in, 107–108
 immediate loading in, 107–114
 mandible of, 108–110, 110f–114f
 maxilla of, 108–109
 periodontal disease risks, 107
Soft tissue
 adherence of, 1
 augmentation of, single-tooth implants with, 140f–141f, 140–141
 contouring of, 167f–170f, 167–168
 peri-implant
  in maxilla, 113f
  response of, 46–48, 86f
Splinting, 20
Static osteogenesis, 5–6
Strain, 3f, 3–4
Stratified squamous epithelium, 46
Straumann implants, 40, 40t, 136, 136f
Subcrestal placement, 132
Surface of implant. *See* Implant surface.

# T
Tapered implants
 in alveolar ridge, 143
 case reports of, 51–52, 136, 136f–137f
 description of, 17, 40f, 41
 single-tooth, 136, 136f–137f
Telescopic abutments, 61, 61f–62f
Telescopic-retained overdentures, in anterior mandible, 56, 57b, 57f–60f, 58
Threaded implants
 advantages of, 17
 description of, 7
 fixed restorations on, 14
Titanium plasma-sprayed implants, 13, 17, 20, 30, 31f
Titanium-free implant, 7
Trabecular bone, 44, 45f
Transitional implants, 15

# V
Vascular endothelial growth factor receptor, 3
Vertical augmentation. *See* Lateral and vertical augmentation, advanced.

# W
Wolff's law, 3
Woven bone, 4, 5f